# Medical Clinic
# ⇒ *Workflow* ⇒

## 2nd Edition • Rick Schanhals

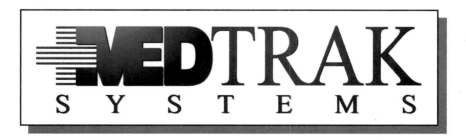

MEDTRAK SYSTEMS

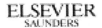

3251 Riverport Lane

St. Louis, Missouri 63043

Medical Clinic Workflow                    ISBN: 978-1-4557-1083-6

**Copyright © 2012 by Saunders, an imprint of Elsevier Inc.**

**Notices**

Knowledge and best practice in this field are constantly changing. As new research and experience broaden our understanding, changes in research methods, professional practices, or medical treatment may become necessary.

Practitioners and researchers must always rely on their own experience and knowledge in evaluating and using any information, methods, compounds, or experiments described herein. In using such information or methods they should be mindful of their own safety and the safety of others, including parties for whom they have a professional responsibility.

With respect to any drug or pharmaceutical products identified, readers are advised to check the most current information provided (i) on procedures featured or (ii) by the manufacturer of each product to be administered, to verify the recommended dose or formula, the method and duration of administration, and contraindications. It is the responsibility of practitioners, relying on their own experience and knowledge of their patients, to make diagnoses, to determine dosages and the best treatment for each individual patient, and to take all appropriate safety precautions.

To the fullest extent of the law, neither the Publisher nor the authors, contributors, or editors, assume any liability for any injury and/or damage to persons or property as a matter of products liability, negligence or otherwise, or from any use or operation of any methods, products, instructions, or ideas contained in the material herein.

**International Standard Book Number: 978-1-4557-1083-6**

*Acquisitions Editor:* Susan Cole
*Developmental Editor:* Laurie Vordtriede
*Editorial Assistant:* Helen O'Neal
*Publishing Services Manager:* Pat Joiner-Myers
*Project Manager:* Stephen Bancroft

Printed in Canada

Last digit is the print number: 9 8 7 6 5 4 3 2 1

Rick Schanhals, BSE

University of Michigan, College of Engineering

President, MedTrak Systems, Inc.

North Muskegon, Michigan

## Software licensed by:

## MedTrak Systems, Inc.

Development Lab

1847 Ruddiman Drive

North Muskegon, MI 49445

## Publications in the MedTrak Educational Series include:

Medical Clinic Workflow • Second Edition

Billing and Reimbursement • Second Edition

Care Pathways • Second Edition

# Acknowledgements

**Shelley Beckett**
Center Manager and EMR Liaison
US HealthWorks
Carlsbad, California

**Ranelle Brew, Ed.D, CHES**
Assistant Professor
College of Health Professions
Grand Valley State University
Grand Rapids, Michigan

**David A. Blaszak, BS Mathematics**
Senior Program Developer
MedTrak Systems, Inc.
North Muskegon, Michigan

**Fred Butler, MD, MPH**
Murrieta, California

**Barbara Carr, MD**
Diplomate
American Board of Emergency Medicine
US Army

**Eric Gatmaitan**
Industrial Management Consulting
SMConsulting LLC

**John Klaes**
Creative Director
MedTrak Systems, Inc.
North Muskegon, Michigan

**Maureen Marston**
Senior Director
Western Regional Business Office
US HealthWorks
Valencia, California

**Synthia Laura Molina, MBA**
Managing Partner
Central IQ, Inc.

**Laurie Pierce, MD, MPH**
Carlsbad, California

**Marybeth Pieri-Smith, MBA, RHIA, CCS-P, CPC, CMA**
Assistant Professor
Davenport University
Battle Creek, Michigan

**Nick Schanhals**
Author's 5th grade, 11-year-old grandson
North Muskegon Elementary School
North Muskegon, Michigan

**Susan Slajus, RHIA**
Associate Dean and Assistant Professor
Davenport University
Holland, Michigan

**Rick Valentine**
Healthcare Management Consulting
Centennial, Colorado

**Larisa West**
Directory of Physician Services and Billing
American Occupational Network
Carlsbad, California

**Michelle Wilson**
Center Manager
US HealthWorks
Murrieta, California

# Contents

Chapter **1**   **Medical Clinic Workflow** (15 minutes)                    7

Chapter **2**   **Logging into MedTrak**                                    13

Chapter **3**   **Adding Patients** (45 minutes)                            14

Chapter **4**   **Helpful Tips and Navigation** (30 minutes)                20

Chapter **5**   **Attaching Payers to a Patient** (30 minutes)              25

Chapter **6**   **Scheduling** (60 minutes)                                 33
                 Work product produced

Chapter **7**   **Patient Registration** (45 minutes)                       49

Chapter **8**   **Clinic Status Screen** (15 minutes)                       73

Chapter **9**   **Nursing Intake** (30 minutes)                             81

Chapter **10**  **Physician - Initial Contact** (30 minutes)                99

Chapter **11**  **Open Orders Processing** (30 minutes)                     108

Chapter **12**  **Out the Door - Overview** (15 minutes)                    119

Chapter **13**  **Physician - Additional Orders** (15 minutes)              131

Chapter **14**  **Physician - Referrals** (15 minutes)                      138

Chapter **15**  **Physician - Diagnosing** (15 minutes)                     147

Chapter **16**  **Physician - Patient History
                and Physical Exam** (30 minutes)                            156

# Contents

Chapter **17**  **Physician - Prescribing** (15 minutes)     172

Chapter **18**  **Physician - Aftercare Instructions** (30 minutes)     181

Chapter **19**  **Physician - Evaluation and Management** (15 minutes)  198

Chapter **20**  **Nursing Discharge** (15 minutes)     206

Chapter **21**  **Front Desk - Payment Collection** (15 minutes)     214

Chapter **22**  **Pending Results** (60 minutes)     219

Chapter **23**  **Unbilled Charges** (30 minutes)     247

Chapter **24**  **Posting Charges to a Bill** (20 minutes)     259

Chapter **25**  **Printing Bills** (15 minutes)     268
    Work product produced

Chapter **26**  **Payment Processing** (45 minutes)     275

Chapter **27**  **Accounts Receivable** (20 minutes)     295
    Work product produced

Chapter **28**  **Collection Activity** (20 minutes)     309

# CHAPTER

# 1

# Medical Clinic Workflow

**Estimated time needed to complete this chapter - 15** minutes

## Learning outcomes gained from this chapter

- ♦ A brief understanding of clinical workflow systems and their complications
- ♦ An understanding of the categories of clinical workflow and their major processes
- ♦ An introduction to MedTrak's rules-based methodology for clinical workflow

## Key concepts in this chapter

*clinical workflow systems*

*collaboration of the clinical staff*

*improving communications*

*automating paperwork*

*medical processes*

*detailed clinical step*

*presenting problems*

*track each patient*

*rules-based*

*specialized dashboards*

*screen sequences*

*clinical objects*

*evidence-based*

## Medical Clinic Workflow

*Clinical workflow systems* can be a significant factor in both lowering the cost and increasing the quality of medical care at every level of delivery by increasing the efficiency of the healthcare facility, reducing patient throughput time, and integrating rules-based problem solving with evidence-based actions.

> ### Clinical workflow efficiencies focus on:
>
> - Supporting the *collaboration* of the clinical staff.
>
> - *Improving communications* both inside and outside the medical clinic.
>
> - *Automating paperwork* through the completion and approval processes.
>
> - *Fully integrating rules-based problem solving* that triggers evidence-based actions at every step of treatment.

*Medical processes* are like business and manufacturing processes that can be broken down into the detailed steps needed for completion. By performing these *detailed clinical steps* the same way each time, the clinical staff is able to diagnose and treat their patients in a consistent, thorough, and efficient manner. A clinical workflow system, like MedTrak, enables clinicians to always complete every step in the patient's care. Whether a clinician is experienced or new on the job, using a clinical workflow system will help ensure that the patient's care is always to the standards set by the clinic.

> ### Clinical workflow systems enable the clinical staff to know:
>
> - What clinical *process step* (action) the patient needs next
>
> - How long the patient has been *waiting for the step*
>
> - *Who is responsible* for performing the step

Clinical workflow systems also help reduce the stress level in a clinic by providing up-to-the-second tracking information for each patient in the medical facility. This makes it easier for new employees to perform their jobs with the same consistency and efficiency as experienced clinicians.

Responsibilities, skills, and medical knowledge in the healthcare setting clearly separate the medical disciplines into a hierarchical structure:

- The physician has direct responsibility for the patient's care.
- The nursing staff supports the physician by carrying out the physician's orders.
- The front desk personnel schedule, register, and collect payments.
- The administrative staff monitors patient charts and outside communications.
- The billing staff prepares and sends out bills and records payments.

Clinical workflow is further complicated by the very nature of the patient's *presenting problems*. While some medical clinics see predominately one type of presenting problem, others see patients for everything from a drug screen collection, a sports physical, chronic asthma, a broken arm, a laceration of the foot, to a sore throat. Many of these patients are scheduled, but some are walk-ins without an appointment. The clinic needs to efficiently treat each one of these types of patient encounters without missing a single necessary process. In order to do this, the clinic needs to be able *track each patient* from registration through discharge. This tracking needs to include all physician orders for diagnostics and treatments. Additionally, the clinical staff needs to coordinate their actions to ensure that each step in the patient's care is done efficiently and in the proper order.

## Clinical Workflow Categories

### Major Categories of Clinical Workflow

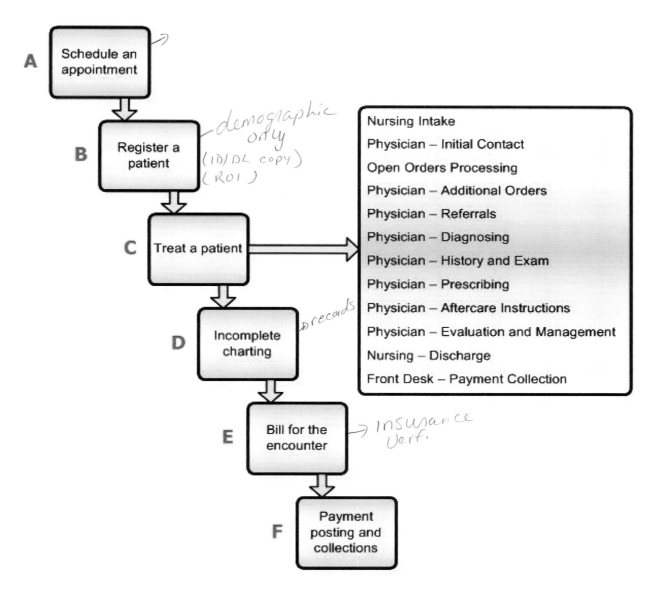

A — Schedule an appointment

B — Register a patient

*demographic only*
*(ID/DL copy)*
*(ROI)*

C — Treat a patient

Nursing Intake
Physician – Initial Contact
Open Orders Processing
Physician – Additional Orders
Physician – Referrals
Physician – Diagnosing
Physician – History and Exam
Physician – Prescribing
Physician – Aftercare Instructions
Physician – Evaluation and Management
Nursing – Discharge
Front Desk – Payment Collection

D — Incomplete charting

*records*

E — Bill for the encounter

*Insurance Verf.*

F — Payment posting and collections

Each one of these major categories can be broken down into processes that can be further broken down into the detailed steps that make up the processes.

## A - Schedule an appointment (processes):

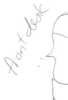

- Add appointment for a new patient
- Schedule appointment for an existing patient
- Change appointment's time and/or day
- Block time for meetings, lunch, etc. on physician's schedule
- Add note concerning the patient to an appointment

## B - Register a patient (processes):

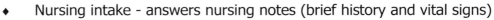
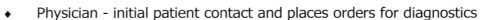

- Register patient from the Scheduler
- Add patient's demographic information
- Register patient using the Patient Registration process
- Add new patient
- Select existing patient
- Select company (if it is an occupational medicine case)
- Create new case for the patient
- Select patient's payers (for patient responsibility patients)
- Select type of patient visit (primary doctor, orthopedic, rehab, etc.)
- Select presenting problems to initiate the problem-focused clinical workflow

## C - Treat a patient (processes):

- Nursing intake - answers nursing notes (brief history and vital signs)
- Physician - initial patient contact and places orders for diagnostics
- Order processing of open diagnostic orders
- Physician places orders for treatments (including referrals to specialists)
- Physician selects patient's diagnoses
- Physician documents patient's history
- Physician documents patient's physical examination
- Physician orders medications - both dispensed and prescription
- Physician selects patient's aftercare instructions
- Physician confirms level of service (evaluation and management)
- Nursing staff delivers paperwork to patient
- Front desk collects any payments due

## D - Pending results (processes):

- ◆ Track patients waiting for physician to finish the history and exam
- ◆ Track patients waiting on lab results
- ◆ Track patients waiting on imaging results
- ◆ Track patients referred to specialists for treatment
- ◆ Track surgery authorization requests

## E - Bill for the encounter (processes):

- ◆ Review encounters needing additional information
- ◆ Edit charges for the encounter
- ◆ Post charges to create the invoice
- ◆ Send bill electronically or by mail

## F - Payment posting and collections (processes):

- ◆ Create payment batches
- ◆ Record payments
- ◆ Post payments and adjustments to invoices
- ◆ Monitor aged accounts receivable
- ◆ Record collection activities
- ◆ Process refunds

## *Rules-Based*

To achieve effective clinical workflow, the processes need to be broken down into their individual steps using a *rules-based* methodology. MedTrak's clinical rules-based methodology is comprised of a combination of four basic components:

**1** *Specialized dashboards* designed to model clinical workflow, such as:

- ◆ Clinic status screen
- ◆ Incomplete visit screens (pending chart completion)
- ◆ Unbilled charges dashboard
- ◆ Accounts receivable dashboard
- ◆ Referrals dashboard
- ◆ Surgeries needing authorization dashboard

**2** *Screen sequences* that automatically step users through data capture such as:

- Scheduling appointments
- Registration processing for private pay (group health)
- Registration processing for workers' compensation and employee health
- Payment processing

**3** Functionality attached to *clinical objects* to complete their characteristics, such as:

- Attaching payers with subscriber information to patients
- Attaching worker's compensation insurance to companies
- Attaching initial injury drug screens and physical examinations to companies
- Attaching company contacts by responsibility to companies
- Building employee health rules for companies
- Building specific care rules for a patient
- Rates assigned by billing codes to specific procedures

**4** Orders that trigger sequences of questions to enable *evidence-based* actions, such as:

- Imaging orders including x-rays, MRIs, and CT scans
- Laboratory orders including drug screens and blood tests
- Ancillary orders including hearing tests, eye tests, and pulmonary function test
- Treatments for injuries including surface traumas and orthopedics
- Treatments for systems including HEENT, cardiology, and dermatology
- Follow-up treatments including dressing changes and suture removals
- Medication treatments including injections and vaccinations
- Referrals to outside specialists
- Dispense and prescribe medications
- Administrative orders including form completion and extra services

Chapters 2, 3, 4, and 5 of this book describe how to log into MedTrak, add patients, use the **On-line User Guide**, attach payers to a patient, and schedule patients.

The chapters after 5 train you how to use MedTrak's clinical workflow system to process a patient responsibility (private pay) patient with Blue Cross/Blue Shield insurance who sprained his or her left ankle while walking down some stairs.

# CHAPTER 2

# Logging into MedTrak

**What you need to know before doing this chapter**

- ◆ How to use a computer and access the Internet
- ◆ Follow the directions provided by your instructor for logging into MedTrak.

# CHAPTER

# 3

# Adding Patients

**Estimated time needed to complete this chapter - 45** minutes

**What you need to know before doing this chapter**
- How to sign into MedTrak

**Learning outcomes gained from this chapter**
- How to add a new patient to the database

## Adding a Patient

From the MedTrak <u>Main Menu</u>, the front desk person clicks the *Patient Registration* button. The <u>Patients</u> screen (shown below) appears.

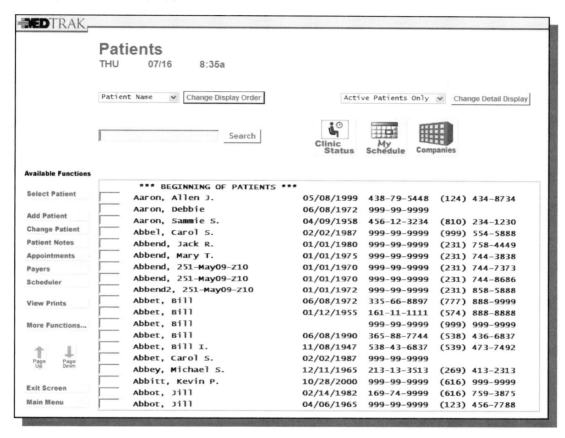

To add a new patient to the patient database, the front desk person clicks the *Add Patient* button. The next screen to appear is the <u>Patient: Add by SSN</u> screen (shown below).

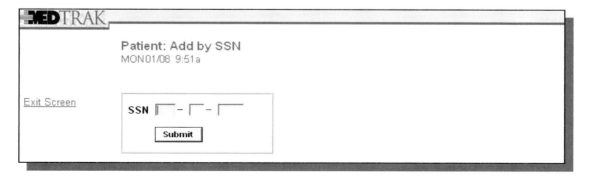

The front desk person enters the patient's social security number on this screen and clicks the *Submit* button. If the social security number is unavailable, the front desk enters **999-99-9999** in this field. Some patients will not provide their social security number and some patients do not have one.

The <u>Patient</u> demographics screen (shown below) appears.

If the social security number is already in the database, the patient's demographic information is shown for review. Otherwise, only the social security number field is pre-populated.

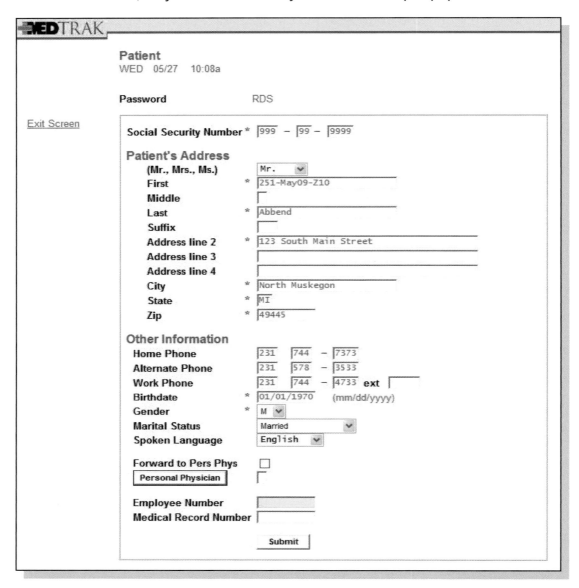

On the <u>Patient</u> demographics screen, **red asterisks** appear next to the fields that *must be answered*. If a required field is not filled in, a message appears (**in red**) below the date and time at the top of the screen, and sets the cursor in the field that needs information.

The front desk person enters the information using *appropriate punctuation and capitalization*.

For example, when entering a street name, the front desk enters "**123 South Main Street**" instead of "**123 south main street**" or "**123 SOUTH MAIN STREET**."

When finished, the front desk person clicks the *Submit* button.

MedTrak freezes all of the fields on the <u>Patient</u> demographics screen and requests verification that the information is correct. If the information is correct, the front desk person presses the *ENTER* key or clicks the *Submit* button. If some of the information needs correcting, he or she clicks the *Exit Screen* button to refresh the <u>Patient</u> demographics entry screen with the fields opened up for data entry.

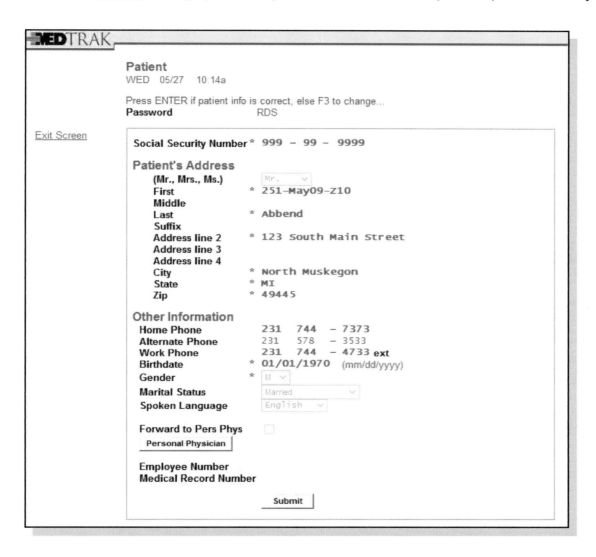

If simply adding a new patient, company selection is not necessary. When the <u>Company</u> selection screen (shown on the next page) appears, the front desk person clicks the *Exit Screen* button. The <u>Patients</u> screen appears again, with the new patient added to the list.

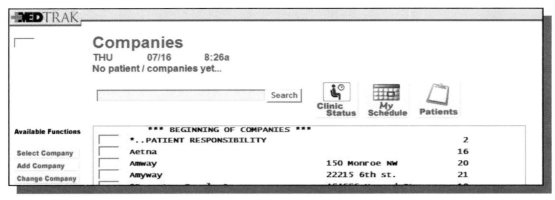

**Do This ▶**   **3.01** - Sign in to MedTrak

      **3.02** - Click the *Patient Registration* button on the MedTrak <u>Main Menu</u>
           (you should be on the <u>Patients</u> screen)

      **3.03** - Click the *Add Patient* button on the <u>Patients</u> screen
           (you should be on the <u>Patient: Add by SSN</u> screen)

      **3.04** - Enter all **9**'s for the social security number (**999-99-9999**)

      **3.05** - Click the *Submit* button
           (you should be on the <u>Patient</u> screen)

---

**Do This ▶**   **3.06** - On the <u>Patient</u> screen

         In the **first name** field enter the following with dashes in between:

           **Course number** - For example, for HINT201, just use the **201**
           **Month** (first three letters) and **year** (last two digits) - **Jan10**
           Your **employee initials** (provided by MedTrak) - **ABC**
              First name should look like this - **201-Jan10-ABC**

         In the **last name** field enter your last name
         Enter data in the rest of the **required fields** on the screen
         Be sure the birthdate results in an age greater than 18 years.

## Do Not Use Your Own Address or Phone Numbers

      **3.07** - Click the *Submit* button - review your patient's information

      **3.08** - Click the *Submit* button again to confirm your patient's information

      **3.09** - On the <u>Companies</u> screen, click the *Exit Screen* button to return
           (you should be on the <u>Patients</u> screen)

**Do This** ▶ **3.10** - Add two more new patients

- Use your first name as you built it in **3.06**
- Use your last name again plus a number
- Add patient numbers 3 and 4 (see examples in box below)
- Record your patient names on the lines below

  (or on another sheet of paper)

_____

_____

_____

(You will also use these patients in **Chapter 6 – Scheduling**)

## See the example names in the box below this one.

**For the examples in this book, the patients' names are:**

**Abbend, 251-May09-Z10**

**Abbend3, 251-May09-Z10**

**Abbend4, 251-May09-Z10**

# CHAPTER

# 4

# Helpful Tips and Navigation

**Estimated time needed to complete this chapter  -  30** minutes

**What you need to know before doing this chapter**

- ♦ How to log into MedTrak
- ♦ How to access the <u>Patients</u> screen

**Learning outcomes gained from this chapter**

- ♦ How to identify the common elements on a MedTrak screen
- ♦ How to use the function keys
- ♦ How to use the tab key
- ♦ How to select an item in a list
- ♦ How to use a button
- ♦ How to select a command from the <u>Help</u> screen
- ♦ How to enter a command
- ♦ How to use multiple commands on the same screen
- ♦ How to search
- ♦ How to use selection boxes
- ♦ How to adjust the text size on the screen
- ♦ How to view the full screen without the menu bars showing

**Key concepts in this chapter**

*User Guide*

*common elements*

*function keys*

*basic navigation*

*selecting items*

*entering commands*

*selection boxes*

*searching*

## MedTrak's On-Line User Guide

This exercise utilizes the *User Guide* located on the <u>Main Menu</u>. Because you will reference the *User Guide* throughout this exercise, keep it open on your desktop (it is in its own window).

**Do This** ▶ **4.01** - Sign in to MedTrak

**4.02** - Click the *User Guide* button on the <u>Main Menu</u>

**4.03** - Keep the **User Guide** window open

**4.04** - Access **Patient Registration** from the <u>Main Menu</u>

# 1  Common Screen Elements

**Do This** ▶ **4.05** - In the **User Guide,** read **Section 1 - Common Elements**

**4.06** - Review the different elements on this screen

# 2  Function Keys

**Do This** ▶ **4.07** - In the **User Guide,** read **Section 2 - Function Keys**

**4.08** - Try the different function keys on this screen

# 3  Basic Navigation

**Do This** ▶ **4.09** - In the **User Guide,** read **Section 3 - Basic Navigation**

**4.10** - Press the *TAB* key to move the cursor down the screen

**4.11** - Hold the *SHIFT* key and press the *TAB* key to move up

## 3.1   Selecting Items

**Do This** ▶   **4.12** -  Place the cursor next to a patient

**4.13** -  Press the *ENTER* key

**4.14** -  On the next screen, click the *Exit Screen* button (*F3* key)

**4.15** -  Click the *Select Patient* button

**4.16** -  On the next screen, click the *Exit Screen* button (*F3* key)

**4.17** -  Type an x and press the *ENTER* key

**4.18** -  On the next screen, click the *Exit Screen* button (*F3* key)

## 3.2   Entering Commands

**Do This** ▶   **4.19** -  Place the cursor next to another patient

**4.20** -  Click the *Change Patient* button in **Available Functions**

**4.21** -  On the next screen, click the *Exit Screen* button (*F3* key)

**Do This** ▶   **4.22** -  Place the cursor next to another patient

**4.23** -  Click the *More Functions* button (*F1* key)

**4.24** -  Click the *Change* checkbox, then click the *Select Function* button

**4.25** -  Press the *ENTER* key on the Patient screen

**4.26** -  On the next screen, click the *Exit Screen* button (*F3* key)

**Do This** ▶ **4.27** - Place the cursor next to another patient

**4.28** - Click the *More Functions* button (*F1* key)

**4.29** - Click the *Change* button

**4.30** - Press the *ENTER* key on the <u>Patient</u> screen

**4.31** - On the next screen, click the *Exit Screen* button (*F3* key)

---

**Do This** ▶ **4.32** - Place the cursor next to another patient

**4.33** - Type the command **ch** for change

**4.34** - Press the *ENTER* key

**4.35** - On the next screen, click the *Exit Screen* button (*F3* key)

## Multiple Commands on a Screen

Manual entry offers an additional benefit of being able to run several commands on records consecutively. To change three patient's records using the change command, type "**ch**" in three command fields (see below) and press the *ENTER* key. The change program processes three times in a row — once for each selected record — thus saving time.

You can do *mouseless control* on every screen and your hands need never leave the keyboard.

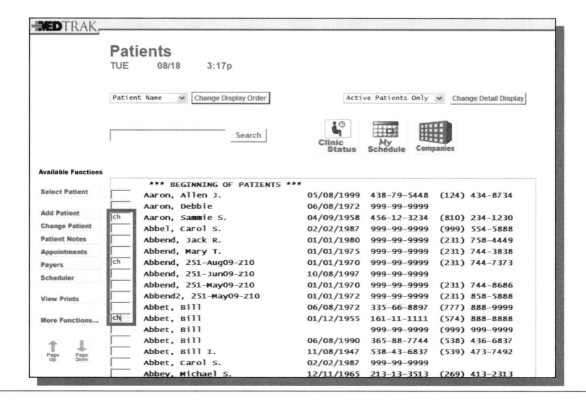

**Do This** ▶ **4.36** - Type the **ch** command next to three patients

**4.37** - Press the *ENTER* key

**4.38** - When the **1st** screen appears, click the *Exit Screen* button (*F3* key)

**4.39** - When the **2nd** screen appears, click the *Exit Screen* button (*F3* key)

**4.40** - When the **3rd** screen appears, click the *Exit Screen* button (*F3* key)

## 4   Selection Boxes

**Do This** ▶ **4.41** - In the **User Guide**, read **Section 4 - Selection Boxes**

(You will use selection boxes during patient registration and clinical processing)

## 7   Searching

**Do This** ▶ **4.42** - In the **User Guide**, read **Section 7 - Searching**
**4.43** - Practice searching for some names

The following Helpful Tips will make it easier to view MedTrak's screens.

## 8   Helpful Tips

**Do This** ▶ **4.44** - In the **User Guide**, read **Section 8 - Helpful Tips**

**4.45** - Click the *Patient Registration* button on the Main Menu

**4.46** - Adjust your text size to **Larger**

**4.47** - Adjust your screen to **Full Size** mode

**To reset your browser from Full Size mode, move the cursor to the top of the screen and click the boxes in the upper right corner.**

# CHAPTER 5

# Attaching Payers to a Patient

**Estimated amount of time to complete this chapter  -  30** minutes

## What you need to know before doing this chapter

- ♦ How to log into MedTrak
- ♦ How to access the <u>Patients</u> selection screen
- ♦ How to add a new patient or locate an existing patient

## Learning outcomes gained from this chapter

- ♦ A brief understanding of the different types of payers
- ♦ How to add a payer to a patient
- ♦ How to add multiple payers to a patient
- ♦ How to add a guarantor
- ♦ How to prioritize the payer order  -  primary, secondary, tertiary, quaternary
- ♦ How to add the subscriber information

## Key concepts in this chapter

*patient responsibility*

*financial classes*

*financial viability*

*mix of patients*

*self pay*

*guarantor*

*payer*

*subscriber*

*primary payer*

*secondary payer*

*tertiary payer*

*quaternary payer*

## *Attaching Payers to a Patient*

For *patient responsibility* patients (either the patient or guarantor or their health insurance will be paying for the medical services), MedTrak allows up to four simultaneous payers to be associated with the patient.

Payers are categorized by *financial classes*. These financial classes (to name just a few) include the following:

- ◆ Self pay
- ◆ Guarantor
- ◆ Commercial insurance
- ◆ Medicare
- ◆ Medicaid
- ◆ Tricare (formerly known as Champus)

Healthcare organizations track their financial information by the individual payers and by the financial class of the payer. It is important to the *financial viability* of the healthcare organization that the *mix of patients* that visit their facilities are in the financial classes based on their budget projections. Just like an airline company that needs to sell a certain portion of its seats to the last-minute travelers at a higher rate than the passengers who booked their seats well in advance, healthcare organizations need to meet their budget based on the mix of patients by financial class.

Some financial classes of patients pay for their medical services at a higher rate than do other financial classes. The rates paid by Medicare and Medicaid are based on national payer tables that vary by geographic location and are typically the lowest rates. The rates paid by commercial insurance carriers vary from one company to another and are higher rates than paid by the government. Usually the highest rates for medical care are for *self pay* and *guarantor* patients. A guaranteed patient is under the age of 18 or incapable of paying for his or her own medical care, and the guarantor is the person who takes responsibility for paying for the patient's care.

In this chapter, you will add three payers to the first patient that you added into MedTrak. This is the patient with your last name and the first name composed of your class number, month and year, and your employee initials.

## *Locating the Patient*

From the MedTrak Main Menu click the *Patient Registration* button. The Patient Registration screen (shown below) will appear.

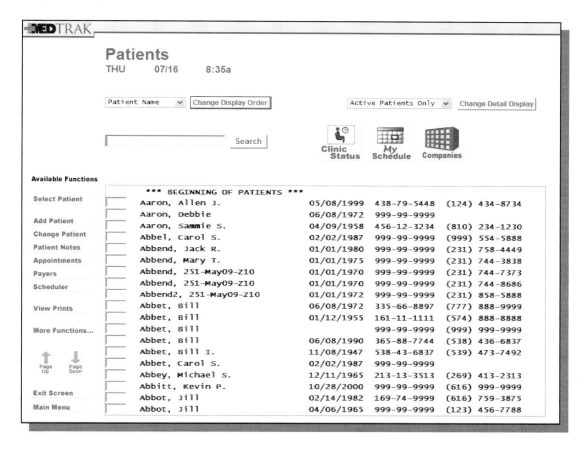

To locate a patient, type the last name in the search field and click the *Search* button. If there are a number of patients with the same last name, then put a comma at the end of the last name, then a space, and then type the first name before clicking the *Search* button.

To attach payers to a patient, place the cursor in the command field next to the patient and click the *Payers* button.

If the patient does not have any payers attached, the next screen to appear is the Entity/Payers: Select screen (shown on the next page). If the patient already has payers attached, the Patient Payers screen will appear.

## Selecting the Payer

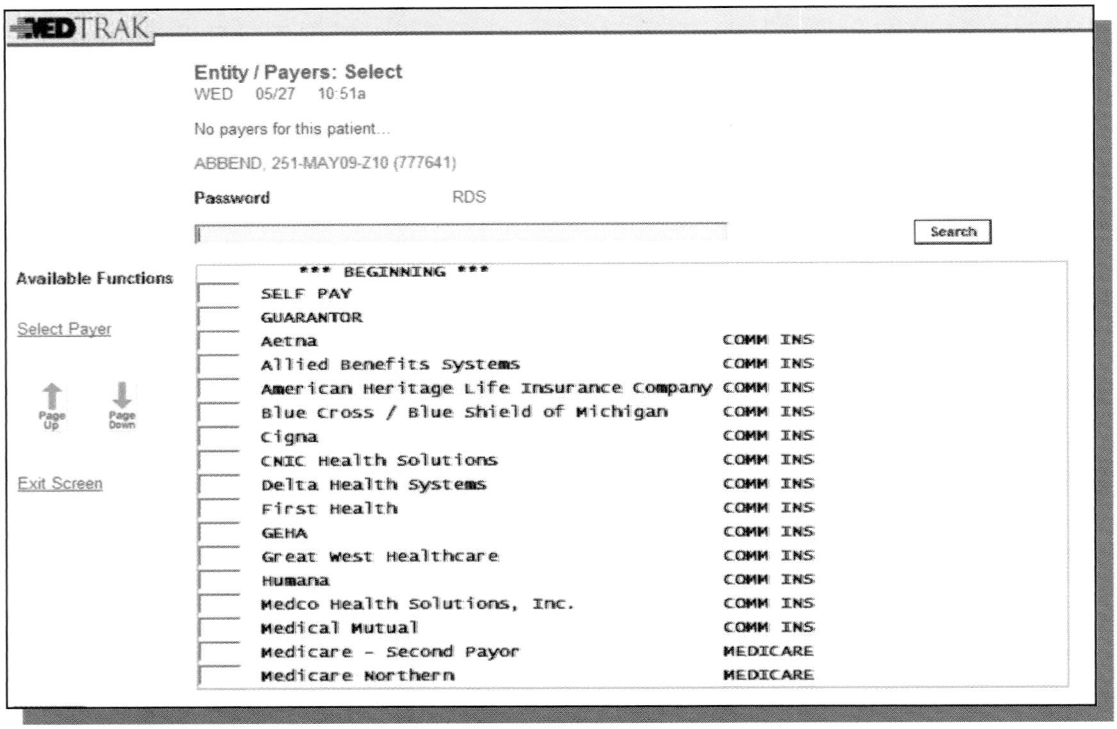

```
MEDTRAK

Entity / Payers: Select
WED   05/27   10:51a

No payers for this patient...

ABBEND, 251-MAY09-Z10 (777641)

Password                    RDS

[                                        ]          [ Search ]

Available Functions          *** BEGINNING ***
                             SELF PAY
Select Payer                 GUARANTOR
                             Aetna                              COMM  INS
                             Allied Benefits Systems            COMM  INS
    ↑        ↓               American Heritage Life Insurance Company  COMM  INS
  Page     Page             Blue Cross / Blue Shield of Michigan      COMM  INS
   Up      Down             cigna                              COMM  INS
                             CNIC Health Solutions              COMM  INS
Exit Screen                  Delta Health Systems               COMM  INS
                             First Health                       COMM  INS
                             GEHA                               COMM  INS
                             Great West Healthcare              COMM  INS
                             Humana                             COMM  INS
                             Medco Health Solutions, Inc.       COMM  INS
                             Medical Mutual                     COMM  INS
                             Medicare - Second Payor            MEDICARE
                             Medicare Northern                  MEDICARE
```

This screen displays all of the authorized payers for the entity that owns the healthcare facility.

To attach a payer, place the cursor in the command field next to the payer and click the *Select Payer* button.

For payers other than **Self Pay** and **Guarantor**, the next screen to appear is the Patient/Payer screen (shown on the next page). Enter the subscriber and insurance policy information on this screen.

If the subscriber is the patient, type in "**self**" in the **Relationship** field and click the *Submit* button. The following fields will be automatically filled in by MedTrak from the patient's demographic record:

> **Last name**
> **First name**
> **Middle initial**
> **Birth date**
> **Gender**

To see the other subscriber relationships, click on the *Relationships* button.

Any subscriber relationship other than **Self Pay** will require the demographics of last name, first name, middle initial, birth date, and gender of the subscriber.

## Entering the Subscriber and Policy Information

```
MEDTRAK

                    Patient / Payer
                    WED  05/27  11:03a


                    ABBEND, 251-MAY09-Z10 (777641)

                    Blue Cross / Blue Shield of Michigan (132)

                    Password          RDS

Available Functions
                    Subscriber
Relationships           Relationship     self              [ Relationships ]
                        Last name        [                ]
Exit Screen             First name       [                ]
                        Middle initial   [  ]
                        Birth date       [        ]  (mm/dd/yyyy)
                        Gender           [  v ]

                    Policy
                        Effective date   010108    (mm/dd/yy)
                        Termination date [     ]    (mm/dd/yy)

                        ID number        37257272
                        Group name       MedTrak Systems, Inc.
                        Group number     G34733
                        Plan type        ppo

                        Co-insurance %   [  ]

                        Co-pay amount    25.00
                        Co-pay note      [                        ]
                                         [                        ]
                                         [                        ]

                                    [ Submit ]
```

The *ID number* is the individual subscriber's contract number assigned by the payer and appears on the front of the insurance card.

The *Group name* is the name of the subscriber's insurance group. In this example, it is MedTrak Systems, Inc., the subscriber's employer.

The *Group number* is the number assigned by the insurance company to the subscriber's group.

The *Plan type* identifies the type of insurance purchased by the group. In this example, the plan type is *PPO*. PPO stands for preferred provider organization and is the most common type of managed care insurance. The managed care company contracts with a network of physicians to provide services at a discounted rate. If the subscriber chooses to see a provider that is not part of the network, the subscriber will be responsible for the portion of the fees that are higher than the contracted rate of the network. The plan type might also be a number as indicated on the front of the insurance card.

The *Co-insurance %* is the portion of the charges that the subscriber must pay for the services.

The *Co-pay amount* is the amount that the subscriber must pay for each office visit. The co-pay amount is applied to the charge for the provider's time to see the patient. Use the *Co-pay note* field for any special notes about the co-payment amount.

**Do This** ▶ **5.01** - Sign into **MedTrak**

**5.02** - Click the *Patient Registration* button on the MedTrak <u>Main Menu</u>

**5.03** - Place the cursor next to the first patient with your last name
(that you added in Chapter 3 - **Adding Patients**)

**5.04** - Click the *Payers* button

**5.05** - Place the cursor next to <u>Blue Cross/Blue Shield of Michigan</u>

**5.06** - Click the *Select Payer* button
(you should be on the Patient/Payer screen for Blue Cross)

**5.07** - Type **self** in the **Relationship** field and click the *Submit* button

**5.08** - Enter an **Effective date** of the beginning of this year

**5.09** - Skip the **Termination date** field

**5.10** - Make up an **ID number**, **Group name**, and **Group number**

**5.11** - Type in a **Plan type** of **PPO**

**5.12** - Skip the **Co-insurance** field

**5.13** - Enter **25** as the **Co-pay amount** (MedTrak will fill in the cents)

**5.14** - Skip the **Co-pay note** field

**5.15** - Click the *Submit* button

## Attaching a Secondary Payer

MedTrak returns to the <u>Entity Payers: Select</u> screen (shown below) with the message at the top "**Payer attached to patient.**" If the patient has more than one payer, you can now select the next payer and fill in the subscriber information.

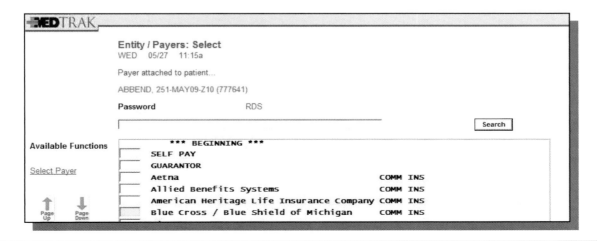

**Do This** ▶ **5.16** - Place the cursor next to <u>Nationwide Insurance</u>

**5.17** - Click the *Select Payer* button

(you should be on the Patient/Payer screen for Nationwide)

**5.18** - Type "**spouse**" in the **Relationship** or select it from the drop-down menu

**5.19** - Fill in the spouse's name, birth date, and gender

**5.20** - Enter an **Effective date** of the beginning of last year

**5.21** - Skip the **Termination date** field

**5.22** - Make up an **ID number**, **Group name**, and **Group number**

**5.23** - Type in a **Plan type** of **PPO**

**5.24** - Skip the **Co-insurance** field

**5.25** - Enter **10** as the **Co-pay** amount

**5.26** - Skip the **Co-pay note** field

**5.27** - Click the *Submit* button

## Attaching a Tertiary Payer

**Do This** ▶ **5.28** - Select <u>Self Pay</u> as the tertiary payer

**5.29** - Click the *Exit Screen* button

After attaching the payers, exit the <u>Entity Payers: Select</u> screen by clicking the *Exit Screen* button. The <u>Patient/Payers</u> screen (shown below) will appear displaying the three payers that you selected.

```
MEDTRAK

                    Patient / Payers
                    WED    05/27    3:41p


                    ABBEND, 251-MAY09-Z10 (777641)

                    Password              RDS
Available Functions
Confirm Payers          P  COMM INS - Blue Cross / Blue Shield of Michigan (01/01/08 -  ? )
                        S  COMM INS - Nationwide Insurance (01/01/08 -  ? )
Primary                 T  SELF PAY
Secondary             ---------------------------------------------------------------
Tertiary                  *** BEGINNING ***
Remove Payer            P  COMM INS - Blue Cross / Blue Shield of Michigan (01/01/08 -  ? )
                       S  COMM INS - Nationwide Insurance (01/01/08 -  ? )
Add Payer              T  SELF PAY
Change Payer              *** END ***
Delete
Show all Payers
Un-delete

More Functions
```

If the payers are not the right ones or they are not in the right order, use the buttons to correct them.

There must always be a primary payer. Secondary, tertiary, and quaternary payers are optional. If there is more than one payer, then the payers must be ordered in the primary, secondary, tertiary, and quaternary order based on who is responsible for paying the claim first, second, third, and fourth. Again, use the buttons to put the payers in their proper order of responsibility.

## Guarantors

For patients under the age of 18, there must be a guarantor attached to the patient, even if there is a group health plan.

To attach a guarantor, select the **Guarantor** option on the Payer: Select screen. The next screen to appear is the listing of patients. On this screen, locate the guarantor using the *Search* function. If the guarantor is not in the patient list, then add the guarantor just like you added a patient.

If the payers are correct, click the *Exit Screen* button or press the *F3* key to return to the list of patients.

---

**Do This** ▶ **5.30** - Review the payers that you attached to your patient (fix, if necessary)

**5.31** - Click the *Exit Screen* button

---

# CHAPTER

# 6

# Scheduling

**Estimated time needed to complete this chapter  -  60** minutes

## What you need to know before doing this chapter

- ◆ How to log into MedTrak
- ◆ How to access the Scheduler screen off the Main Menu

## Learning outcomes gained from this chapter

- ◆ An understanding of how to use the MedTrak Scheduler
- ◆ How to block out time in the schedule
- ◆ How to clear a time segment that was blocked
- ◆ How to schedule a new patient
- ◆ How to schedule an existing patient
- ◆ How to add a note to a patient

## Key concepts in this chapter

*location's schedule*
*time increment*
*location structure*
*location level*
*division level*
*staff level*
*calendar icon*
*block out time*
*clear blocked time*
*established patient*
*new patient*
*patient responsibility*
*occupational medicine*
*payers*
*order of responsibility*
*authorization number*
*appointment note*

## Scheduling

### Major Categories of Clinical Workflow

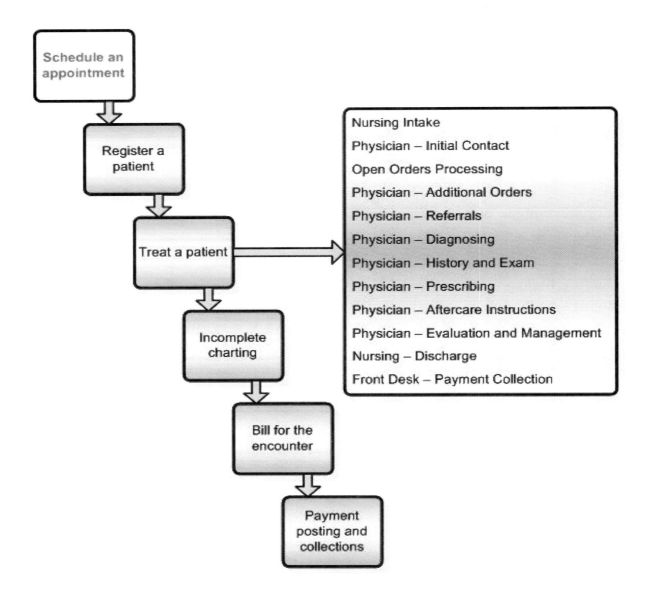

## Scheduling

Medical facilities use a scheduling system to help control their patient flow. Physicians plan their days based on seeing a certain number of patients, returning phone calls, or meeting with patients outside of the office. The medical facility does not want a waiting room full of unhappy patients due to long waiting times.

Depending on the type of patient mix, scheduled patients and walk-ins, a medical facility will set up its schedule according to the availability of the physicians to see patients. Some physicians will only be available to see patients in the office when they are not visiting patients in the hospital, in a care facility, or in surgery.

For this chapter, the scheduling staff accesses the MedTrak Scheduling module from the MedTrak Main Menu by clicking the *Scheduler* button. The Scheduling screen will appear (shown below). This screen displays the *location's schedule* for the days of the week (and the business hours of each day) that the location is open. Each scheduling line will be based on the *time increment* that the location uses for scheduling each appointment. Use the *Page Down* and *Page Up* buttons to view the whole day that the clinic is open.

This clinic location is open Monday through Friday from 8 AM to 5 PM and schedules appointments every 15 minutes.

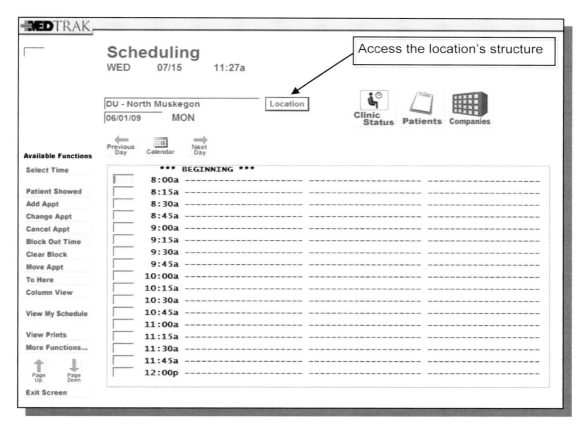

| Do This ▶ | 6.01 - Sign in to MedTrak |
|---|---|
| | 6.02 - Click the *Scheduler* button on the MedTrak Main Menu |

## Setting to a Staff Member's Schedule

The MedTrak **Scheduler** uses a three-tier *location structure*:

1. The first level is the *location level*. This level is used to define a physical location, such as the clinic name.

2. The second level is the *division level* (first indentation), usually defined by departments within the clinic (injury/physical, rehab services, orthopedics, etc.).

3. The third level is the *staff level* (second indentation), where physicians' and/or specialists' names appear.

The scheduling staff accesses the location's structure by clicking on the *Location* button at the top of the Scheduling screen.

The Location/Division: Select screen (shown below) appears.

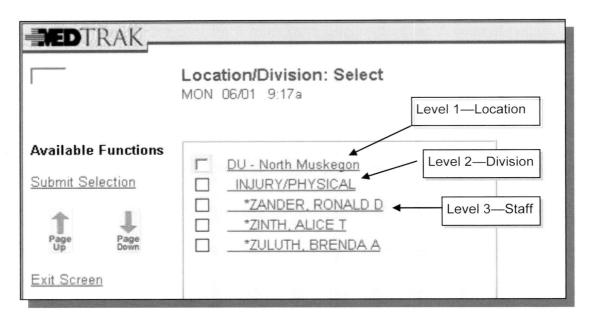

To select a **Staff** member's schedule to use for scheduling patients, the scheduling staff clicks on the staff member's name. MedTrak then resets the Scheduling screen to the staff member's schedule selected.

---

**Do This** ▶   **6.03** - Click the *Location* button on the Scheduling screen

**6.04** - Click on a staff member's name to set to his or her schedule
(remember the staff member's name that you selected)

### Appointments can only be added to a staff member's schedule

---

## Setting to the Appointment Date and Time

The Scheduling screen allows resetting the schedule to any day that the clinic location is open and the provider is in the clinic and available to see patients.

To access the correct day for the appointment, the scheduling staff can use the *calendar icon* at the top of the Scheduling screen to display the calendar for the month (shown below) and then click on the day to see the schedule for that day.

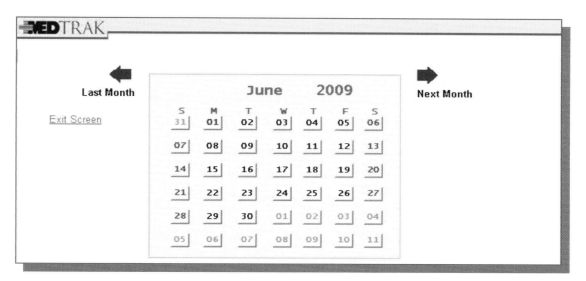

Or, the scheduling staff can manually change the date field (mmddyy) at the top of the Scheduling screen and press the *ENTER* key.

Or, the scheduling staff can move from one day to the next on the Scheduling screen, using the *Next Day* and *Previous Day* buttons.

MedTrak will only display days of the week that the clinic location is open for seeing patients.

**Do This** ▶   **6.05** - Set the Scheduling screen to Monday of this week

## Blocking Out Time in the Schedule for Meetings, Lunch, etc.

To *block out time* in the schedule, the scheduling staff uses the *Block Out Time* button to display the Block screen as shown on the next page. The scheduling staff places the cursor in the starting time field for the block before clicking the *Block Out Time* button.

After entering the **ending time** and the **reason** for the block, the scheduling staff clicks the *Submit* button to set the block. The ending time must be entered using the correct format – **hh:mm** followed by either an **a** for "AM" or a **p** for "PM." MedTrak automatically returns to the Scheduling screen showing the blocked time.

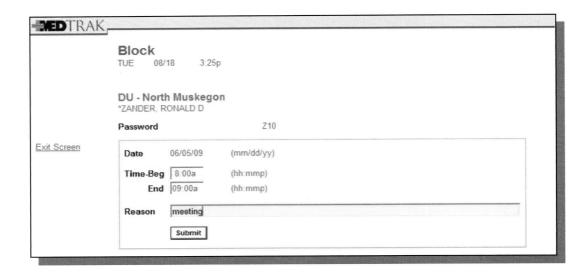

MEDTRAK

**Block**
TUE     08/18     3:25p

**DU - North Muskegon**
*ZANDER, RONALD D

Password                              Z10

Exit Screen

Date        06/05/09      (mm/dd/yy)

Time-Beg  | 8:00a |       (hh:mmp)
      End | 09:00a |      (hh:mmp)

Reason    | meeting |

Submit

---

**Do This** ▶  **6.06** - Block out lunch from 12p to 1p for each day of the week

**6.07** - Block Monday, Wednesday, and Friday at 8a for 1-hour meetings

**6.08** - Block each day from 4p to 5p for walk-in patients

---

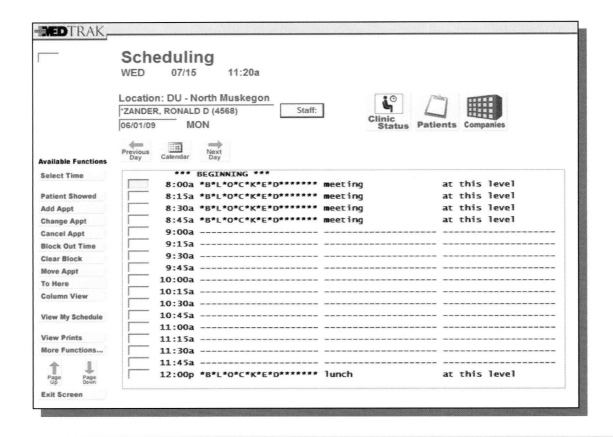

MEDTRAK

**Scheduling**
WED     07/15     11:20a

Location: DU - North Muskegon
*ZANDER, RONALD D (4568)      Staff:

06/01/09     MON

Clinic Status    Patients    Companies

Previous Day    Calendar    Next Day

**Available Functions**

Select Time

Patient Showed

Add Appt

Change Appt

Cancel Appt

Block Out Time

Clear Block

Move Appt

To Here

Column View

View My Schedule

View Prints

More Functions...

Page Up    Page Down

Exit Screen

```
        *** BEGINNING ***
    8:00a *B*L*O*C*K*E*D******* meeting        at this level
    8:15a *B*L*O*C*K*E*D******* meeting        at this level
    8:30a *B*L*O*C*K*E*D******* meeting        at this level
    8:45a *B*L*O*C*K*E*D******* meeting        at this level
    9:00a --------------------- --------------------- ---------------------
    9:15a --------------------- --------------------- ---------------------
    9:30a --------------------- --------------------- ---------------------
    9:45a --------------------- --------------------- ---------------------
   10:00a --------------------- --------------------- ---------------------
   10:15a --------------------- --------------------- ---------------------
   10:30a --------------------- --------------------- ---------------------
   10:45a --------------------- --------------------- ---------------------
   11:00a --------------------- --------------------- ---------------------
   11:15a --------------------- --------------------- ---------------------
   11:30a --------------------- --------------------- ---------------------
   11:45a --------------------- --------------------- ---------------------
   12:00p *B*L*O*C*K*E*D******* lunch          at this level
```

## *Clearing Time Blocked on the Schedule*

To *clear blocked time* in the schedule, the scheduling staff places the cursor in the starting time for the block and clicks the *Clear Block* button. To confirm the clearing of the block, then they click the *Submit* button. All of the fields on this screen are frozen because they reflect the blocking of the time period.

MedTrak will automatically return to the Scheduling screen showing the schedule is now clear for that time period.

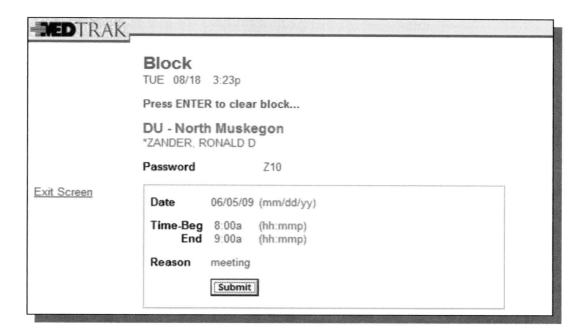

**Do This** ▶ **6.09** - Clear the block for Friday's meeting at 8a

**6.10** - Create a new block for Friday's meeting at 9a for 1 hour

## Scheduling Patient Appointments

To schedule patients for appointments, the scheduling staff sets to the right staff's schedule and appointment date, then clicks the *Add Appt* button.

**Do This** ▶ **6.11** - Set the scheduling date back to your Monday for your staff member

### Be sure that you are on your staff member's schedule

**6.12** - Place the cursor in the command field for the time for the appointment
(set to 9:15a time slot - it should be available)

**6.13** - Click on the *Add Appt* button

### If you get an error on this screen, review steps 6.03 and 6.04

## Selecting or Adding the Patient to a Schedule

The next screen to appear is the <u>Patient: Select</u> screen (shown below) for locating the patient's name.

If this is an *established patient* (their name will be in the list), the scheduling staff uses the **Search** field to locate the patient, then places the cursor next to the patient's name, and clicks the *Select* button.

If this is a *new patient* (their name will not appear in the list), the scheduling staff clicks the *Add* button to add the new patient.

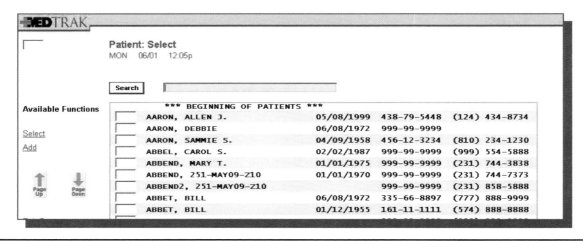

**Do This** ▶ **6.14** - Click the *Add* button
(assume this is a new patient)

## *Adding Partial Patient Information*

The next screen is the <u>Partial Patient Add</u> (shown below). When scheduling an appointment for a new patient, the only patient demographic information needed is the patient's name and phone numbers. Full demographic information will be collected at the front desk during registration when the patient arrives for the clinical visit.

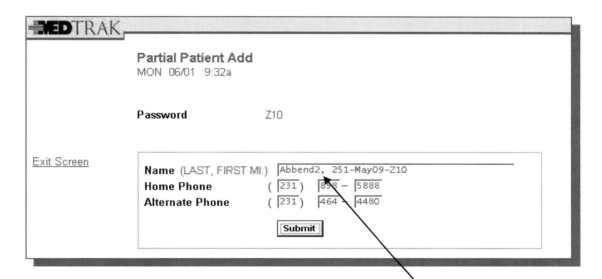

The scheduling staff enters the patient's name in last name, comma, first name, and middle initial order and clicks the *Submit* button.

The <u>Patient Partial Add</u> screen will reappear for verification of correct information. The scheduling staff clicks the *Submit* button again to confirm the accuracy of the data.

**Do This** ▶ **6.15** - Add a new patient with your last name plus the number **2**

**6.16** - Use the same first name that you did in <u>Chapter 3, Adding Patients</u>

**6.17** - Make up a home phone number

**6.18** - Make up an alternate phone number

**6.19** - Click the *Submit* button

**6.20** - Verify the information, then click the *Submit* button again

## *Selecting the Patient/Company*

MedTrak is designed to handle *patient responsibility* cases (self pay, guarantor, group health, Medicare, Medicaid, etc.), where the patient is responsible for payment of services through his or her group health coverage or out of his or her own pocket; and *occupational medicine* cases (workers' compensation and employee health), where the employer is responsible for payment of services through the employer's workers' compensation insurance or the employer's checkbook.

Because this is a new patient, there are no existing Patient/Company relationships. Therefore, after entering the patient's demographic information, the next screen to appear is the Company: Select screen (shown below). In this example, the patient is responsible for the payment of services so the scheduling staff places the cursor next to the "**..Patient Responsibility**" selection and clicks the *Select* button.

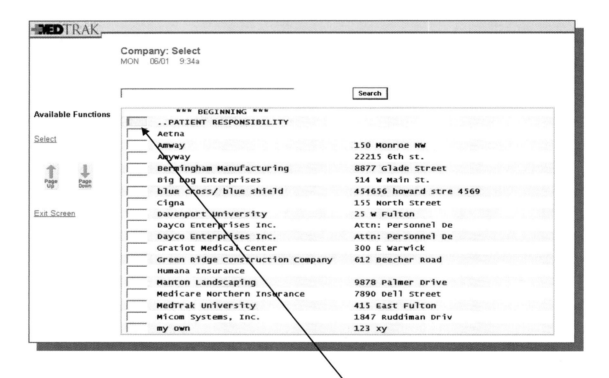

**Do This** ► **6.21** - Place the cursor next to **..Patient Responsibility**

**6.22** - Click the *Select* button

## Selecting the Patient's Payer(s) for Patient Responsibility Cases

Again, because this is a new patient who is responsible for payment of the services, the next screen to appear is the <u>Entity/Payers: Select</u> screen (shown below). This screen displays all of the authorized *payers* for the entity that owns the clinic. This screen will not appear if this is a work comp or employee health case since the employer is responsible for paying for those types of visits.

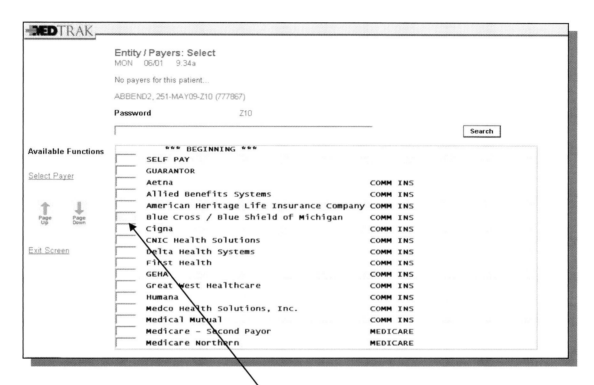

For this example, our patient has Blue Cross/Blue Shield of Michigan as his group health insurance coverage. The scheduling staff places the cursor next to Blue Cross/Blue Shield of Michigan and clicks the *Select Payer* button.

MedTrak shows a message at the top of the screen in red:   Payer attached to patient (as incomplete). There were no other payers for our patient, so we exit this screen by clicking the *Exit Screen* button.

When the patient arrives for the appointment, the front desk will gather the rest of the patient's demographic information including subscriber and policy data for Blue Cross.

---

**Do This** ▶ **6.23** - Place the cursor next to Blue Cross/Blue Shield of Michigan

**6.24** - Click the *Select Payer* button (only one payer for this exercise)

**6.25** - Click the *Exit Screen* button

---

## Reviewing the Patient's Payer(s)

The next screen to appear is the <u>Patient/Payers</u> screen (shown below).

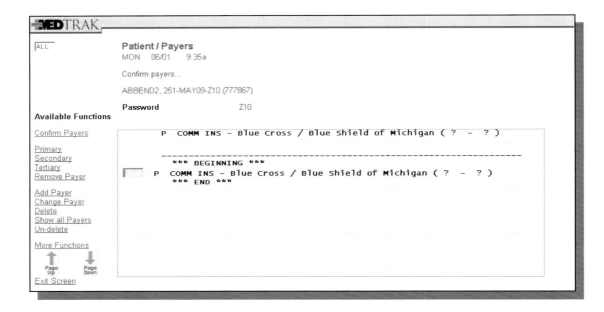

As you learned in **Attaching Payers to a Patient**, Chapter 5, there can be up to four payers attached to a patient. In this example, there is only one payer — Blue Cross/Blue Shield of Michigan.

If there were multiple payers, the payers would need to be attached to this patient in the order of responsibility for paying any claims. If you loaded the payers in the *order of responsibility* for payment, the primary, secondary, tertiary, and quaternary indicators will be attached to the patient in the right order. If the payer priority order is not correct, change the order by using the Primary, Secondary, Tertiary, and Quaternary buttons to switch the order.

**Do This** ▶ **6.26** - Review the payer (in this case there is only one)

**6.27** - Click the *Confirm Payers* button

## *Appointment Scheduling Screen*

The next screen is the appointment <u>Scheduling</u> screen (shown below).

For this example, the reason for the appointment is **lower back pain**. There was no *authorization number* needed, so the scheduling staff enters **not needed**.

For work comp or employee health cases, MedTrak requires the person's name who authorized the visit for the employer.

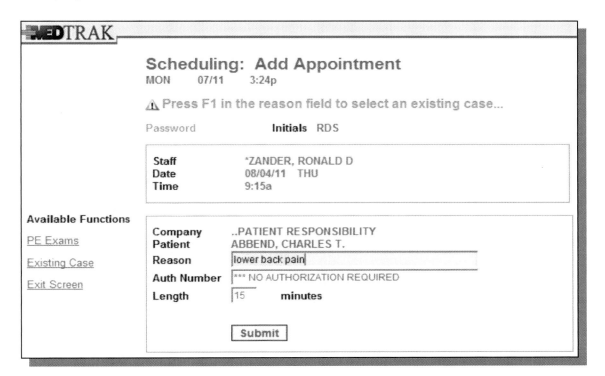

---

**Do This** ▶ **6.28** - Enter **lower back pain** as the reason for the appointment

**6.29** - (No authorization number is needed for this insurance carrier, and the length of the appointment defaults to 15 minutes.)

**6.30** - Click the *Submit* button

## *Appointment Note Screen*

The next screen is the Appointment Note screen (shown below). On this screen, the scheduling staff enters an *appointment note* for the physician to read. Most appointments will not have a note attached.

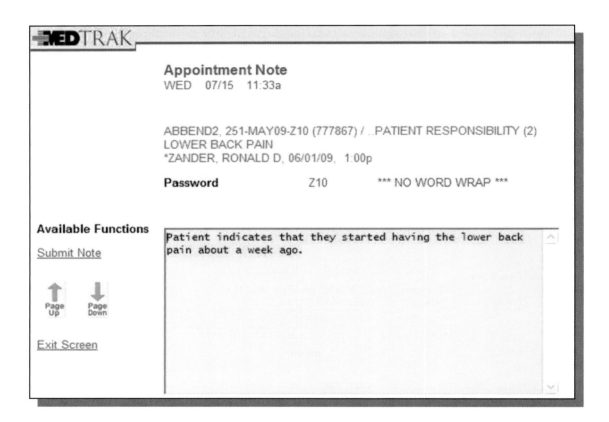

To attach the note, the scheduling staff clicks the *Submit Note* button.

---

**Do This** ▶ **6.31** - Enter a note for the appointment (it can be the same one as above)

**6.32** - Click the *Submit Note* button

---

MedTrak will return to the Scheduling screen (shown below) displaying this appointment.

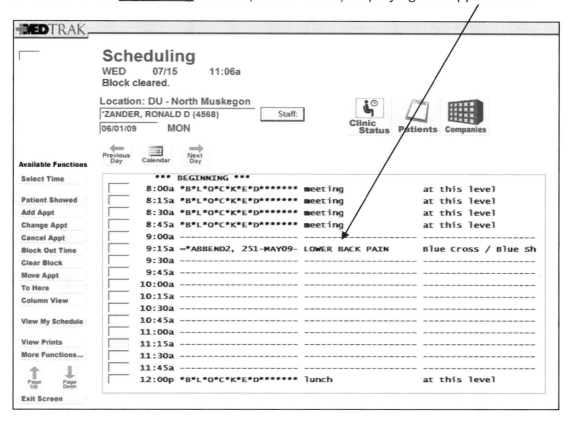

**Do This** ▶ **6.33** - **Schedule three new patient appointments for Monday**

(use the processing starting with **Step 6.15**)

(create your own **new** patient names)

**6.33.1** - A patient responsibility patient at 9:30a with a sore throat

**6.33.2** - A Bermingham employee at 10:00a with right hip pain

**6.33.3** - A Sampson employee at 10:30a for an annual physical

**Do This** ▶ **6.34** - **Schedule established patient appointments for Monday**

(use patients that you added in Chapter 3 – **Adding Patients**)

**6.34.1** - Schedule your patient #3 for 1:15p with a sore neck

(select patient responsibility as the company with payer of self pay)

**6.34.2** - Schedule your patient #4 for 2:00p with right arm pain

(select South Padre as the company)

**Do This** ▶ **6.35** - *Cancel* the 10:00a Bermingham employee with right hip pain

                       **Reason**: *Employee went to the emergency room.*

**Do This** ▶ **6.36** - *Move* the 2:00p patient #4 with right arm pain to 10:00a

                       Use the *Move Appt* and *To Here* buttons.

**Do This** ▶ **6.37** - *Print* the schedule for your Monday showing your appointments

                       (make sure to set the scheduler to your Monday)

**6.38** - Place the cursor in any one of the command fields

**6.39** - Type the print command - **PR**

**6.40** - Press the **ENTER** key

**6.41** - Click the **PRINT** button

                       (look for "Report sent to printer/queue" message)

**6.42** - Click the **EXIT SCREEN** button

**6.43** - MedTrak creates PDF's of your prints and places them in a queue

**6.44** - To view your print queue, click the **View Prints** button

                       (this will open another window displaying your PDF print queue)

                       (this screen is called Available User Reports)

**6.45** - Place the cursor next to the print that you want to view

**6.46** - Click the **View Print** button

                       (this will open Adobe displaying the PDF of your chart)

**6.47** - Click the *diskette* icon at the top left of the PDF

**6.48** - Save PDF to a folder for your class assignments

**6.49** - Attach the PDF to your assignment from this folder

**6.50** - Close the *Adobe* window displaying your chart

**6.51** - Close the Available User Reports window

**6.52** - Click the *Main Menu* button

                       (you should be on the Clinic Status screen)

# CHAPTER 7

# Patient Registration

**Estimated time needed to complete this chapter  -  45** minutes

## What you need to know before doing this chapter

- How to log into MedTrak
- How to access the <u>Scheduler</u> off the <u>Main Menu</u>
- How to access <u>Patient Registration </u>off the <u>Main Menu</u>

## Learning outcomes gained from this chapter

- An understanding of how to register a patient from the Scheduler
- An understanding of how to register a patient from <u>Patient Registration</u>
- How to add the patient's demographic information
- How to select the patient's company (payer responsibility relationship)
- How to create a new case
- How to confirm the patient's payers
- How to add a visit
- How to select the presenting problem(s)

## Key concepts in this chapter

*scheduled patients*
*walk-in patients*
*disciplines of medicine*
*problem-focused system*
*blended checklists*
*multiple presenting problems*
*add a new patient*
*established patient*
*patient responsibility*
*occupational medicine*
*payer responsibility relationship*

## Patient Registration

### Major Categories of Clinical Workflow

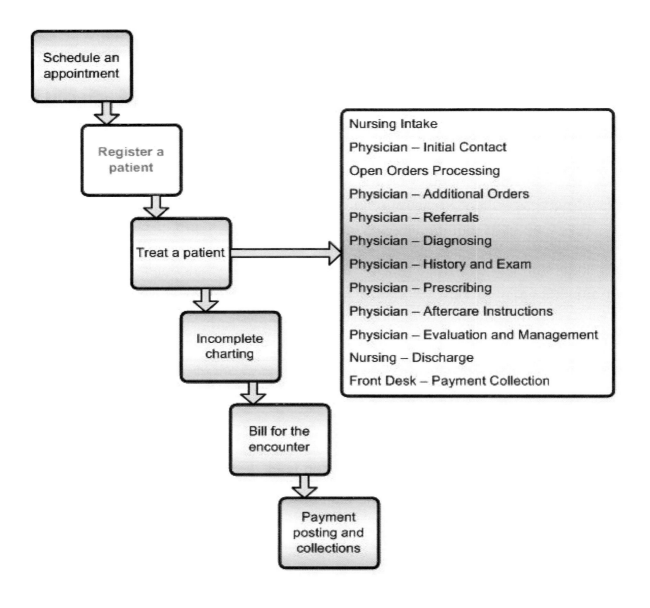

## Patient Registration

When a patient arrives at the front desk of a healthcare facility for registration, the front desk person typically asks who the person is and whether he or she has an appointment. Additionally, the front desk person will ask the patient to sign the check-in register. The mix of *scheduled patients* versus *walk-in patients* (those who do not have an appointment) ranges from 100% scheduled and 0% walk-ins to 0% scheduled and 100% walk-ins.

When registering a scheduled patient, the front desk person will "mark" on the schedule that the patient arrived for the appointment and then register him or her.

In this chapter, you will use 2 different processes to register a patient in MedTrak:

1. For patients who have scheduled appointments, the front desk person will access the Scheduler module from the MedTrak Main Menu by clicking the *Scheduling* button.

2. For patients who do not have an appointment (walk-in patients), the front desk person will access the Patient Registration module from the MedTrak Main Menu by clicking the *Patient Registration* button.

## Registering a Patient from the Scheduler

If the patient has an appointment, MedTrak enables the front desk person to register a patient directly from the Scheduler. The front desk person accesses the Scheduler screen (shown below). The Scheduler screen automatically sets to the location view for that day's schedule.

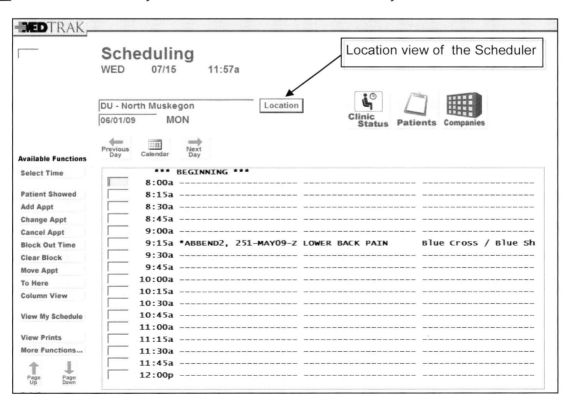

To register the patient, the front desk person locates the patient's name on the day's schedule, places the cursor next to the patient's name, and clicks the *Patient Showed* button.

---

**Do This** ▶ **7.01** - Sign in to MedTrak

         **7.02** - Access the MedTrak Scheduler from the Main Menu

         **7.03** - Set to the Monday that you scheduled in Chapter 6

         **7.04** - Place the cursor next to the lower back pain patient (number 2)

         **7.05** - Click the *Patient Showed* button

---

## Adding the Patient's Demographic Information

The next screen to appear is the <u>Patient</u> demographic screen (shown below), since the **lower back pain** patient is a <u>new</u> patient. Remember, for <u>new</u> patients, the only patient demographic information recorded when scheduling the visit was the patient's name, phone numbers, and primary payer (for patient responsibility visits).

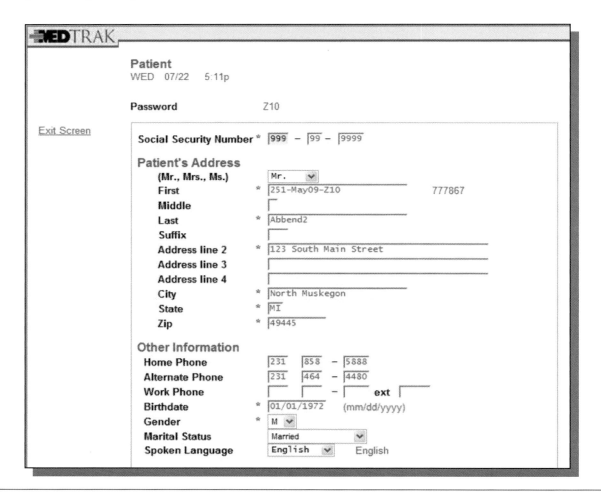

> **Do This** ▶ **7.06** - Enter the patient's demographic information
>
> **7.07** - Click the **Submit** button

## Creating a New Case

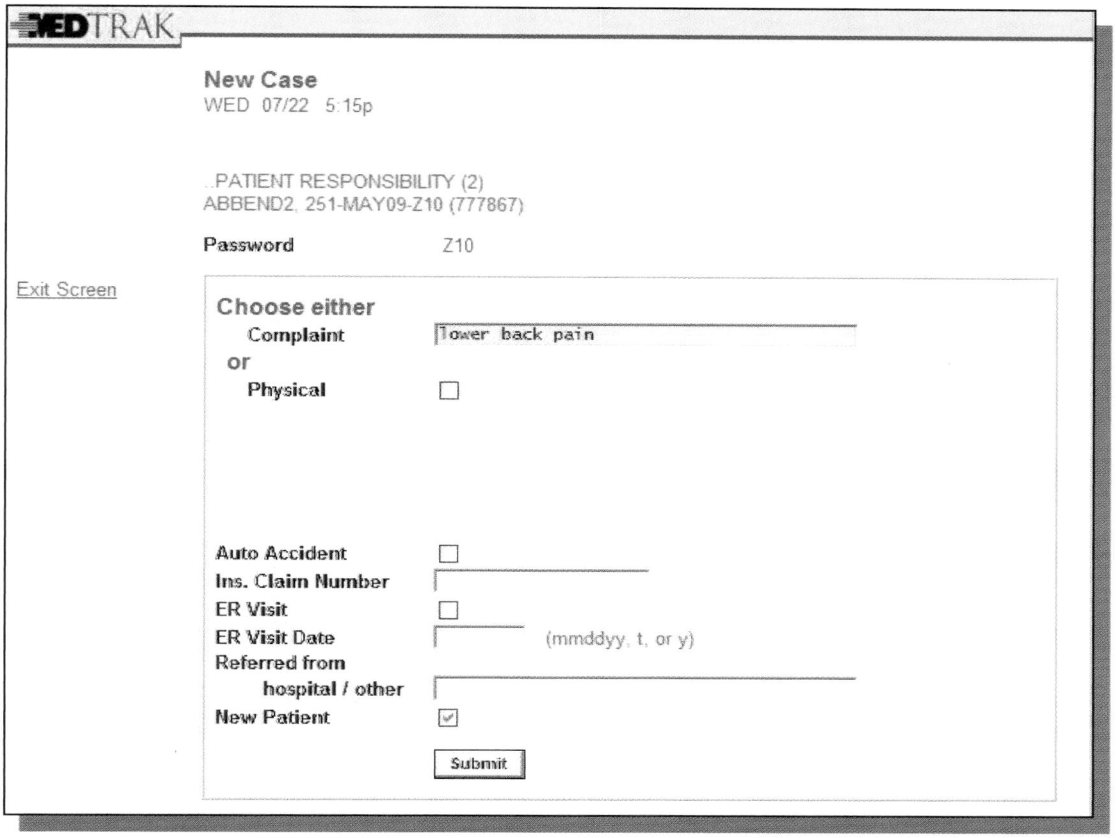

> **Do This** ▶ **7.08** - Enter **lower back pain** in the **Complaint** field
>
> **7.09** - Click the **Submit** button

## Confirming the Patient's Payers

The next screen to appear is the Patient/Payers screen (shown on the next page), as this is a *patient responsibility* visit (meaning that either the patient or the patient's health insurance will pay for the visit).

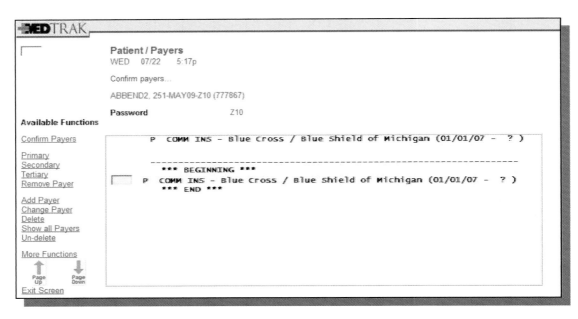

The front desk person scans the patient's insurance card and driver's license, and attaches the scanned information to the case in MedTrak. Using the data from the insurance card, the front desk person clicks the *Change Payer* button to access the Patient/Payer screen (shown below). Remember, for new patients, the only payer information recorded during scheduling was the name of the payer. The front desk person enters the subscriber and policy information.

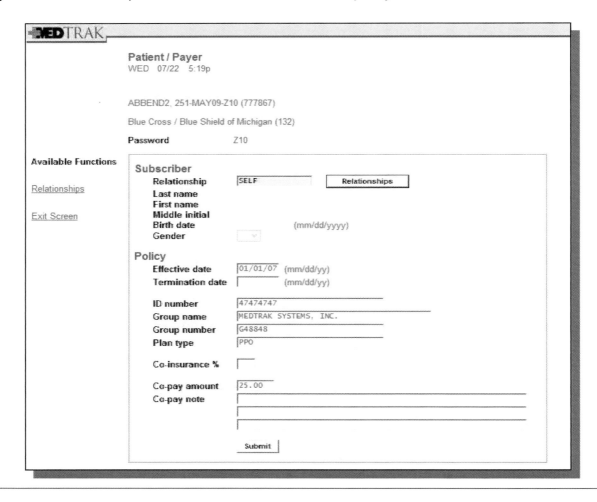

For more information about attaching payers to a patient, refer to **Chapter 5 – Attaching Payers to a Patient**. After filling in all of the payer information, MedTrak returns to the <u>Patient/Payers</u> screen (shown below) for confirmation of the payers. After updating the payers or adding new payers, the front desk person clicks the *Confirm Payers* button.

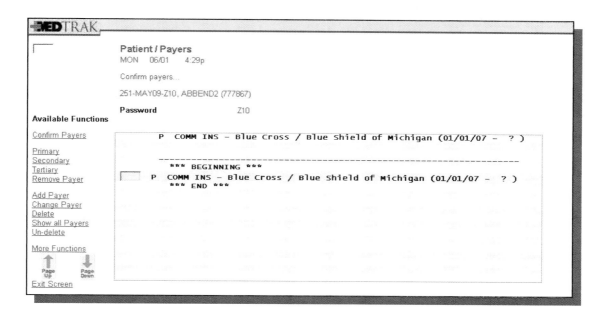

**Do This ▶**   **7.10** - Click the *Change Payer* button

**7.11** - Make up the <u>Subscriber</u> and <u>Policy</u> information - put **25** in the co-pay

**7.12** - Click the *Submit* button on the <u>Patient/Payer</u> screen

**7.13** - Click the *Confirm Payers* button to confirm the payers

## *Adding the Visit*

The next screen to appear is the <u>Visit Add</u> screen (shown on the next page). MedTrak is designed to support a variety of *disciplines of medicine* including:

- ♦ Primary care doctors
- ♦ Urgent care doctors
- ♦ Occupational medicine doctors (workers' compensation and employee health)
- ♦ Orthopedic doctors
- ♦ Rehab services (physical therapy and occupational therapy)
- ♦ Emergency room doctors
- ♦ Chiropractic doctors

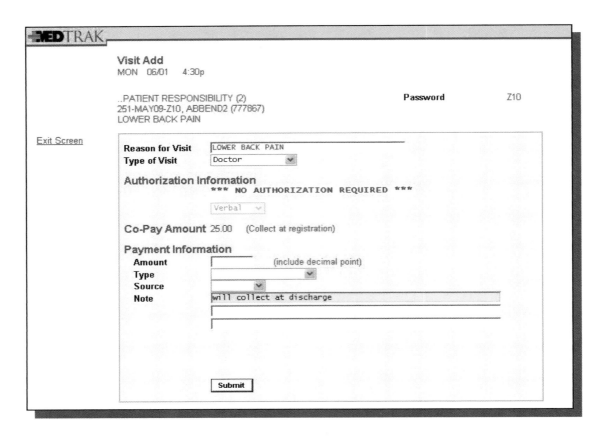

For this visit, the patient is in the clinic to see the doctor for **lower back pain**.

This patient's payer requires a $25 co-payment amount for the doctor visit. Because a payment from the patient is needed, MedTrak requires the front desk person to enter an amount collected (or a note about the payment collection) to exit this screen. In this example, the front desk person enters a note that the co-payment will be collected at discharge.

| | |
|---|---|
| **Do This** ▶ | **7.14** - Confirm that the **Reason for Visit** is for **lower back pain** |
| | **7.15** - Select **Doctor** for the **Type of Visit** |
| | **7.16** - Enter a **Note** about the payment for the visit |
| | **7.17** - Click the *Submit* button |

## *Selecting the Presenting Problem*

MedTrak is a *problem-focused system*. As such, the front desk person selects from a list of presenting problems (shown below) the reason(s) that the patient is visiting the clinic. For this visit, the patient is here to see the doctor for **lower back pain**.

The front desk person clicks the check box for Injury-Bones/Jts and then clicks the *Submit* button.

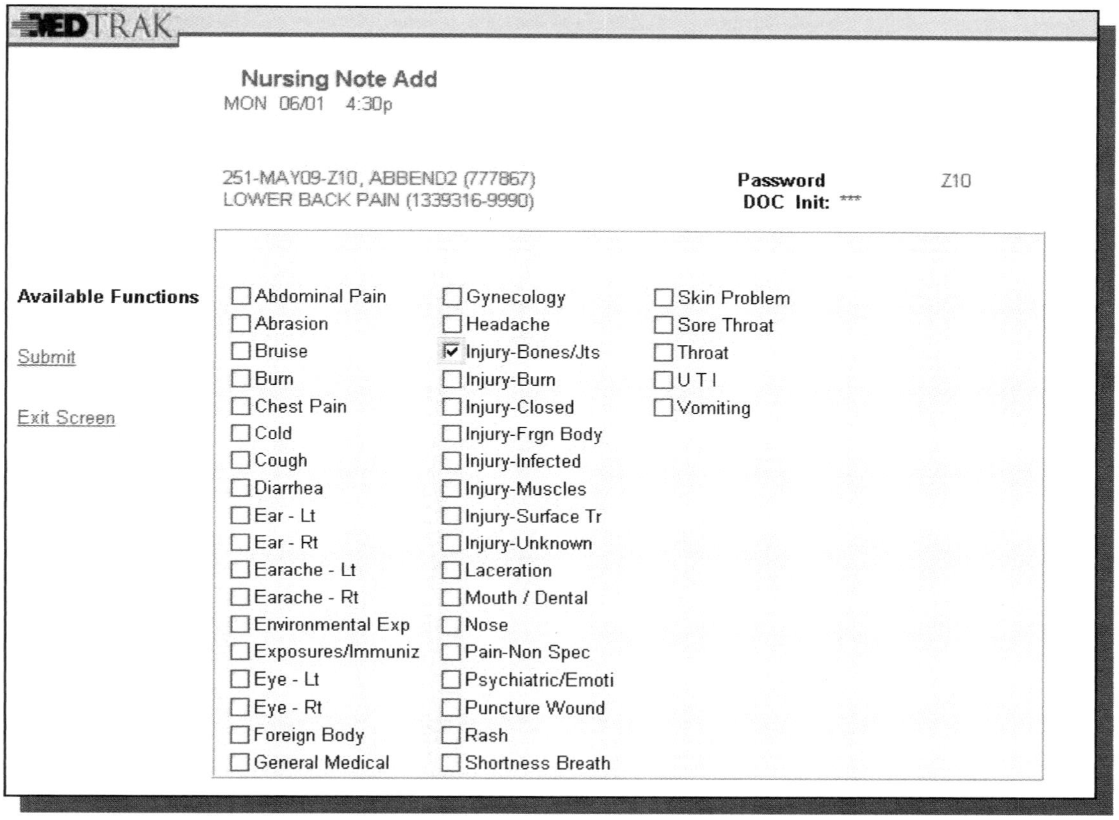

**MED**TRAK

**Nursing Note Add**
MON  06/01   4:30p

251-MAY09-Z10, ABBEND2 (777867)          **Password**          Z10
LOWER BACK PAIN (1339316-9990)          **DOC  Init:** ***

**Available Functions**

Submit

Exit Screen

| ☐ Abdominal Pain | ☐ Gynecology | ☐ Skin Problem |
| ☐ Abrasion | ☐ Headache | ☐ Sore Throat |
| ☐ Bruise | ☑ Injury-Bones/Jts | ☐ Throat |
| ☐ Burn | ☐ Injury-Burn | ☐ U T I |
| ☐ Chest Pain | ☐ Injury-Closed | ☐ Vomiting |
| ☐ Cold | ☐ Injury-Frgn Body | |
| ☐ Cough | ☐ Injury-Infected | |
| ☐ Diarrhea | ☐ Injury-Muscles | |
| ☐ Ear - Lt | ☐ Injury-Surface Tr | |
| ☐ Ear - Rt | ☐ Injury-Unknown | |
| ☐ Earache - Lt | ☐ Laceration | |
| ☐ Earache - Rt | ☐ Mouth / Dental | |
| ☐ Environmental Exp | ☐ Nose | |
| ☐ Exposures/Immuniz | ☐ Pain-Non Spec | |
| ☐ Eye - Lt | ☐ Psychiatric/Emoti | |
| ☐ Eye - Rt | ☐ Puncture Wound | |
| ☐ Foreign Body | ☐ Rash | |
| ☐ General Medical | ☐ Shortness Breath | |

The next screen to appear is the body part selection screen for an injury to the bones or joints (shown on the next page). The front desk person selects the affected body part(s) for the injury on this screen.

**Nursing Note Add**
MON 06/01 4:31p

251-MAY09-Z10, ABBEND2 (777867)          Password          Z10
LOWER BACK PAIN (1339316-9990)          DOC Init: ***

INJURY-BONES/JTS

**Available Functions**

Submit

Exit Screen

| | | | |
|---|---|---|---|
| ☐ Abdomen | ☐ Digit-Rt #1-Thumb | ☐ Hip/Buttock - Rt | ☐ Thumb - Lt |
| ☐ Ankle - Lt | ☐ Digit-Rt #2-Index | ☐ Inguinal - Lt | ☐ Thumb - Rt |
| ☐ Ankle - Rt | ☐ Digit-Rt #3-Middl | ☐ Inguinal - Rt | ☐ Toes - Lt |
| ☐ Arm - Lt (upper) | ☐ Digit-Rt #4-Ring | ☐ Knee - Lt | ☐ Toes - Rt |
| ☐ Arm - Rt (upper) | ☐ Digit-Rt #5-Littl | ☐ Knee - Rt | ☐ Wrist - Lt |
| ☐ Axilla - Lt | ☐ Elbow - Lt | ☐ Leg - Lt | ☐ Wrist - Rt |
| ☐ Axilla - Rt | ☐ Elbow - Rt | ☐ Leg - Rt | |
| ☑ Back - Lower | ☐ Face | ☐ Mouth | |
| ☐ Back - Upper | ☐ Flank - Lt | ☐ Neck | |
| ☐ Breast - Lt | ☐ Flank - Rt | ☐ Nose | |
| ☐ Breast - Rt | ☐ Foot - Lt | ☐ Pelvis | |
| ☐ Chest - Lt | ☐ Foot - Rt | ☐ Ribs - Lt | |
| ☐ Chest - Rt | ☐ Forearm - Lt | ☐ Ribs - Rt | |
| ☐ Digit-Lt #1-Thumb | ☐ Forearm - Rt | ☐ Scalp | |
| ☐ Digit-Lt #2-Index | ☐ Hand - Lt | ☐ Shoulder - Lt | |
| ☐ Digit-Lt #3-Middl | ☐ Hand - Rt | ☐ Shoulder - Rt | |
| ☐ Digit-Lt #4-Ring | ☐ Head | ☐ Thigh - Lt | |
| ☐ Digit-Lt #5-Littl | ☐ Hip/Buttock - Lt | ☐ Thigh - Rt | |

For this example, the front desk person checks the box for **Back - Lower** and then clicks the *Submit* button.

MedTrak is designed to create *blended checklists* of history and exam questions for the nurse and the doctor of the presenting problems from head to toe. When a patient has *multiple presenting problems*, the front desk selects all of them. The *Nursing Note* and *Physician's Checklist* contain suggested questions about those presenting problems in one list of questions, starting at the head and working down to the toes.

Additionally, MedTrak displays the most likely orders for the types of presenting problems on the order entry screens for physicians to select from by checking off the ones that they want. This saves physicians valuable time in searching for orders to place.

In this example, there is one presenting problem, so the lists will only contain questions related to **lower back pain**. If there had been presenting problems for a sore throat, lower back pain, and right knee pain, the Nursing Note and Physician's Checklist would contain questions starting with the head, then the lower back, and finally the right knee.

The Nursing Note Add screen (shown on the next page) refreshes with the message "**Back - Lower Injury-Bones/Jts selected**" in red at the top of the screen.

After selecting the presenting problems, the front desk person exits the Nursing Note Add screen to return to the Scheduling screen to register the next patient.

**MED**TRAK

Nursing Note Add
MON  06/01   4:31p

Back - Lower Injury-Bones/Jts selected...

251-MAY09-Z10, ABBEND2 (777867)                    Password                Z10
LOWER BACK PAIN (1339316-9990)                     DOC  Init:  ***

INJURY-BONES/JTS

Available Functions

☐ Abdomen          ☐ Digit-Rt #1-Thumb    ☐ Hip/Buttock - Rt    ☐ Thumb - Lt
☐ Ankle - Lt       ☐ Digit-Rt #2-Index    ☐ Inguinal - Lt       ☐ Thumb - Rt
Submit             ☐ Ankle - Rt           ☐ Digit-Rt #3-Middl    ☐ Inguinal - Rt       ☐ Toes - Lt
☐ Arm - Lt (upper) ☐ Digit-Rt #4-Ring     ☐ Knee - Lt           ☐ Toes - Rt
Exit Screen        ☐ Arm - Rt (upper)     ☐ Digit-Rt #5-Littl    ☐ Knee - Rt           ☐ Wrist - Lt
☐ Axilla - Lt      ☐ Elbow - Lt           ☐ Leg - Lt            ☐ Wrist - Rt

**Do This** ▶   **7.18** - Click the **Injury - Bones/Jts** check box

**7.19** - Click the *Submit* button

**7.20** - Click the **Back - Lower** check box

**7.21** - Click the *Submit* button

**7.22** - Review the message for **Back - Lower Injury - Bones/Jts selected**

**7.23** - Click the *Exit Screen* button
             (you should be back on the first Nursing Note Add screen)

**7.24** - Click the *Exit Screen* button again
             (you should be on the Scheduling screen)

The Scheduling screen (shown below) marks scheduled patients who have been registered for their appointments with an equal sign (=) in front of their name.

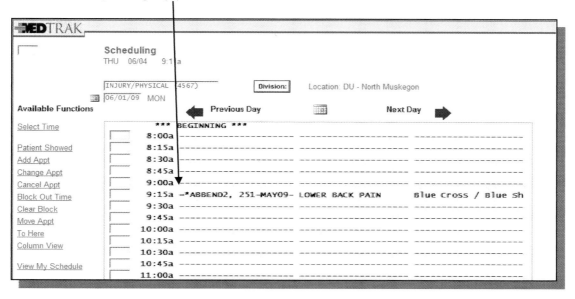

**MED**TRAK

Scheduling
THU  06/04   9:1 a

INJURY/PHYSICAL  (4567)          Division:    Location: DU - North Muskegon
06/01/09  MON

Available Functions              ◀ Previous Day              Next Day ▶

Select Time          ***  BEGINNING ***
                     8:00a ---------------------------------------------
Patient Showed       8:15a ---------------------------------------------
Add Appt             8:30a ---------------------------------------------
Change Appt          8:45a ---------------------------------------------
Cancel Appt          9:00a ---------------------------------------------
Block Out Time       9:15a =*ABBEND2, 251-MAY09- LOWER BACK PAIN    Blue Cross / Blue Sh
Clear Block          9:30a ---------------------------------------------
Move Appt            9:45a ---------------------------------------------
To Here              10:00a ---------------------------------------------
Column View          10:15a ---------------------------------------------
                     10:30a ---------------------------------------------
View My Schedule     10:45a ---------------------------------------------
                     11:00a ---------------------------------------------

## Registering Patients Using Patient Registration

If the patient does not have an appointment (walk-in patient), MedTrak enables the front desk person to register the patient using the **Patient Registration** path. The front desk person accesses the Patients registration screen (shown below) from the Main Menu.

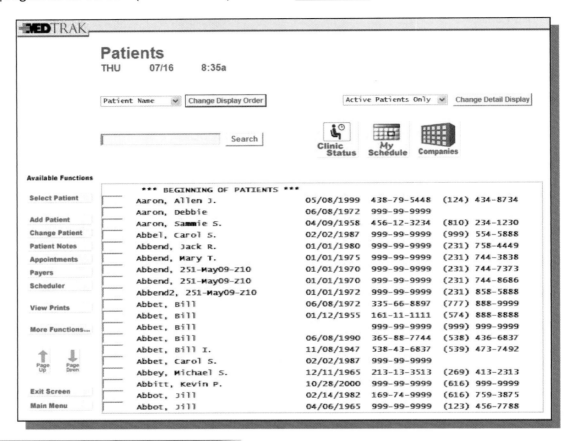

## Adding New Patients

To add a new patient to the patient database, the front desk person clicks the *Add Patient* button. The next screen to appear is the Patient: Add by SSN screen (shown below).

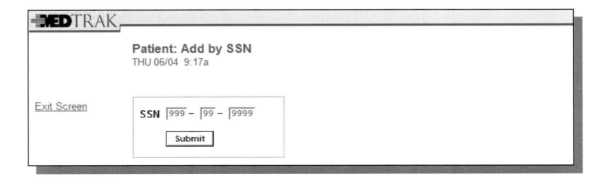

If the patient does not have a social security number or will not provide it, the front desk enters all 9s in the social security number field.

If the patient's social security number is already in the patient database, the Patient demographics screen (shown below) appears with the patient's information filled in.

If the patient's social security number is not in the system, the Patient demographics screen appears with only the social security number filled in.

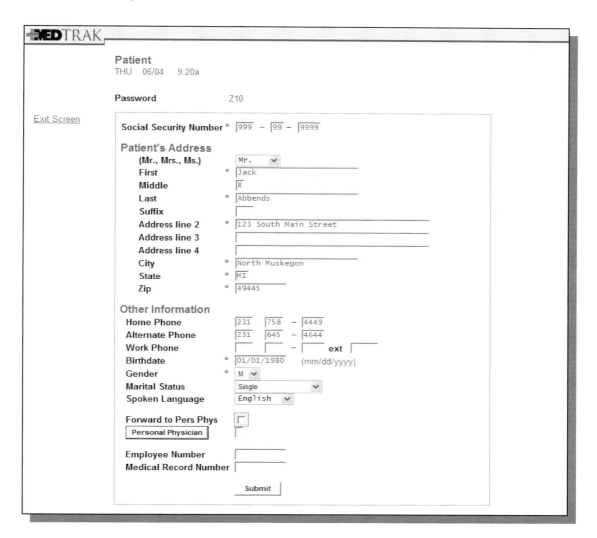

On the Patient demographics screen, red asterisks appear next to the fields that must be answered.

If a required field is not filled in, a message appears (in red) below the date and time at the top of the screen, and the cursor will be set to the field that needs information.

Be sure to enter the information using appropriate punctuation and capitalization.

For example, when entering a street name, the front desk enters "**123 Maple Lane**" instead of "**123 maple lane**" or "**123 MAPLE LANE**."

When finished, the front desk clicks the *Submit* button. MedTrak freezes all of the fields on the <u>Patient</u> demographics screen and requests verification that the information is correct. If the information is correct, the front desk person clicks the *Submit* button again. If some of the information needs correcting, the front desk person clicks the *Exit Screen* button to unlock the <u>Patient</u> demographics entry screen for editing.

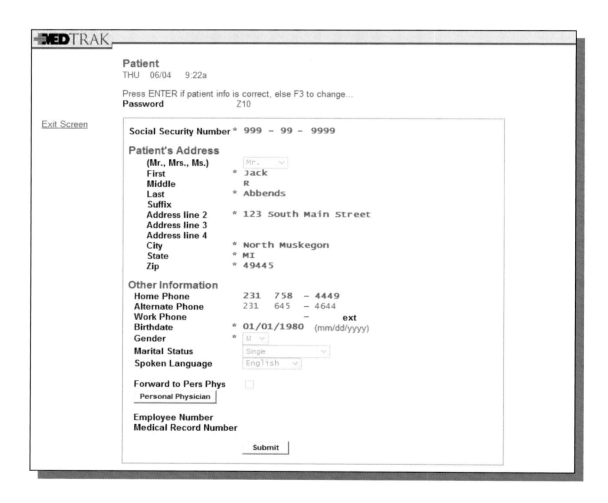

## Selecting Established Patients from the List of Patients

To locate an established patient in the database, the front desk person types in some of the first letters of the patient's last name in the search field and clicks the *Search* button.

For this example (shown below), the search is for **Abbend, 251-May09-Z10.** Since this patient appears on the first screen, we did not need to use the search field.

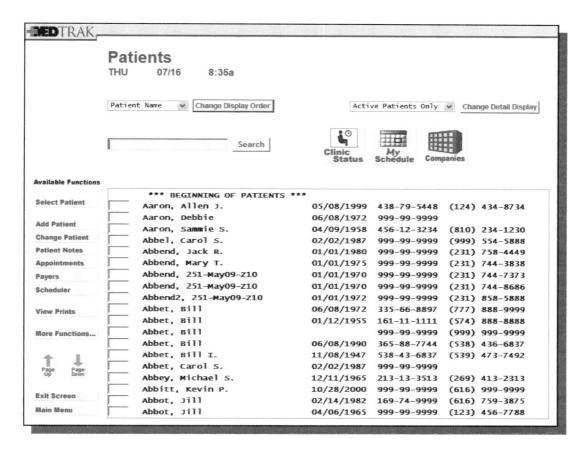

For established patients, the front desk will want to verify the patient's demographic information and make any necessary changes. To review the patient's demographic information, the front desk places the cursor next to the patient and clicks the *Change Patient* button.

The <u>Patient</u> demographics screen (shown on the next page) appears. The front desk verifies with the patient that the information is correct.

If there are changes, the front desk person clicks on the *Submit* button to record the changes and return to the <u>Patients</u> database screen.

If there are no changes, the front desk person can click on the *Exit Screen* button or the *Submit* button to return to the <u>Patients</u> database screen.

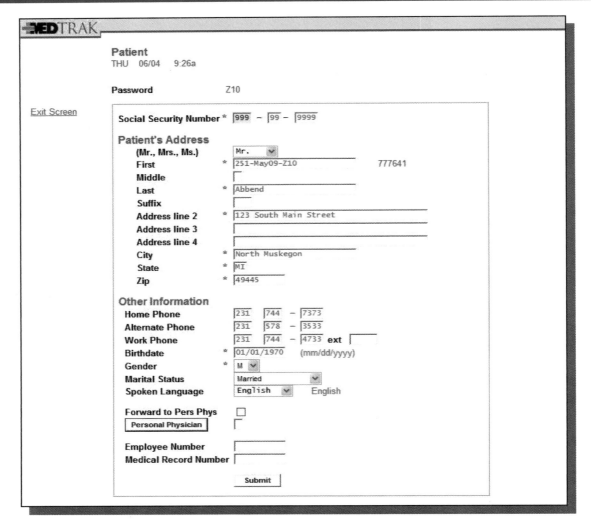

Once the front desk person finishes reviewing the demographic information for the established patient, he or she places the cursor next to the patient and clicks the *Select Patient* button to start the registration process.

**Do This ▶**

**7.25** - Click the *Exit Screen* on the <u>Scheduler</u> screen
(you should be on the MedTrak <u>Main Menu</u>)

**7.26** - Access <u>Patient Registration</u> off the MedTrak <u>Main Menu</u>

**7.27** - Place the cursor next to the **first patient** that you added in **Chapter 3**
(we added Abbend as the first patient for this book)
(you might need to use **Search** to locate your patient)

**7.28** - Click the *Change Patient* button
(review your patient's demographic information)

**7.29** - Click the *Submit* button

**7.30** - With the cursor next to your patient, click the *Select Patient* button

## Selecting the Patient/Company

MedTrak is designed to manage *patient responsibility* cases (self pay, guarantor, group health, Medicare, Medicaid, etc.), where patients are responsible for payment of services through their group health coverage or out of their own pocket, and *occupational medicine* cases (workers' compensation and employee health), where employers are responsible for payment of services through workers' compensation insurance or the employer's checkbook.

Since this is a new patient, there are no existing **Patient/Company** relationships. Therefore, after entering and/or confirming the patient's demographic information, the next screen to appear is the Company selection screen (shown below).

In this example, the patient is responsible for the payment of services, so the front desk person places the cursor next to the "**..Patient Responsibility**" selection and clicks the *Select Company* button.

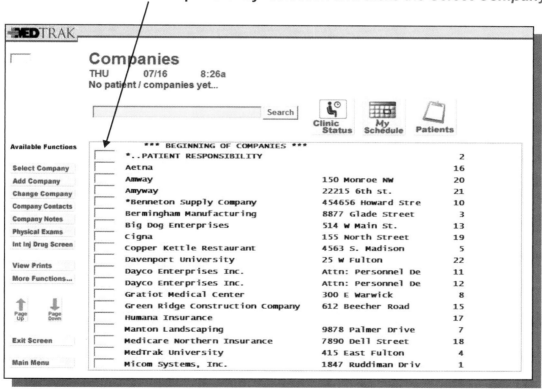

---

**Do This** ▶  **7.31** - Place the cursor next to **..Patient Responsibility**

**7.32** - Click the *Select Company* button

## Creating the New Case

Because this is a new patient, the next screen to appear is the <u>New Case</u> screen (shown below).

In this example, the new patient is at the clinic because he has **left ankle pain**.

The front desk person enters **left ankle pain** in the **Complaint** field, skips the other fields on the screen, and clicks the *Submit* button.

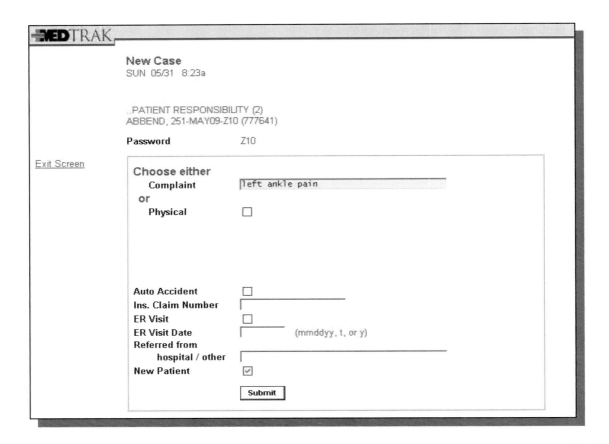

---

**Do This** ▶ **7.33** - Type **left ankle pain** in the <u>Complaint</u> field

**7.34** - Click the *Submit* button

---

## *Selecting the Patient Payer*

The front desk person scans the patient's insurance cards and driver's license, and will attach the *scanned information* to the case in MedTrak right after registering the patient.

Because this patient's payers were attached to him when he was added to MedTrak in Chapter 5 - **Attaching Payers to a Patient**, the next screen to appear is the Patient/Payers screen (shown below).

This screen displays all of the payers that we previously attached to the patient. The front desk person reviews the payers by checking them with the insurance card information provided by the patient. To review the subscriber and policy information, the front desk person sets the cursor next to the payer that he or she wants to review and clicks the *Change Payer* button. If the payers are accurate and in the right *payer order*, the front desk person clicks the *Confirm Payers* button. Remember the payer order is the order that the payers will be billed. The primary payer will be the first one to receive the bill for the encounter, the secondary payer will be *balance billed* the remainder of the bill not paid by the primary payer, and so on.

If the payer's subscriber and policy information does not match the insurance card information, the front desk person corrects the information by adding, changing, deleting, or changing the payer order before clicking the *Confirm Payers* button.

In this example, the payer information is accurate since we built it in **Chapter 5**, so the front desk person will click the *Confirm Payers* button to continue with registration.

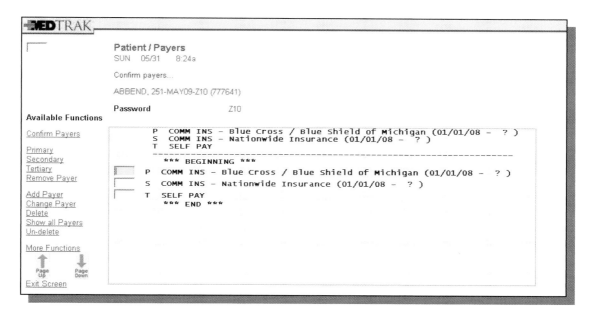

---

**Do This** ▶  **7.35** - Click the *Confirm Payers* button to confirm the payers

---

## Adding the Visit (Encounter)

The next screen to appear is the Visit Add screen (shown below).

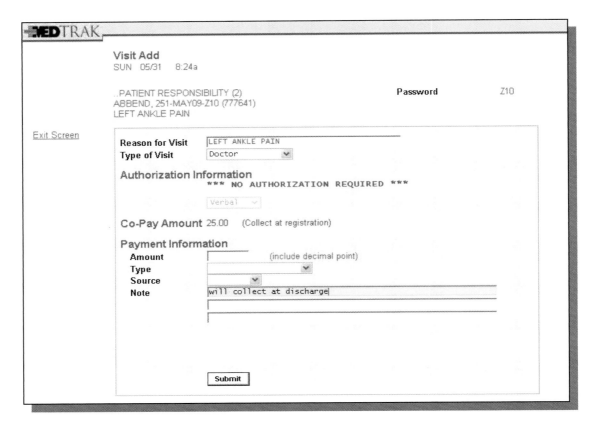

For this visit, the patient is in the clinic to see the **doctor** for **left ankle pain**.

This patient's primary payer requires a $25 co-payment amount for the doctor visit. Because a payment from the patient is needed, MedTrak requires the front desk person to enter an amount collected (or a note about the payment collection) to exit this screen. In this example, the front desk person enters a note that co-payment will be collected at discharge at the end of the patient's visit.

---

**Do This** ▶  **7.36** - Confirm that the Reason for Visit is **LEFT ANKLE PAIN**

**7.37** - Select **Doctor** for the Type of Visit

**7.38** - Enter a Note about the payment for the visit

**7.39** - Click the *Submit* button

---

## Selecting the Presenting Problem

As you learned in the Scheduling chapter, MedTrak is a problem-focused system. The front desk person selects from a list of *presenting problems* (shown below), the reasons that the patient is visiting the clinic. For this visit, the patient is here to see the doctor for **left ankle pain**.

The front desk person clicks the check box for **Injury-Bones/Jts** and then clicks the *Submit* button.

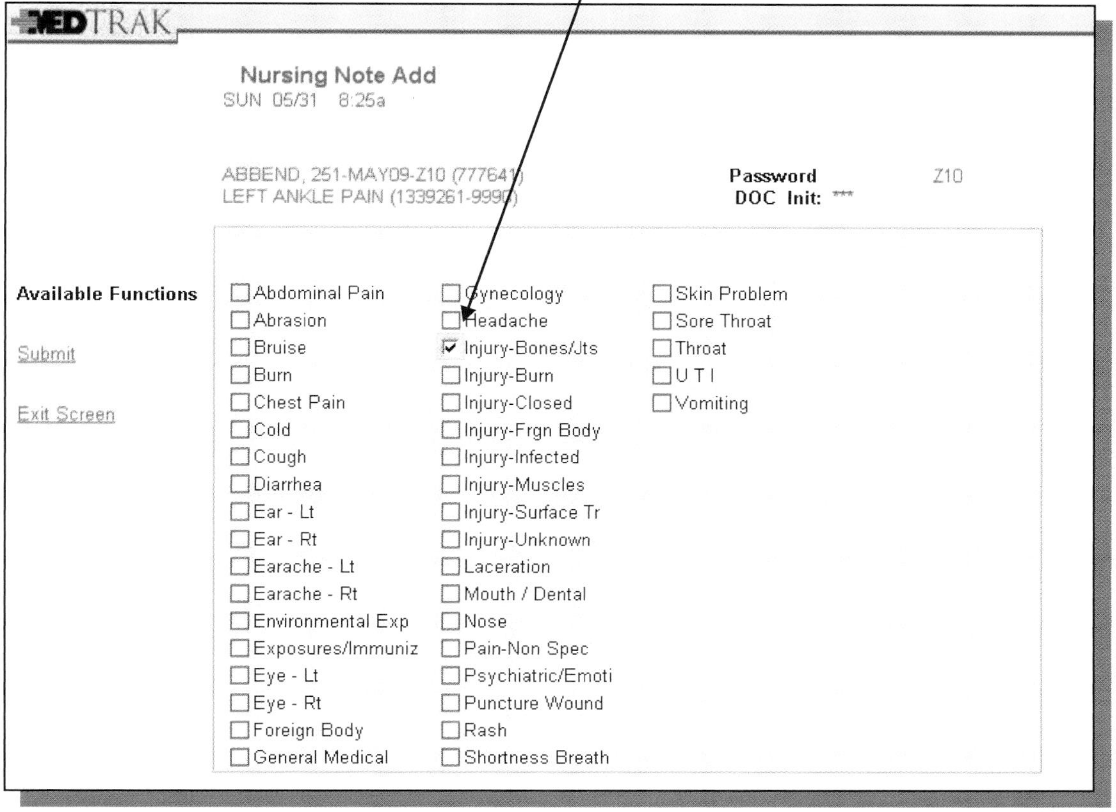

The next screen to appear is the body part selection screen for an injury to the bones or joints (shown on the next page). The front desk person selects the affected body part(s) for the injury on this screen.

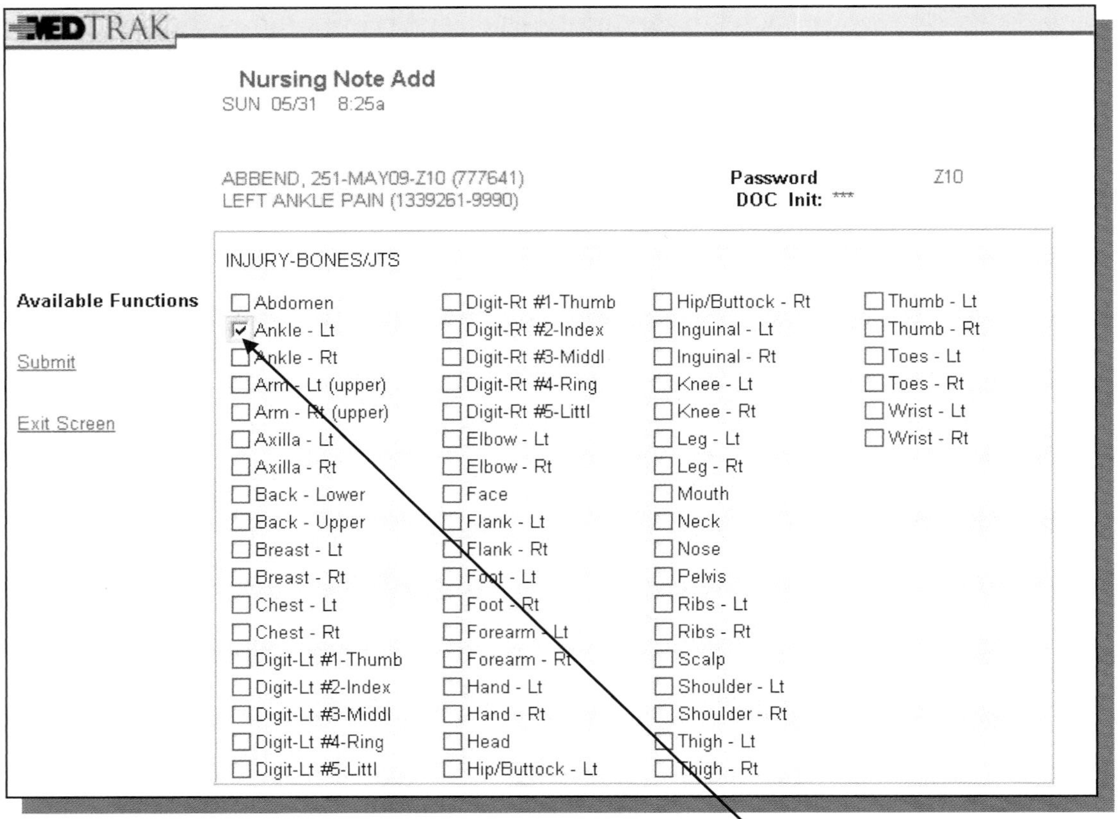

**Nursing Note Add**
SUN 05/31 8:25a

ABBEND, 251-MAY09-Z10 (777641)        Password        Z10
LEFT ANKLE PAIN (1339261-9990)        DOC Init: ***

INJURY-BONES/JTS

For this example, the front desk person checks the box for **Ankle - Lt** and then clicks the *Submit* button. The Nursing Note Add screen (shown below) for body part selection of an injury to the bones or joints refreshes with the message "**Ankle - Lt Injury - Bones/Jts selected**" appearing at the top of the screen.

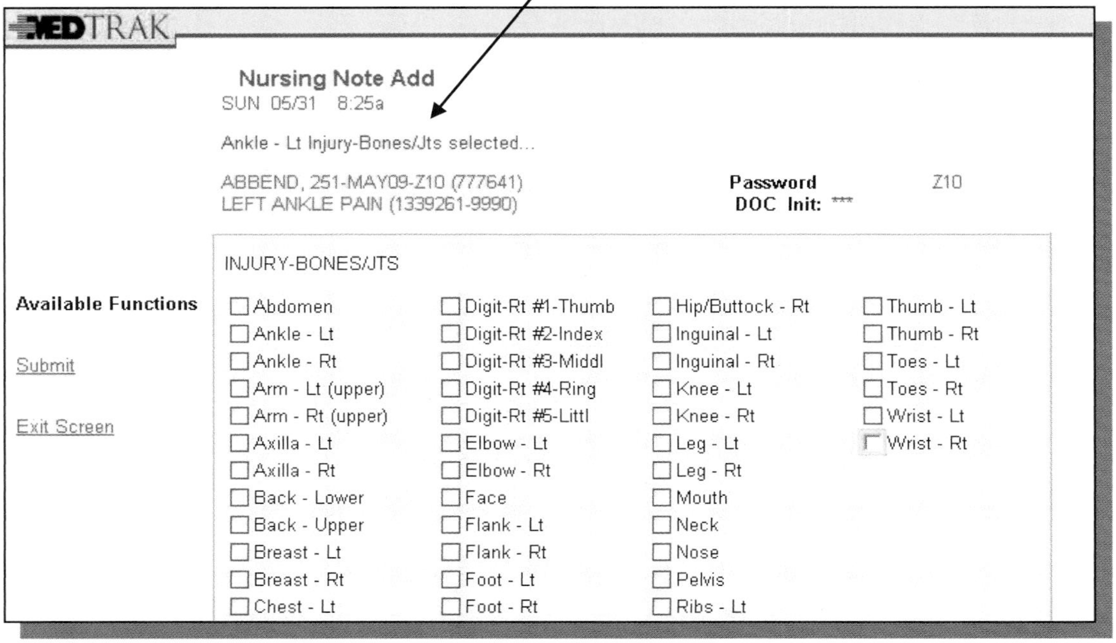

After selecting the body part(s) affected, the front desk person exits the <u>Nursing Note Add</u> screen for body part selection to return to the <u>Nursing Note Add</u> screen for presenting problems to select the next presenting problem, if there are any.

MedTrak allows the front desk person to select all of the presenting problems and affected body parts at the same time (in parallel) or one at a time (in series). It just depends on the preference of the front desk person.

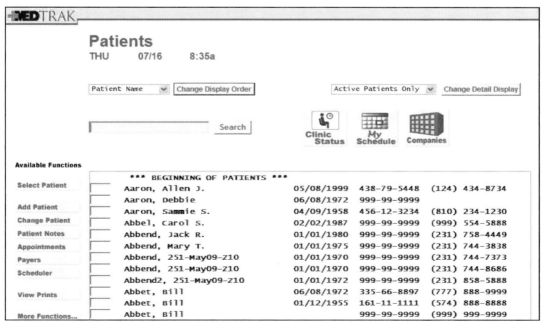

In this example, the front desk is done selecting the problem and body part affected, so the staff member clicks on the *Exit Screen* button to return to the <u>Patients</u> screen (shown below) to register the next patient.

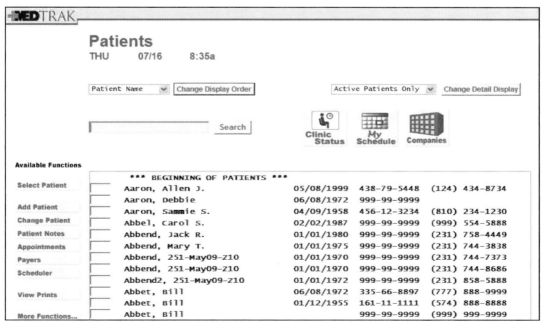

**Do This** ▶   **7.40** - Click the **Injury - Bones/Jts** check box

           **7.41** - Click the *Submit* button

           **7.42** - Click the **Ankle - Lt** check box

           **7.43** - Click the *Submit* button

           **7.44** - Review the message for **Ankle - Lt Injury - Bones/Jts selected**

           **7.45** - Click the *Exit Screen* button

                  (you should be on the Presenting Problems screen)

           **7.46** - Click the *Exit Screen* button

                  (you should be on the Patient Registration screen)

           **7.47** - Click the *Exit Screen* button again to return to the Main Menu

For efficient clinical operations, the front desk person needs to be able to register scheduled patients and walk-in patients with minimal effort.

Your patient is now on the <u>Clinic Status</u> screen that is used by the medical staff (physicians, nursing, lab, x-ray, therapy, and administration) to control the workflow of the registered patients through the clinic.

# CHAPTER

# 8

# Clinic Status Screen

**Estimated time needed to complete this chapter  -  15** minutes

## What you need to know before doing this chapter

- ◆ How to log into MedTrak
- ◆ How to access Clinic Status off the Main Menu

## Learning outcomes gained from this chapter

- ◆ How to switch divisions within a location
- ◆ How to toggle between the patient names and ages with chief complaints
- ◆ How to read the symbols in the patient orders column
- ◆ How to read the terms in the clinical workflow status column
- ◆ How to read the discipline waiting times
- ◆ How to identify the last clinical staff and physician to see the patient
- ◆ How to read the total time for the patient's visit

## Key concepts in this chapter

*real-time workflow*

*workflow status*

*location*

*division*

*ages with reasons*

*status of the patient's orders*

*next step*

*discipline waiting times*

*current clinical staff and physician*

*total elapsed time*

## Clinic Status Screen Overview

**Major Categories of Clinical Workflow**

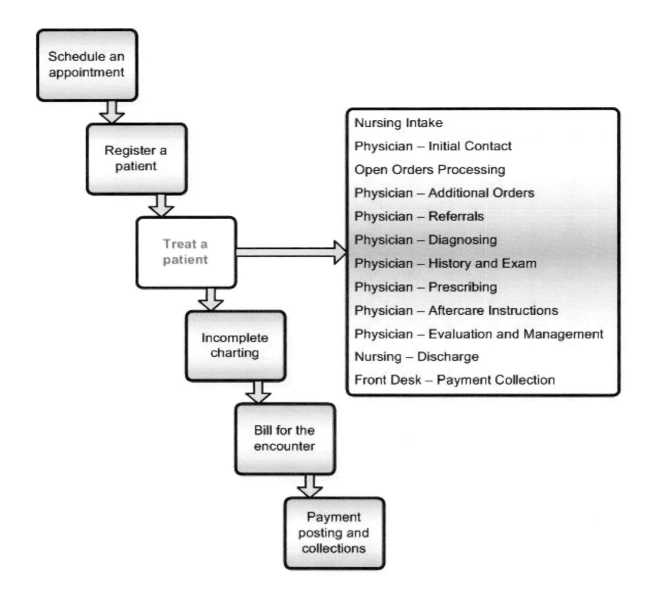

## Clinic Status Screen Overview

The Clinic Status screen (shown below) displays a *real-time workflow* view of the medical facility.

Each member of the clinical staff uses this screen to access his or her portion of the documentation screens for the clinical care of the patient.

Registered patients, both scheduled and walk-ins, appear on this screen with the *workflow status* of **Room**.

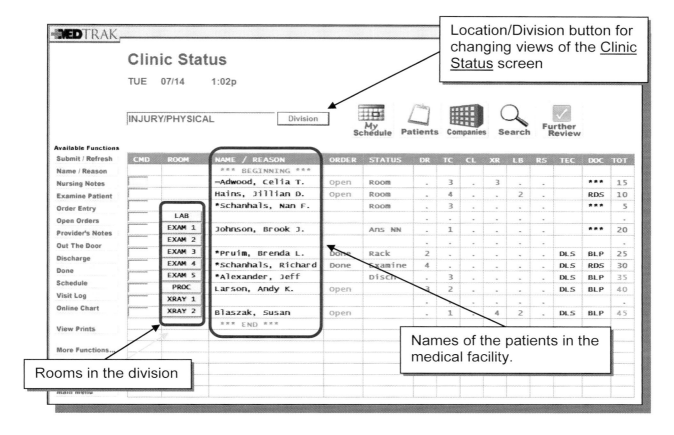

At the top of the screen is the *location* or *division* name. By clicking the *Location/Division* button, the user can switch the view of the location from viewing the whole location and all of its divisions to viewing just one division. In this example, the Clinic Status screen is set to the **Injury/Physical** division.

Also, the initial view of the Clinic Status screen displays the names of the patients currently in the medical facility.

## Toggling Between Patient Names and Ages with Reasons for Visits

Users can toggle the <u>Clinic Status</u> screen between displaying the patients' names to displaying their *ages with reasons* by clicking the *Name/Reason* button (*F6* key). The <u>Clinic Status</u> screen (shown below) now displays the patient's ages with reasons for the visits. To reset the screen to display patient names, the front desk person clicks the *Name/Reason* button (*F6* key) again.

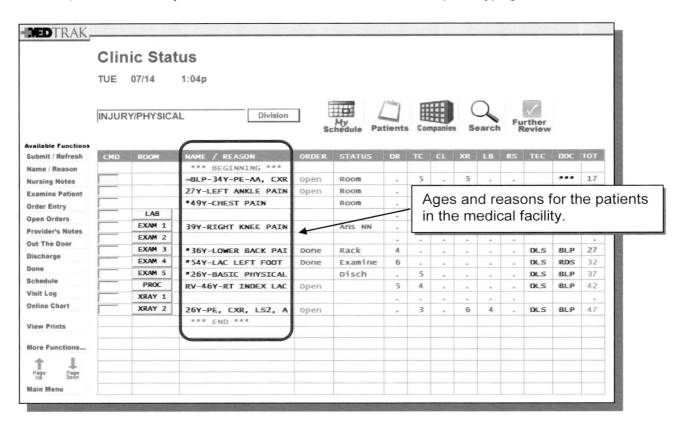

**Notes about special formatting for the name field (age and reason field):**

| Indicator | Meaning | Example |
|---|---|---|
| = | Patient registered for a scheduled appointment. | =45Y-RT INDEX LACER |
| physician initials | Physician scheduled to see the patientor who saw the patient at the last visit. | =BLP-33Y-PE-AA<br>BLP-30Y-RT KNEE PAIN |
| * | Notes are attached to the patient. | *25Y-BASIC PHYSICAL |
| RV | This is a return visit (follow-up). | RV-BLP-25Y-LEFT LEG |

## *Patient Orders*

To the right of the **NAME/REASON** column on the <u>Clinic Status</u> screen (shown below) is the **ORDER** column, which displays the *status of the patient's orders* for the current visit. If the column displays:

| **(blank)** | The patient does not have any orders. |
|---|---|
| Open | Open orders are present. |
| Done | There are no remaining open orders. |

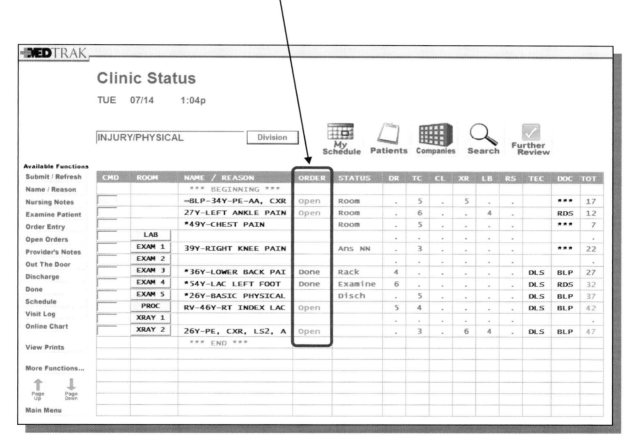

## Clinical Workflow Status

To the right of the **ORDER** column is the **STATUS** column (shown below), which displays the *next step* in the clinical workflow for each patient. The patient workflow statuses are:

| | |
|---|---|
| **Room** | Waiting to be placed into an exam/treatment room. Currently in the reception area. |
| **Ans NN** | Waiting for the clinical staff to answer the nursing notes. |
| **Prt CL** | Waiting for the clinical staff to put the chart in the rack (or print the physician's checklist). |
| **Call** | Waiting for the physician to call the company before seeing the patient (*work comp only*). |
| **Rack** | Waiting for the physician to pick up the chart and examine the patient. |
| **Examine** | The physician is currently examining the patient. |
| **Disch** | The patient has all the necessary paperwork and is ready to be discharged. |
| **Done** | The patient is done and has returned to the front desk to pay (*patient responsibility only*). |
| **Blank** | The patient currently has open orders that were placed by the physician. |

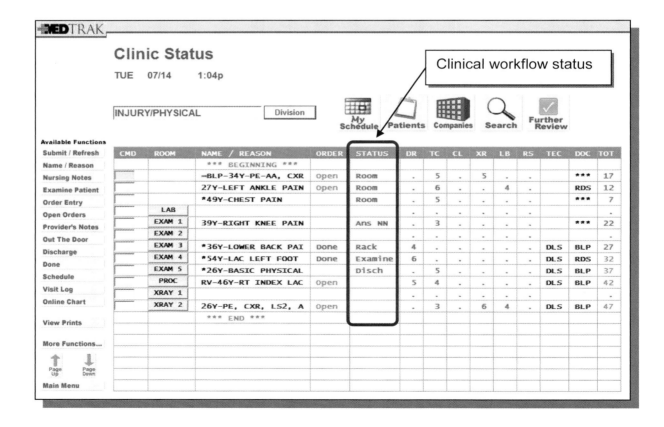

## Waiting Times by Discipline

To the right of the **STATUS** column on the <u>Clinic Status</u> screen (shown below) are columns displaying the **patient waiting times** for each discipline. The *discipline waiting times* in minutes are:

| DR | Waiting for the physician. |
|----|----------------------------|
| TC | Waiting for the clinical staff. |
| CL | Waiting for the front desk/clerical staff. |
| XR | Waiting for an x-ray. |
| LB | Waiting for lab. |
| RS | Waiting for rehab services. |

The discipline waiting times are color coded as follows:

| Green | 15 minutes or less. |
|-------|---------------------|
| Yellow | 16 to 30 minutes. |
| Red | 31 minutes or more. |

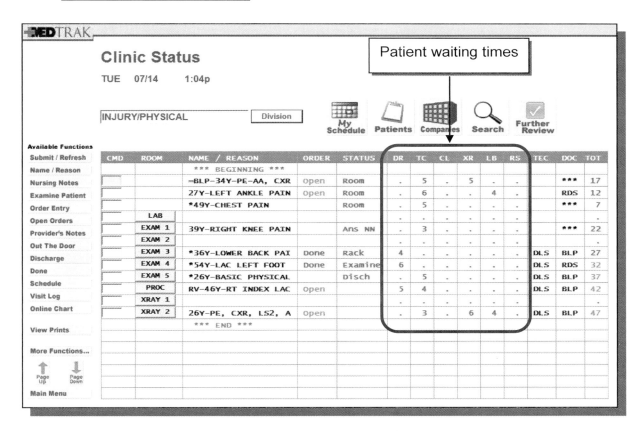

## Current Tech and Physician to See the Patient

To the right of the **patient waiting times** columns on the Clinic Status screen are columns displaying the *current clinical staff and physician* to see the patient at this visit.

- **TEC** - current clinical staff
- **DOC** - current physician

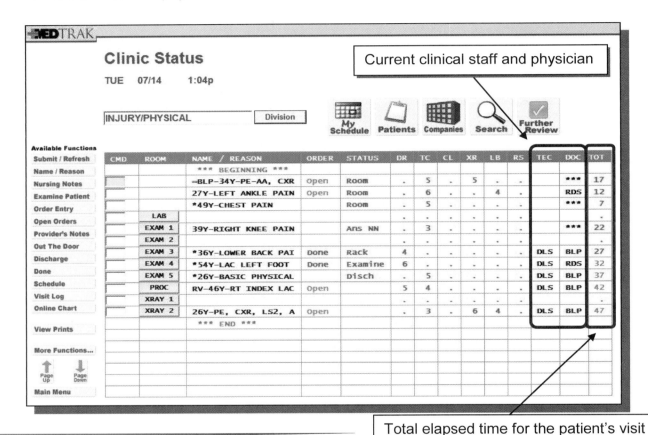

Current clinical staff and physician

Total elapsed time for the patient's visit

## Total Time for the Patient Visit

The last column on the right contains the *total elapsed time* for the patient's visit from the time that he registered at the front desk.

The total waiting times are color coded as follows:

| Green | 30 minutes or less. |
|---|---|
| Yellow | 31 to 60 minutes. |
| Red | 61 minutes or more. |

# CHAPTER
# 9
# Nursing Intake

**Estimated time needed to complete this chapter - 30** minutes

**What you need to know before doing this chapter**

- ♦ How to log into MedTrak
- ♦ How to register a patient
- ♦ How to access <u>Clinic Status</u> off the <u>Main Menu</u>

**Learning outcomes gained from this chapter**

- ♦ How to locate a patient on the <u>Clinic Status</u> screen
- ♦ How to move a patient to a room
- ♦ How to review the Nursing Note Processor
- ♦ How to add and/or delete Nursing Note Lists
- ♦ How to answer an expanded answer question
- ♦ How to answer a question with a stored response
- ♦ How to answer a question with a normal answer
- ♦ How to view the on-line chart
- ♦ How to put the chart in the rack for the physician

**Key concepts in this chapter**

*reason(s) for visiting*
*medical history*
*vital signs*
*real reason for their visit*
*presenting problem*
*data entry field*
*expanded answer*
*standard answers*
*triggers*
*stored responses*
*normal answers*
*on-line chart*
*rack*

## Nursing Intake

**Major Categories of Clinical Workflow**

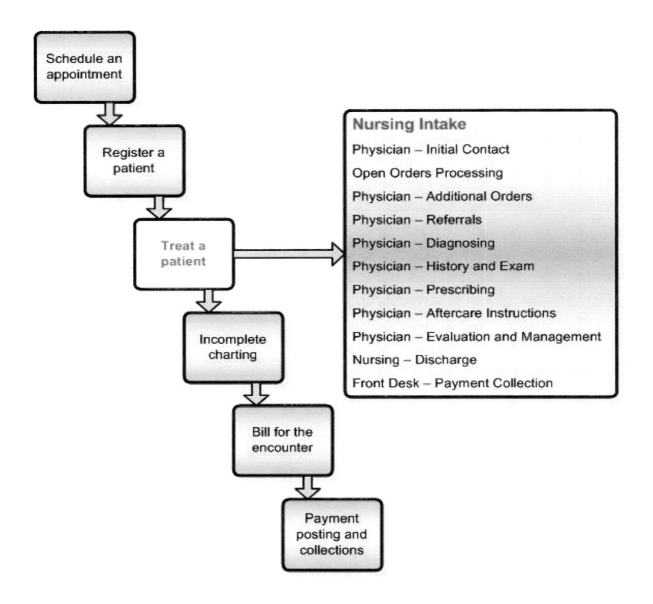

## Nursing Intake

After registration, the patient waits in the reception area for the clinical staff to place him or her into an examination room and ask some preliminary nursing questions prior to the physician seeing him or her.

In most clinical situations, these preliminary nursing questions include:

- Reason(s) for seeing the physician - chief complaint(s)
- History of the chief complaint(s)
- Symptoms
- Previous medical history including similar injuries or illnesses
- Current prescription and over-the-counter medication information
- Allergies (including medication allergies)
- Vital signs, including blood pressure, heart rate, respiration, and temperature
- Other nursing observations

The patient that you registered in **Chapter 7, Patient Registration,** is now on the Clinic Status screen and ready for clinical processing.

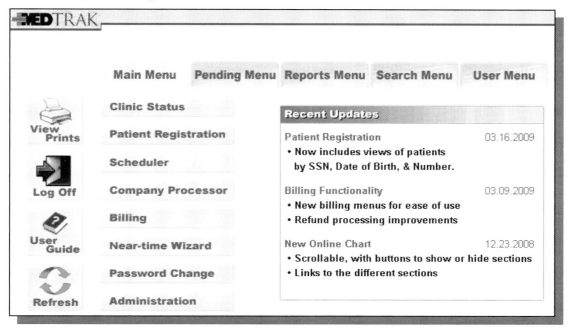

**Do This** ▶ **9.01** - Sign in to MedTrak

**9.02** - Click the *Clinic Status* button on the MedTrak Main Menu

## *Checking for Room Availability*

Prior to moving the patient into an exam room, the clinical staff visually checks to see which rooms are available, and then checks the <u>Clinic Status</u> screen (shown below) for confirmation of availability. The clinical staff then goes to the front desk/waiting room to get the patient's paperwork (some clinics continue to use paper charts to supplement the electronic medical record and/or to store papers that they do not want to store in the electronic chart).

On the way to the front desk to get the patient, the clinical staff moves the patient on the <u>Clinic Status</u> screen from the waiting room to an exam room.

To move a patient to a room on the <u>Clinic Status</u> screen, the clinical staff places the cursor next to the patient and then clicks an exam room button.

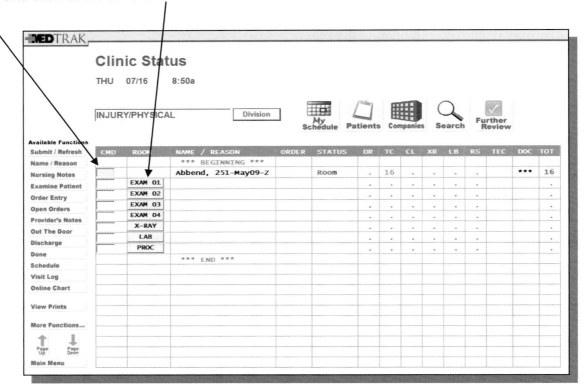

## Moving the Patient to a Room

In this example (shown below), the clinical staff moves the patient into **Exam Room 03** by placing the cursor in the command field next to the patient and clicking the *Exam 03* room button.

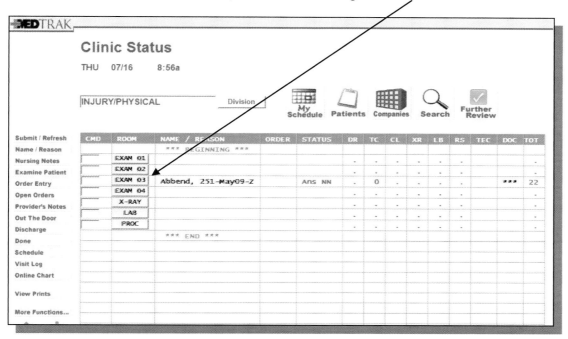

**Do This** ▶ **9.03** - Click the *Name/Reason* button

(the Clinic Status screen now displays the ages and reasons)

**9.04** - Place the cursor next to your patient with the **lower back pain**

**9.05** - Click on the **PROC** room button

(your lower back patient should now be in **PROC** room)

**9.06** - Place the cursor next to your patient with the **left ankle pain**

**9.07** - Click on the **EXAM 03** room button

(your left ankle patient should now be in the **EXAM 03** room)

(the workflow **STATUS** column now indicates **Ans NN**)

**9.08** - Click the *Visit Log* button for your left ankle pain patient

(the visit log is a record of all the clinical steps)

(you might need to review your Visit Log at a later time)

**9.09** - Click the *Exit Screen* button to return to the Clinic Status screen

## *Reason(s) for Visiting the Clinic*

Once the clinical staff moves the patient to an exam room, they ask the patient questions about his or her *reason(s) for visiting* the medical facility. Also, they ask questions about the patient's *medical history* and medication history, and they usually take the patient's *vital signs*.

Depending on the clinical practice, the nursing questions could be printed on a nursing note or answered in real-time directly into MedTrak. If the clinic uses the **Nursing Notes** printout, the clinical staff will write the answers on this form and then go to a computer to enter the answers into MedTrak.

To access the **Nursing Notes**, with the cursor next to the patient, the clinical staff clicks the *Nursing Notes* button.

The next screen to appear is the Nursing Note Processor (shown below). This screen displays the reason(s) for the patient's visit. If the reason(s) selected by the front desk are not accurate, the clinical staff should redirect the nursing note lists to the proper ones by using the *Add List* and *Delete List* buttons.

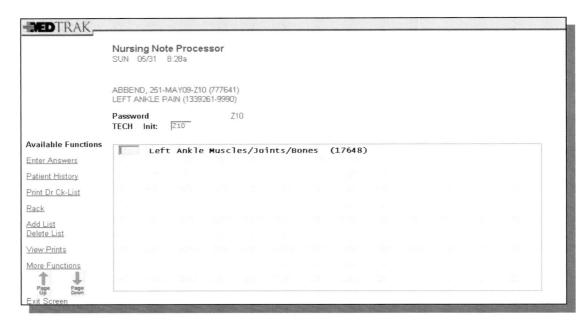

Sometimes patients will not tell the front desk person or the clinical staff the *real reason for their visit* to the clinic. Because MedTrak is problem-focused, the checklist questions for the nurse and the physician are based on the presenting problem(s) selected by the front desk and/or the clinical staff. It is clinically important for the front desk and clinical staff to ensure that the Nursing Note Processor presenting problem(s) are accurate.

---

**Do This ▶**    **9.10** - Place the cursor next to your patient with left ankle pain

(the left ankle pain patient should be in the **Exam 03** room)

        **9.11** - Click the *Nursing Notes* button

---

## *Answering Nursing Questions*

After verifying the accuracy of the presenting problems selected and displayed on the <u>Nursing Notes Processor</u> screen (as shown on the previous page), the clinical staff answers the questions on the nursing note. To answer the questions, with the cursor next to a *presenting problem* (if there are multiple, the cursor can be next to any one of them), the clinical staff clicks the *Enter Answers* button.

**Do This ▶ 9.12** - Click the *Enter Answers* button

The next screen to appear is the <u>Nursing Notes</u> screen (shown below). This screen lists all of the questions for the clinical staff to answer for the presenting problem(s).

**▬ED**TRAK

**Nursing Notes**
MON    07/11    4:07p

Password              **Initials** RDS
**TECH Init**    RDS

ABBEND, CHARLES T. (19908)
LEFT ANKLE PAIN (7295-9990)

| Available Functions | |
| --- | --- |
| On-line Chart | |
| Submit Answers | |
| Normal Answer | |
| Stored Response | |
| Expanded Answer | |
| | |
| Beginning | |
| Patient History | |
| | |
| View Prints | |
| More Functions | |
| ↑ Page Up    ↓ Page Down | |
| Exit Screen | |

```
        * * *   B E G I N N I N G   * * *
      CURRENT PROBLEM
       CHIEF COMPLAINT:   LEFT ANKLE PAIN
       HISTORY CHIEF COMPLAINT:
          History of Injury:
          Symptoms:
        Pain scale:
      PATIENT HISTORY
        MEDICATIONS
           Prescription Meds:
           Over-the-counter substances:
        ALLERGIES
           Medication Allergies:
             If yes, type of allergic reaction:
      PAST MEDICAL HISTORY
          Significant condition:
      PAST SURGICAL HISTORY
          Lower extremity surgery:
      PREVIOUS INJURIES
```

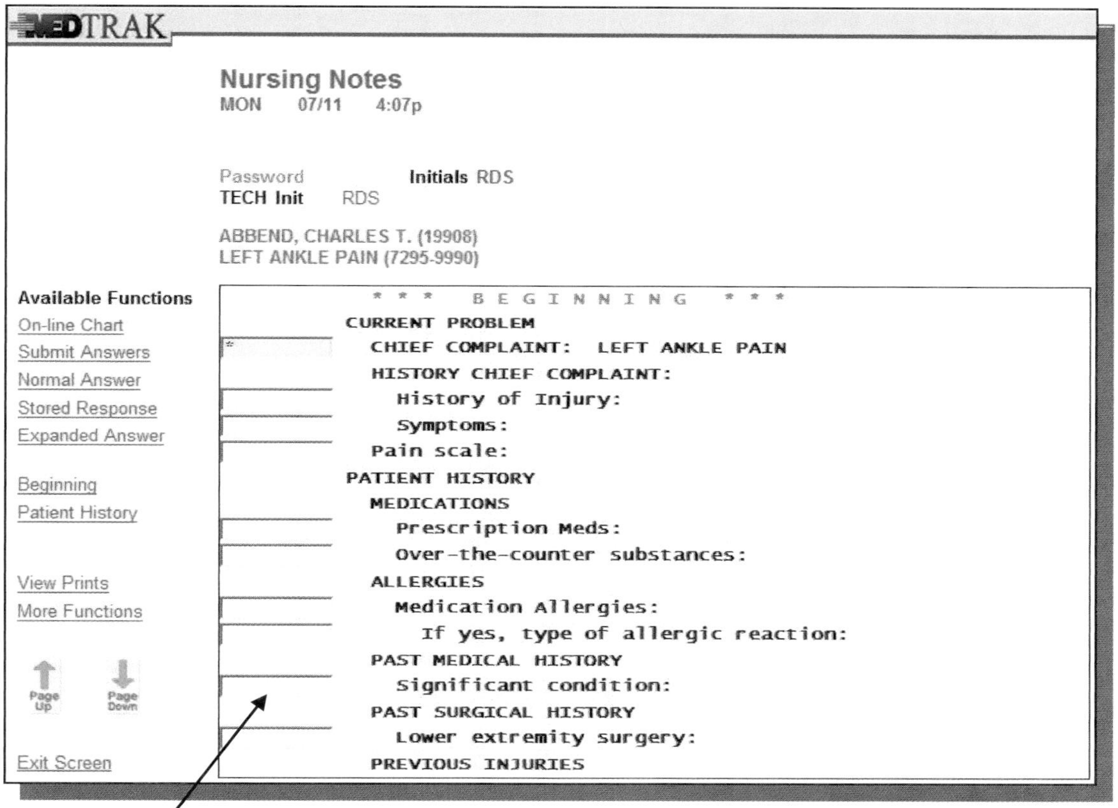

Each question's *data entry field* holds up to 10 characters. Many answers to nursing questions will fit into this 10-character data entry field.

For a question whose answer is longer than 10 characters, the clinical staff clicks the *Expanded Answer* button.

## *Expanded Answers*

In this example, the MA selects the *expanded answer* function to enter the answer for the **Chief Complaint** question.

The next screen to appear is the Expanded Answer screen (shown below). This screen allows entry of information in three ways:

- Typing directly into the field
- Cutting and pasting information from another document (for example a Word document created by a transcriptionist)
- Using voice recognition software and a microphone to dictate directly into the field

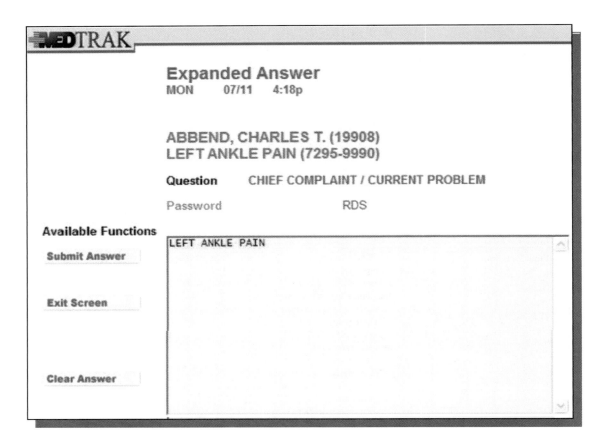

In this example, the clinical staff verifies that "**left ankle pain**" appears in the expanded answer for the **Chief Complaint** question (shown above). After verifying the answer in the Expanded Answer screen, the clinical staff clicks the *Submit Answer* button. The Nursing Notes screen (shown below) reappears, displaying the answer to the right of the **Chief Complaint** question.

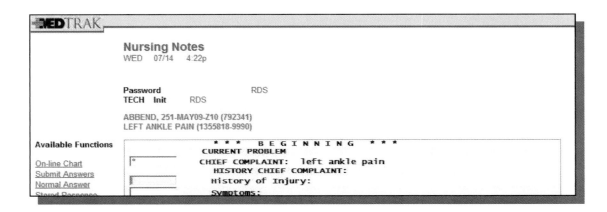

**Do This** ▶ **9.13** - Place the cursor next to the **Chief Complaint** question

**9.14** - Click the *Expanded Answer* button

(the Expanded Answer screen for **Chief Complaint** appears)

**9.15** - Enter an answer for the **Chief Complaint**

**9.16** - Click the *Submit Answer* button

(the Nursing Notes screen reappears, displaying the answer)

In this same manner, the clinical staff uses the expanded answer functionality to answer the **History of Injury** and **Symptoms** questions (as shown below).

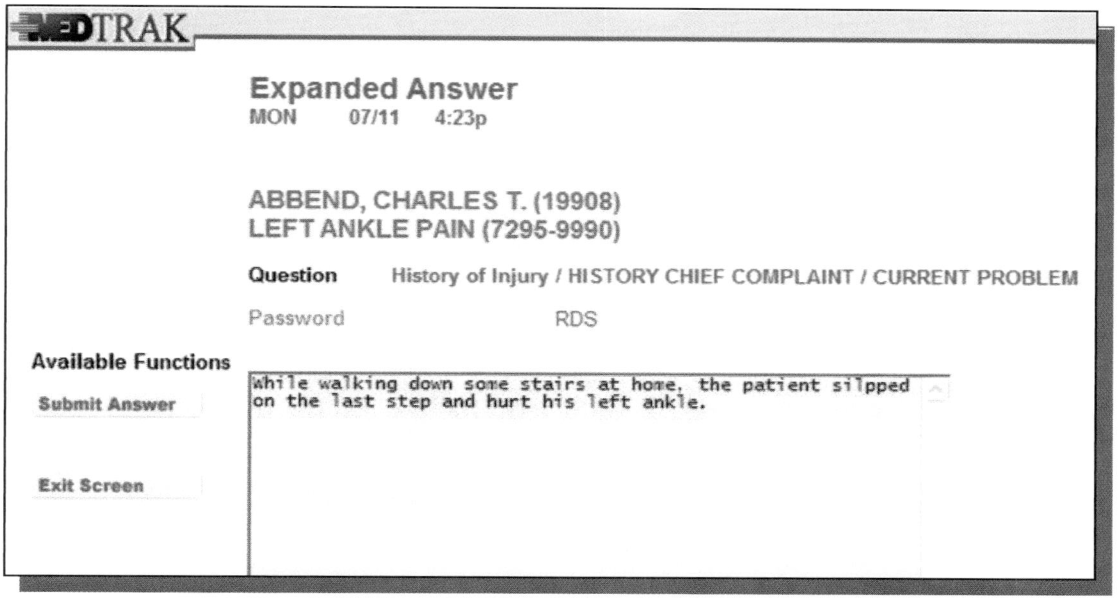

**MEDTRAK**

**Expanded Answer**
MON    07/11    4:23p

ABBEND, CHARLES T. (19908)
LEFT ANKLE PAIN (7295-9990)

Question    History of Injury / HISTORY CHIEF COMPLAINT / CURRENT PROBLEM

Password                RDS

**Available Functions**

Submit Answer

While walking down some stairs at home, the patient slipped on the last step and hurt his left ankle.

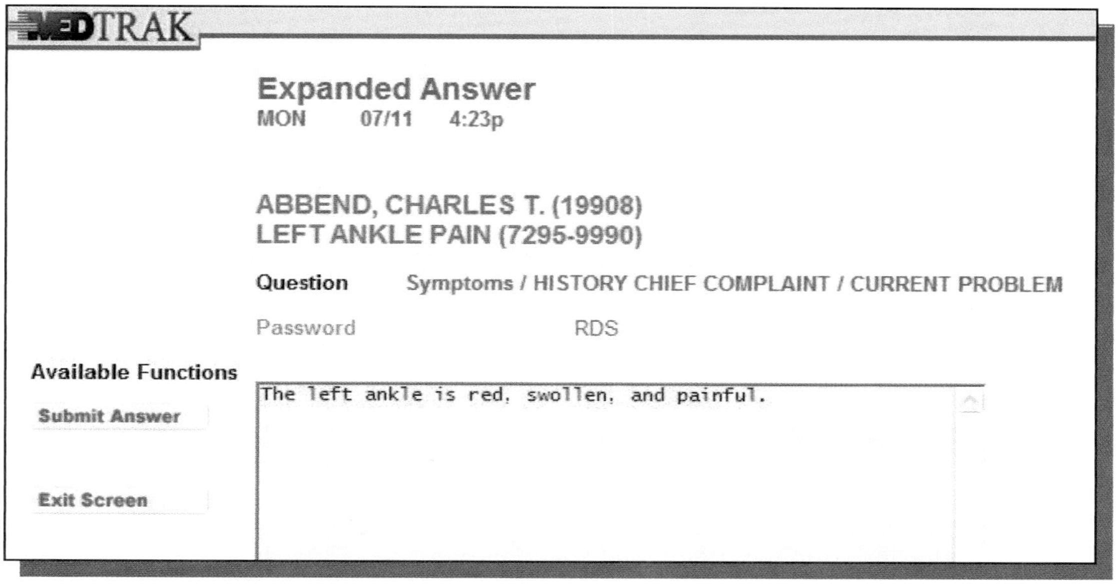

Exit Screen

**MEDTRAK**

**Expanded Answer**
MON    07/11    4:23p

ABBEND, CHARLES T. (19908)
LEFT ANKLE PAIN (7295-9990)

Question    Symptoms / HISTORY CHIEF COMPLAINT / CURRENT PROBLEM

Password                RDS

**Available Functions**

Submit Answer

The left ankle is red, swollen, and painful.

Exit Screen

The <u>Nursing Notes</u> screen (shown below) reappears, displaying the answers to the **History of Injury** and the **Symptoms** questions to the right of the questions.

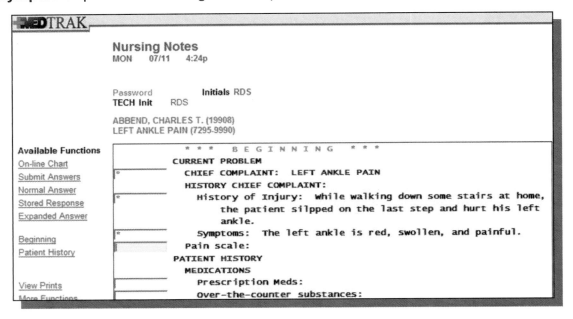

**Do This** ▶   **9.17** - Place the cursor next to the **History of Injury** question

     **9.18** - Click the *Expanded Answer* button

     **9.19** - Enter an answer for the **History of Injury**

     **9.20** - Click the *Submit Answer* button

     **9.21** - Do the same process for the **Symptoms** question
                (the Nursing Notes screen reappears with the answers)

## Stored Responses

Many questions asked by the clinical staff and physician can be answered with *standard answers*. MedTrak allows answering questions with standard answers by using *triggers* to retrieve *stored responses*. Using a trigger to answer a question saves time.

For example, the **Pain Scale** question is typically answered using a scale of 1 to 10.

Experienced users of MedTrak enter these triggers directly into the data entry field next to a question. If the user is not sure what triggers are available for the question, he or she can choose from a list of available triggers by using the *Stored Response* button.

In this example, the clinical staff places the cursor next to the **Pain Scale** question and clicks the *Stored Response* button. The <u>Question Help</u> screen (shown on the next page) appears.

Each question can have its own stored responses; therefore, the <u>Question Help</u> screen will list only the stored responses for that question. Not all questions can be answered using triggers.

The Question Help screen lists all of the available stored responses to the question.

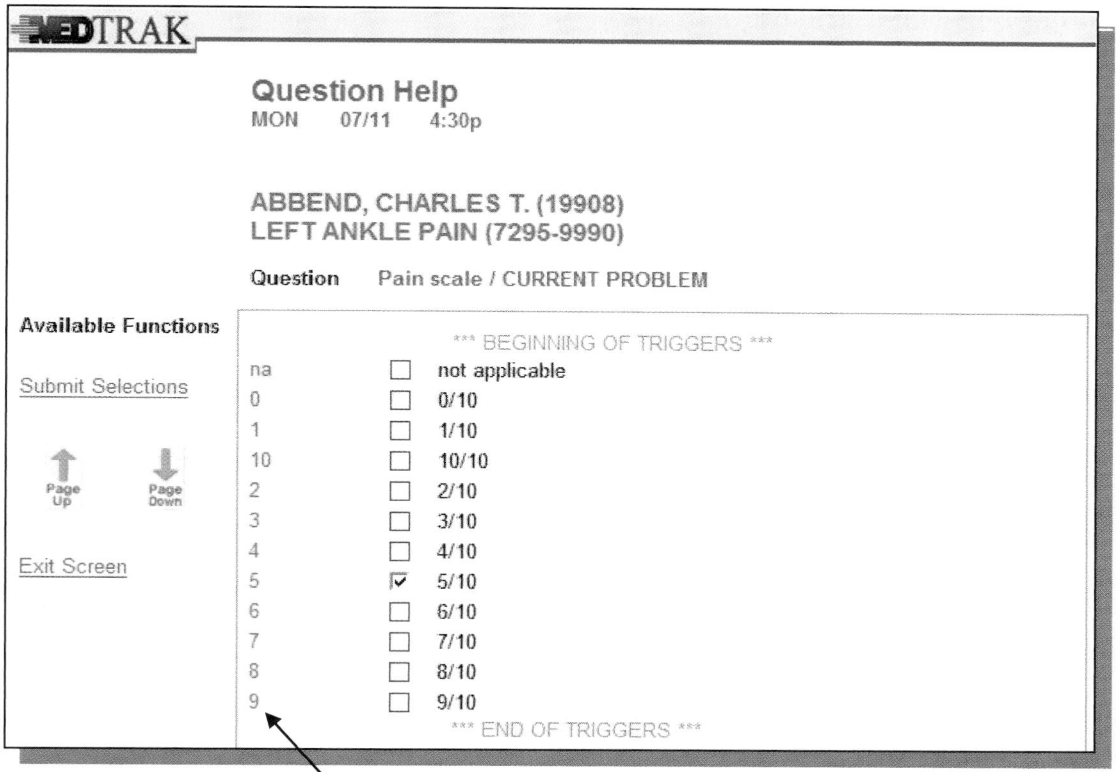

**MEDTRAK**

**Question Help**
MON    07/11    4:30p

**ABBEND, CHARLES T. (19908)**
**LEFT ANKLE PAIN (7295-9990)**

Question    Pain scale / CURRENT PROBLEM

**Available Functions**

Submit Selections

↑ Page Up    ↓ Page Down

Exit Screen

*** BEGINNING OF TRIGGERS ***
| na | ☐ | not applicable |
| 0 | ☐ | 0/10 |
| 1 | ☐ | 1/10 |
| 10 | ☐ | 10/10 |
| 2 | ☐ | 2/10 |
| 3 | ☐ | 3/10 |
| 4 | ☐ | 4/10 |
| 5 | ☑ | 5/10 |
| 6 | ☐ | 6/10 |
| 7 | ☐ | 7/10 |
| 8 | ☐ | 8/10 |
| 9 | ☐ | 9/10 |
*** END OF TRIGGERS ***

The clinical staff could type the *trigger* for the stored response (shown in green on the Question Help screen above) directly into the *data entry field* on the Nursing Notes screen or select it using the check box. Some questions allow for selection of multiple stored responses and some require that the user select only one stored response.

In this example, the clinical staff selects the **5/10** check box. After selection, they click the *Submit Selections* button to accept the stored response as the answer. The Nursing Notes screen (shown below) reappears, displaying the answer to the **Pain Scale** question to the right of the question.

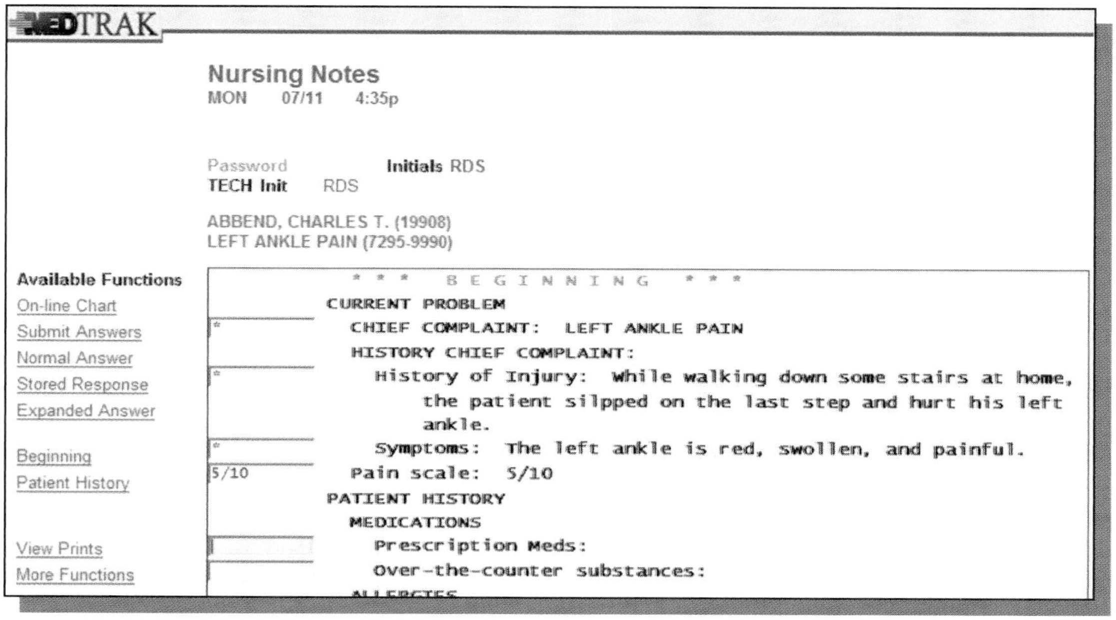

**MEDTRAK**

**Nursing Notes**
MON    07/11    4:35p

Password        **Initials** RDS
**TECH Init**    RDS

ABBEND, CHARLES T. (19908)
LEFT ANKLE PAIN (7295-9990)

**Available Functions**
On-line Chart
Submit Answers
Normal Answer
Stored Response
Expanded Answer

Beginning
Patient History

View Prints
More Functions

* * *    B E G I N N I N G    * * *
CURRENT PROBLEM
    CHIEF COMPLAINT:    LEFT ANKLE PAIN
    HISTORY CHIEF COMPLAINT:
        History of Injury:  While walking down some stairs at home,
            the patient silpped on the last step and hurt his left
            ankle.
        Symptoms:  The left ankle is red, swollen, and painful.
5/10    Pain scale:    5/10
PATIENT HISTORY
    MEDICATIONS
        Prescription Meds:
        Over-the-counter substances:
        ALLERGIES

**Do This** ▶  **9.22** - Place the cursor next to the **Pain Scale** question

**9.23** - Click the *Stored Response* button

**9.24** - Click a check box on the Question Help screen

**9.25** - Click the *Submit Selections* button

(the Nursing Notes screen reappears with the answer selected)

## Normal Answers

Many questions can be answered with *normal answers*. Normal answers are a subset of the standard answers available for a question. MedTrak allows for normal answers by using a trigger of a lowercase **n** to retrieve the normal answer to a question. Not all questions will have a normal answer.

For example, the **Prescription meds** question's normal answer is "**none**," meaning that the patient is not on any prescription medications. The clinical staff can answer this question by clicking the *Normal Answer* button. MedTrak will put a lowercase **n** in this field and automatically move the cursor down to the next question. This also saves time.

Experienced users of MedTrak enter these normal triggers directly into the input field next to a question by typing the lowercase **n** and tabbing down to the next question's *data entry field*. This saves even more time.

In this example, the clinical staff enters normal answers for the rest of the questions on this screen (as shown below) and clicks the *Page Down* button to go to the next screen.

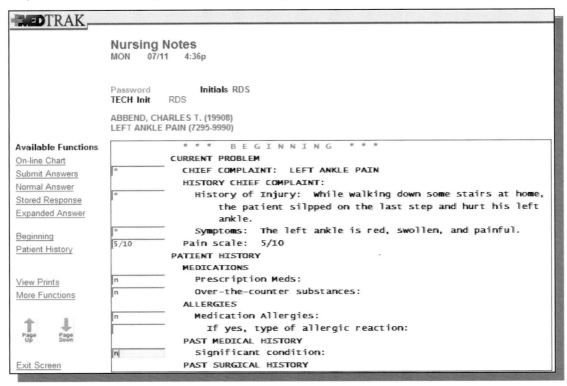

On this screen, the clinical staff again enters normal answers for those questions where a normal answer is applicable (as shown below). Then the clinical staff enters the vital signs directly into the input fields (because the vital signs are 10 characters or fewer in length) and clicks the *Page Down* button to go to the next screen.

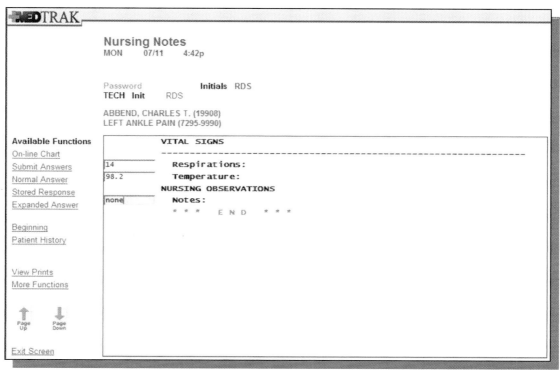

On the next screen, the clinical staff enters the answers for the remaining vital signs. The clinical staff enters "**none**" for the **Nursing Observations  -  Notes** question and clicks the *Submit Answers* button.

The <u>Nursing Notes</u> screen refreshes with the answers to the questions to the right of the questions (as shown below).

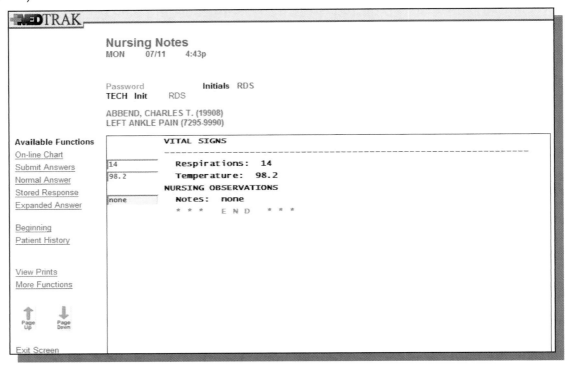

To review the answers to the previous screen of questions, the clinical staff clicks the *Page Up* button (as shown below).

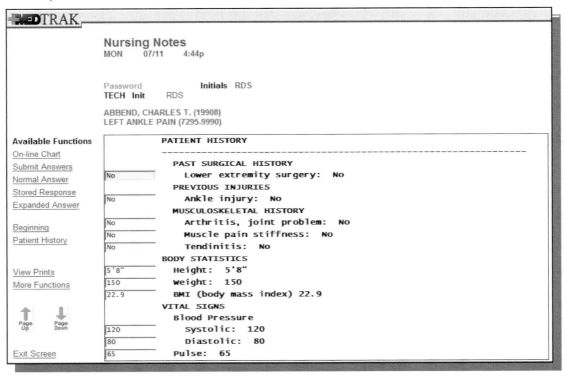

To review the answers to the first screen of <u>Nursing Notes</u> questions, the clinical staff clicks the *Page Up* button again (the first screen is not shown).

At any time during the entering of the <u>Nursing Note</u> answers, the clinical staff can review the *on-line chart* showing the questions and answers for the Nursing Notes.

To review the <u>On-line Chart</u> screen (shown below), the clinical staff clicks the *On-line Chart* button. To exit the <u>On-line Chart</u> screen, the clinical staff clicks the *Exit Chart* button.

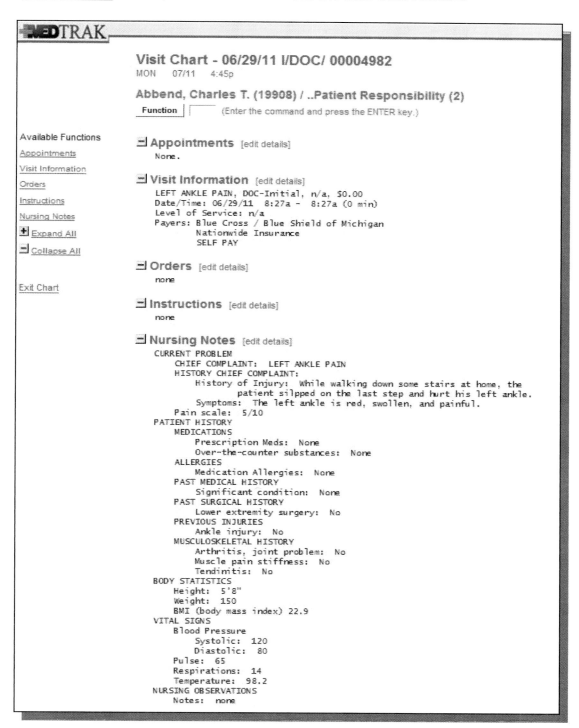

After reviewing the answers, the clinical staff exits the <u>Nursing Notes</u> screen to return to the <u>Nursing Note Processor</u> screen (as shown on the next page).

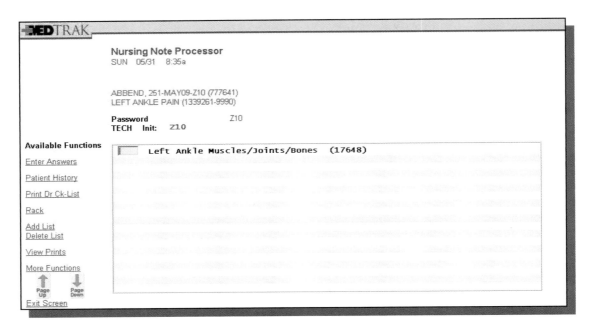

**MED**TRAK

Nursing Note Processor
SUN   05/31   8:35a

ABBEND, 251-MAY09-Z10 (777641)
LEFT ANKLE PAIN (1339261-9990)

**Password**                          Z10
**TECH   Init:**   Z10

**Available Functions**

Enter Answers

Patient History

Print Dr Ck-List

Rack

Add List
Delete List

View Prints

More Functions

Page Up    Page Down

Exit Screen

Left Ankle Muscles/Joints/Bones   (17648)

---

**Do This ▶**

**9.26** - Place the cursor next to the **Prescription meds** question

**9.27** - Click the *Normal Answer* button

**9.28** - Click the *Normal Answer* button for the rest of the questions
  (skip the **If yes, type of allergic reaction** question)

**9.29** - Click the *Page Down* button

**9.30** - Click the *Normal Answer* button for each question down to **Height**

**9.31** - Enter the **Height** and **Weight** (make them up)

**9.32** - Enter the **BMI** (you may calculate this, or make it up)

**9.33** - Enter the vital signs  (make them up)
  **(be sure to answer all of the vital signs)**

**9.34** - Click the *Page Down* button again (finish vital signs)

**9.35** - Enter **none** for the **NURSING OBSERVATIONS - Notes** question

**9.36** - Click the *Submit Answers* button

**9.37** - Click the *On-line Chart* button

**9.38** - Review the *Nursing Notes* section in the on-line chart

**9.39** - Click the *Exit Chart* button

**9.40** - Click the *Exit Screen* button
  (to return to the Nursing Note Processor screen)

## Letting the Physician Know that the Patient is Ready to be Seen

The clinical staff is done with this patient and needs to notify the physician that the patient is ready to be seen. To do so, the clinical staff indicates on the <u>Clinic Status</u> screen that the chart is now in the **Rack,** and the patient is ready to be seen by the physician.

The clinical staff clicks the *Rack* button. The screen refreshes with the "**Rack status set**" message in **red** at the top of the screen.

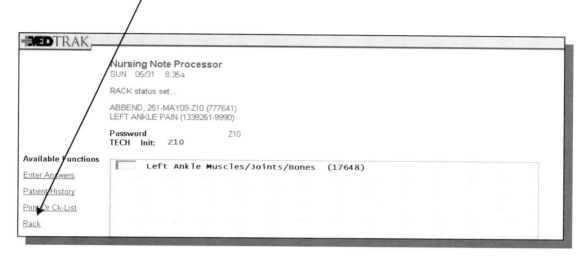

The clinical staff clicks the *Exit Screen* button to return to the <u>Clinic Status</u> screen to see what he or she needs to do for the next patient. The <u>Clinic Status</u> screen now displays that the chart is in the **Rack**, and the patient is ready to be seen by the physician.

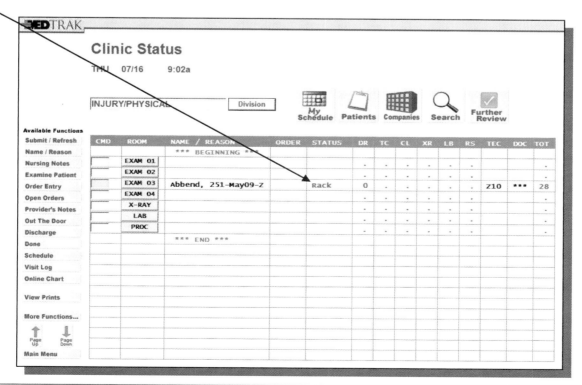

**Do This** ▶  **9.41** - Click the *Rack* button

**9.42** - Review that the "**Rack status set**" message is at the top

**9.43** - Click the *Exit Screen* button

**9.44** - You should be on the <u>Clinic Status</u> screen
(your patient's workflow status should now be **Rack**)

# CHAPTER
# 10

# Physician - Initial Contact

**Estimated time needed to complete this chapter - 30 minutes**

## What you need to know before doing this chapter

- How to log into MedTrak
- How to register a patient
- How to access Clinic Status off the Main Menu
- How to move a patient to a room and answer nursing notes

## Learning outcomes gained from this chapter

- How to pick up the chart by entering the physician's initials
- How to place an order for an x-ray
- How to place an order for a treatment for an injury
- How to move up and down the orders tree

## Key concepts in this chapter

*workflow status*

*chart is in the rack*

*physician access*

*touch-screen*

*voice recognition*

*face time*

*CPOE (computerized patient order entry)*

*problem-focused*

*most likely orders*

*orders tree*

*open orders*

## Physician - Initial Contact

### Major Categories of Clinical Workflow

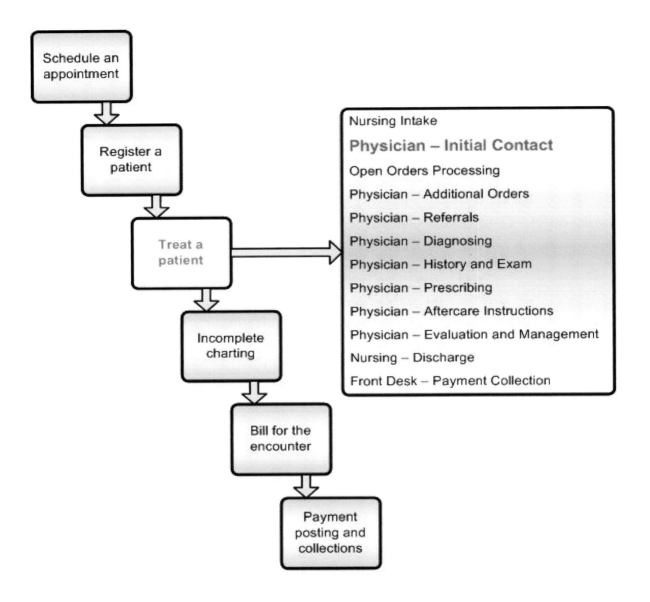

Schedule an appointment

Register a patient

Treat a patient

Incomplete charting

Bill for the encounter

Payment posting and collections

Nursing Intake

**Physician – Initial Contact**

Open Orders Processing

Physician – Additional Orders

Physician – Referrals

Physician – Diagnosing

Physician – History and Exam

Physician – Prescribing

Physician – Aftercare Instructions

Physician – Evaluation and Management

Nursing – Discharge

Front Desk – Payment Collection

## Physician - Initial Contact

After registration by the front desk and intake by the clinical staff, the patient is ready to see the physician.

The patient is on the <u>Clinic Status</u> screen, and the *workflow status* is **Rack**, meaning that the patient's *chart is in the rack* waiting for the physician to pick it up and see the patient.

*Physicians access* MedTrak in several different ways.

◊ Some physicians take a wireless computer tablet with a *touch-screen* and *voice recognition* into the exam room with them and enter their clinical information during their *face time* with the patient.

◊ Some physicians prefer to leave the computer outside the exam room and come out to enter their documentation away from the patient.

◊ Some medical facilities have computers hooked up in each exam room for the physicians to use during their face time.

To indicate that the physician is now seeing the patient for the initial contact, the user places the cursor in the command field on the <u>Clinic Status</u> screen next to the patient (shown below) and clicks the *Examine Patient* button. The physician does this before seeing the patient.

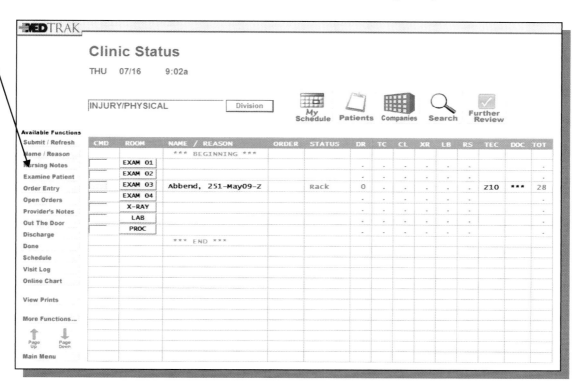

This notifies the medical facility that this patient is now being seen by the physician whose initials appear in the **DOC** column for this patient. MedTrak automatically changes the workflow status on the <u>Clinic Status</u> screen to **Examine** (shown on the next page).

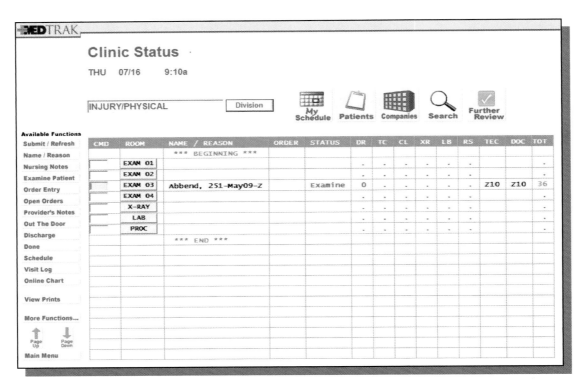

**Do This** ▶  **10.01** - Access the <u>Clinic Status</u> screen off the Main Menu

**10.02** - Place the cursor next to your patient

**10.03** - Click the **Examine Patient** button

(your patient's status should now be **Examine**)

## Initial Contact with the Patient - Placing Orders

In this example, the physician takes the touch-screen tablet into **Exam 03** and examines the left ankle of patient Abbend. The physician discusses the circumstances that caused the ankle injury. Additionally, the physician asks the patient about his medical, social, and family history.

Since the ankle is red, swollen, and painful to walk on, the physician decides to order an x-ray to see whether it is broken and orders an ice pack to help reduce the swelling.

Using the touch-screen tablet, the physician places the cursor next to the patient on the <u>Clinic Status</u> screen and clicks the **Order Entry** button. MedTrak's **CPOE** (**computerized physician order entry**) is part of its integrated EMR system.

The next screen to appear is the <u>Visit Orders</u> screen (shown on the next page).

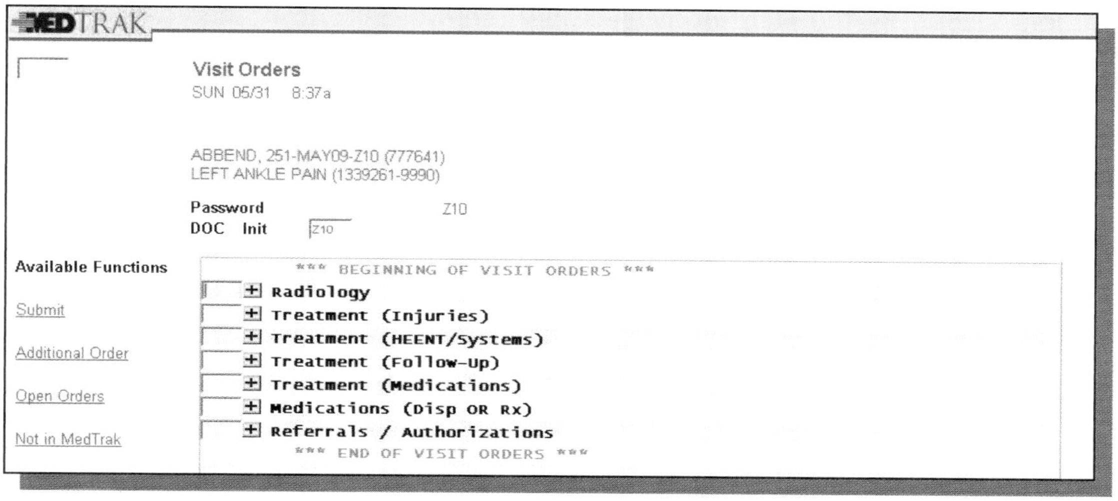

As noted earlier, MedTrak is a *problem-focused* system. This means that when a patient is seen for a left ankle injury, the *most likely orders* for a left ankle injury appear first for the physician to select. If the patient had a right elbow injury, then MedTrak would display the most likely orders that the physician would need for that injury. Since this is a musculoskeletal injury, the order category for **Laboratory** does not appear on the screen. If the physician wants to place an order for a lab, he clicks the *Additional Order* button to display all of the order categories in the *orders tree*.

To locate the order for the left ankle x-ray, the physician clicks the yellow plus sign ➕ next to **Radiology** to see the most likely x-rays for the left ankle. The yellow plus sign ➕ indicates that there are more options available for that selection in the orders tree. The next screen to appear is the

Visit Orders screen for the **Radiology** category (shown below) displaying the most likely left ankle x-rays.

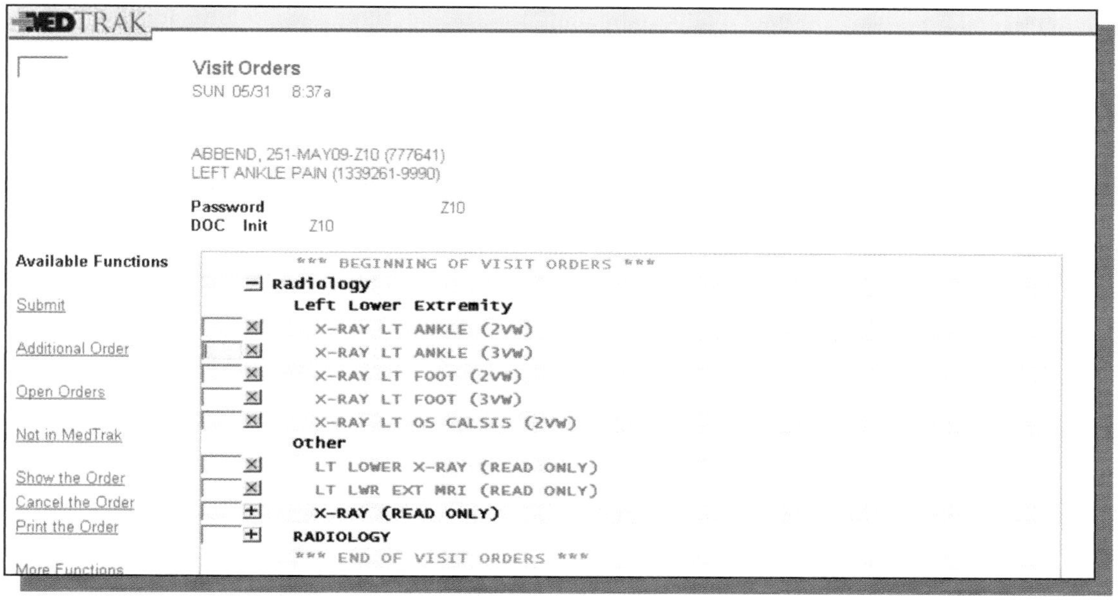

Selectable orders are identified with a **green** ✗ button, and their descriptions are also in **green**. To select the 3-view x-ray for the left ankle, the physician clicks the **green** ✗ button next to it.

The <u>Visit Orders</u> screen for the **Radiology** category (shown below) refreshes, indicating that the physician placed an order for the **3-view left ankle x-ray**.

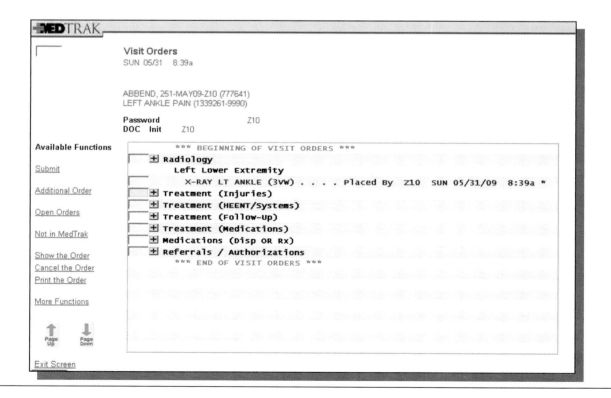

To place the order for the **ice pack**, the physician clicks the yellow minus sign ⊟ next to the **Radiology** category name (on the screen shown above) to go back up the orders tree to display all of the categories on the <u>Visit Orders</u> screen (shown below).

To locate the order for the ice pack, the physician clicks the yellow plus sign ⊞ next to the **Treatment (Injuries)** category to see the most likely treatments for the left ankle. Again, the yellow plus sign ⊞ indicates that there are more options available for that selection in the orders tree. The next screen to appear is the Visit Orders screen for the **Treatment (Injuries)** category (shown below), displaying the most likely left ankle treatments.

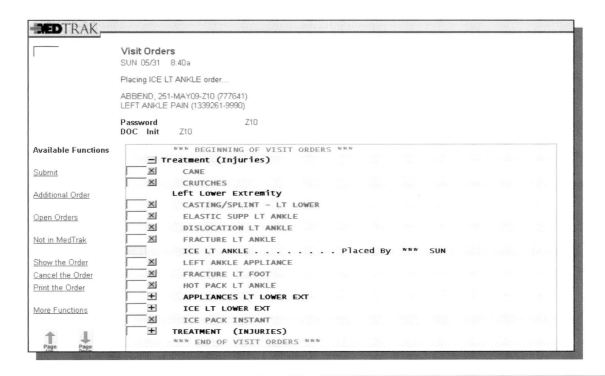

To select the ice treatment for the left ankle, the physician clicks the green ☒ button next to it.

The <u>Visit Orders</u> screen for the **Treatment (Injuries)** category (shown below) refreshes, indicating that the physician placed an order for the **ice treatment**.

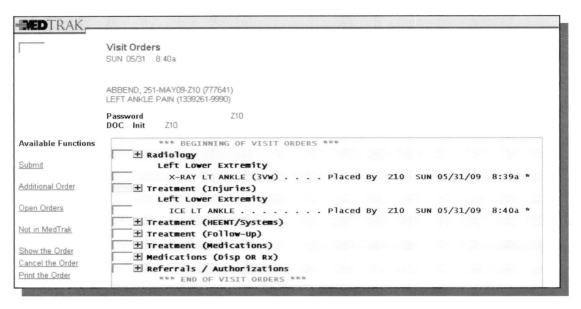

The asterisks next to the x-ray and treatment orders indicate that these are *open orders*, meaning that they are incomplete. In this example, the physician placed orders for the left ankle x-ray and the ice treatment. At this time, these are the only orders that the physician needs for the patient's care. Once the x-ray is completed and the physician does the wet read in the clinic, then the physician will place additional orders for this patient.

The physician clicks the *Exit Screen* button to return to the <u>Clinic Status</u> screen (shown below). The word Open appears in the **ORDER** column next to the patient, and the timer starts in the **TC** and **XR** columns for this patient.

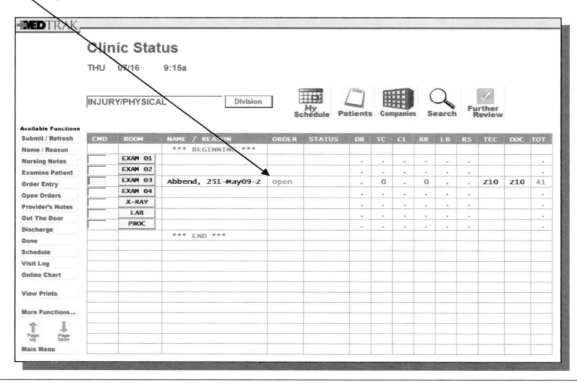

The Clinic Status screen in conjunction with **CPOE** (computerized physician order entry) enables efficient clinical workflow. In MedTrak, each order is broken down into its individual steps and assigned to a discipline for completion.

Once a patient has an open order, he or she cannot be discharged from the healthcare facility without either completing the open order or canceling the order. This ensures that every order placed for a patient is completed before the patient leaves the healthcare facility. It also means that every discipline knows exactly what is needed for each patient at all times. Nothing is missed and everyone is aware of the clinical workload.

---

**Do This** ▶  **10.04** - Place the cursor next to your patient

**10.05** - Click the *Order Entry* button

**10.06** - Click the *Radiology* category plus sign button **+|**

**10.07** - Click the *X-ray LT Ankle (3VW)* order selection button **X|**

**10.08** - Click the *Radiology* category minus sign button **–|**

**10.09** - Click the *Treatment (Injuries)* category plus sign button **+|**

**10.10** - Click the *Ice LT Ankle* order selection button **X|**

**10.11** - Click the *Exit Screen* button
          (to return to the Visit Orders screen)

**10.12** - Click the *Exit Screen* button
          (to return to the Clinic Status screen)

---

# Open Orders Processing

**Estimated time needed to complete this chapter - 30** minutes

## What you need to know before doing this chapter

- How to log into MedTrak
- How to register a patient
- How to access <u>Clinic Status</u> off the <u>Main Menu</u>
- How to move a patient to a room and answer nursing notes
- How to place orders for a patient

## Learning outcomes gained from this chapter

- How to identify a patient with an open order
- How to answer open order's questions
- How to select from a list of procedure options
- An understanding of open orders workflow

## Key concepts in this chapter

*waiting times*
*discipline columns*
*additional question types*
*procedural questions*
*field indicators*
*quality control question*
*age and gender specific*
*procedure selection options*
*cascade of questions*
*workflow steps*
*wet read*
*overread*
*evidence-based medicine completed orders*

## Open Orders Processing

### Major Categories of Clinical Workflow

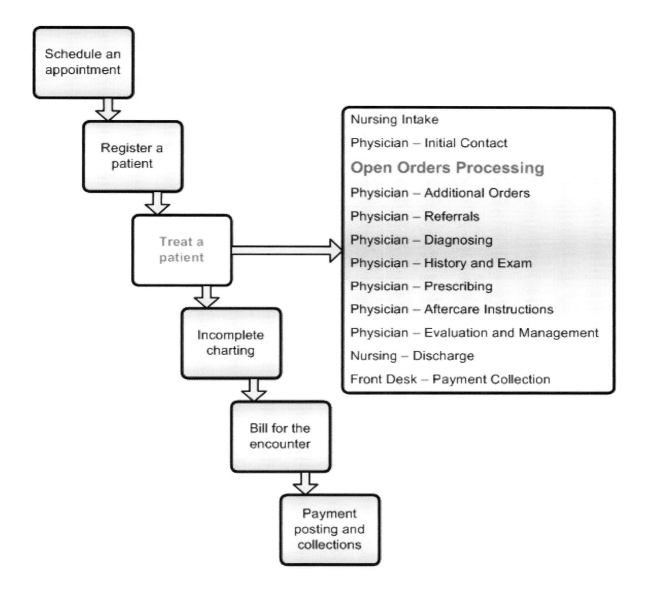

## Identifying Patients with Open Orders

After the physician places orders for the patient based on the examination during the initial contact with the patient, the Clinic Status screen displays the word Open next to the patient to indicate that the patient has open orders.

The *waiting times* in the *discipline columns* indicate which discipline is responsible for performing the next step of the open order.

In this example, the patient in **Exam 03** has open orders for the **TC** (clinical staff) and **XR** (x-ray staff).

The clinical staff (**TC**) and the x-ray personnel (**XR**) see that they have something to do for the patient in **Exam 03** because they have the timer started in their discipline waiting time column on the Clinic Status screen (shown below).

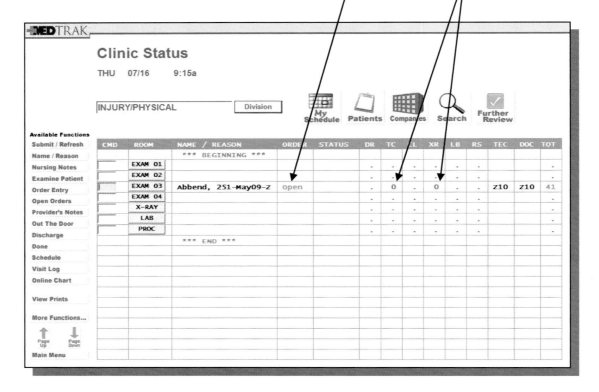

To review what the physician wants them to do for the patient, the clinical and x-ray personnel places the cursor next to the patient and clicks the *Open Orders* button.

The Open Orders processor screen (shown below) appears. The case number and patient name appear at the top of the screen. The location of the patient appears in the message field in red. The discipline responsible for performing the open order and the order name appear in the body of the screen along with the questions to be answered.

On this screen, the clinical staff (**TECH**) and the x-ray personnel (**XRAY**) read the physician orders for the patient in **Room 03**.

The **TECH** needs to provide ice for the left ankle for patient Abbend.

**XRAY** needs to do a 3-view x-ray of the left ankle on patient Abbend.

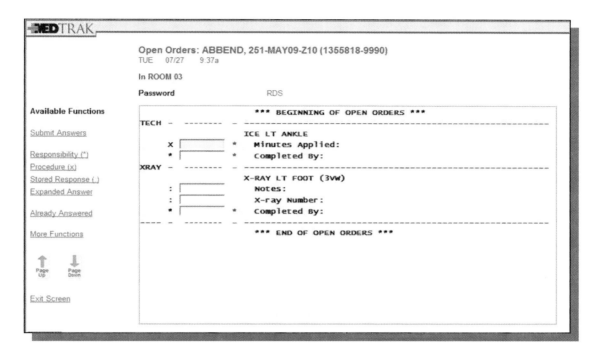

## Answering Open Orders Questions

Open orders questions use the same processes for entering answers that are used on the Nursing Notes screen. *Additional question types* include questions to be answered with someone's initials and procedural questions. *Procedural questions* require the selection of options on another screen.

*Field indicators* (a colon, an X, or an asterisk) appear to the left of the input fields and include:

| | |
|---|---|
| **:** | Question can be answered on the screen with up to 10 characters, <br> or by selecting a stored response (or typing the trigger in the field), <br> or by using the Expanded Answer screen. |
| **X** | Question must be answered with an **X** to access the procedural selection area. |
| **\*** | Question must be answered with the initials of the person responsible for the work. |

The red asterisk * to the right of the input field indicates that this is a *quality control question* and must be answered before the patient can be discharged from the medical facility. Questions without a red asterisk are optional and do not need an answer to complete the order. Questions can be *age and gender specific*. If this patient was female, the x-ray order would include a question related to whether the patient was possibly pregnant; and therefore, should not be exposed to the radiation of an x-ray.

When finished completing the orders:

- The **TECH** needs to document the minutes applied and who completed the ice order. Both of these questions are quality control and must be answered.

- **XRAY** needs to document any special notes about the x-ray, the x-ray number, and who completed the x-ray as shown on the Open Orders processing screen (shown below). The only question for the x-ray that is quality control is who completed the x-ray.

- In this example, the clinical and x-ray staff answer both the **TECH** and **XRAY** questions at the same time. In the actual clinical setting, these questions would probably be answered by different personnel at different times.

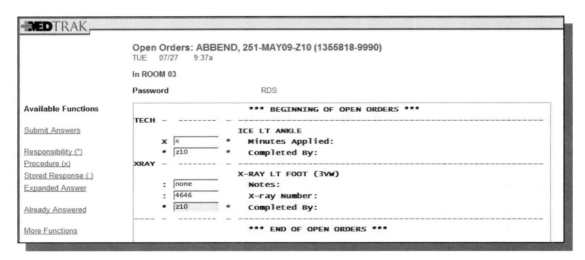

The **X** to the left of the minutes applied question indicates that this is a procedural question and must be answered with an **x**. After answering the minutes applied with the x and entering his or her initials, the **TECH** clicks the *Submit Answers* button. The next screen to appear is the Procedure Options screen (shown below).

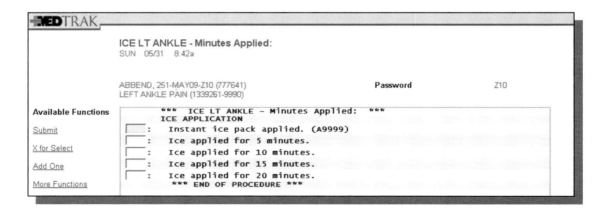

The order name and question appear at the top of the screen in addition to the patient's name and chief complaint. The *procedure selection options* appear in the body of the screen.

On this screen (shown below), the clinical staff (**TC**) selects the option for the application of the ice. In this example, the clinical staff selects the first option (Instant ice pack) by placing the cursor next to the instant ice pack and clicking the *X for Select* button. The clinical staff could have also typed the **x** in the field using the mouse. To indicate that more than one ice pack was used, the clinical staff could type the quantity into the input field. After selecting the procedure options, the clinical staff clicks the *Submit* button.

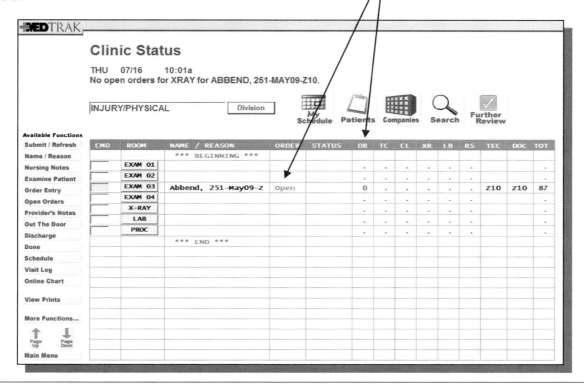

Once all of the open orders questions are answered, MedTrak automatically returns to the Clinic Status screen (shown below). The Open word is still in the **ORDER** column, but now the waiting time is set for the physician (**DR**). The next step in the workflow for the x-ray is for the physician to do the initial read.

**Do This** ► **11.01** - Place the cursor next to your patient

(you should be on the <u>Clinic Status</u> screen)

**11.02** - Click the *Open Orders* button

**11.03** - Answer the *TECH* questions for the **ICE LT ANKLE** order

Type an **x** in the **Minutes Applied** question entry field

Type your employee initials in the **Completed By** entry field

**11.04** - Answer the *XRAY* questions for the **X-RAY LT ANKLE (3VW)** order

Type **none** in the **Notes** question

Type **464646** in the **X-ray Number** question entry field

Type your employee initials in the **Completed By** entry field

**11.05** - Click the *Submit Answers* button

(you should be on **ICE LT ANKLE - Minutes Applied** screen)

**11.06** - Type an **x** in the **Instant Ice pack applied** entry field

**11.07** - Click the *Submit* button

(you will be returned to the <u>Clinic Status</u> screen)

**11.08** - Verify the *ORDER* column still reads *Open*.

## *Open Orders Workflow*

Another aspect of MedTrak's clinical workflow is the processing of open orders. Each order can have its own *cascade of questions* that pass responsibility for the *workflow steps* from one discipline to another. All orders start with the physician placing the order. Then, depending on the workflow steps in the medical facility, the order will appear in the column of the next discipline responsible for completing the task.

In this example, the patient had an x-ray and the x-ray personnel finished taking the x-ray and documenting that they did. As soon as the x-ray staff answers their questions, the <u>Clinic Status</u> screen notifies the physician (DR) that there is an open order that requires a response. The word Open in the **ORDER** column indicates that the patient has at least one open order.

The next step in the x-ray order is for the physician to read the x-ray and document the findings. The initial read of an x-ray by a physician is commonly referred to as a *wet read*. If the physician sees something that appears to be abnormal, he or she will probably ask for an *overread* by a radiologist.

The physician places the cursor next to the patient on the Clinic Status screen and clicks the *Open Orders* button. The next screen to appear is the Open Orders processing screen (shown below).

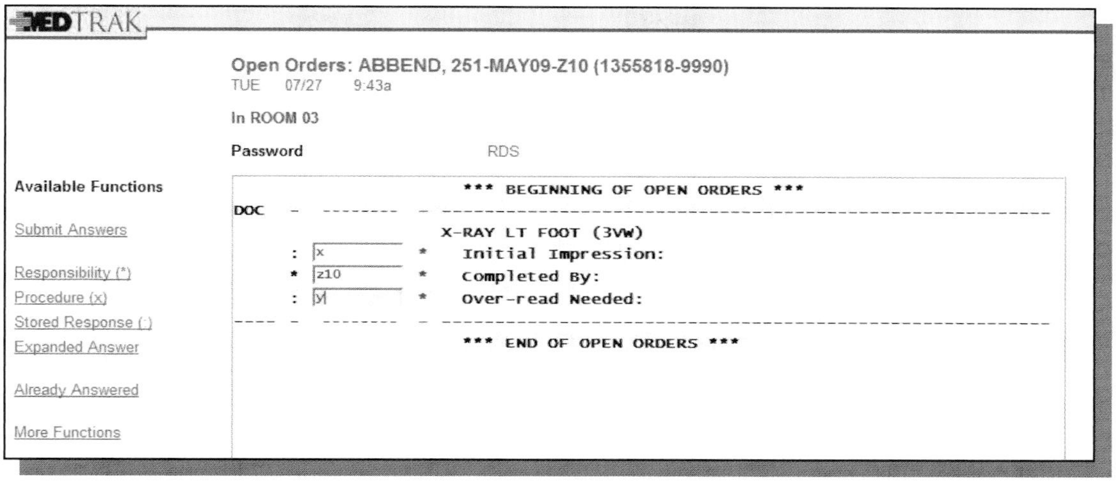

```
MEDTRAK
                    Open Orders: ABBEND, 251-MAY09-Z10 (1355818-9990)
                    TUE   07/27    9:43a

                    In ROOM 03

                    Password              RDS

Available Functions              *** BEGINNING OF OPEN ORDERS ***
                        DOC  -  --------  -  --------------------------------------
Submit Answers                               X-RAY LT FOOT (3VW)
                              :  x       *   Initial Impression:
Responsibility (*)            *  z10     *   Completed By:
Procedure (x)                 :  y       *   Over-read Needed:
Stored Response ( )           ----  -  --------  -  -------------------------------
Expanded Answer                          *** END OF OPEN ORDERS ***

Already Answered

More Functions
```

Using the keyboard, the physician enters an **x** to go to the expanded answer screen for the **Initial Impression** question. Then the physician enters his or her employee initials in the **Completed by** question to indicate that he or she did the wet-read. In the **Over-read needed** question, the physician enters a **y** that is the trigger for the stored response indicating the need for an over-read by a radiologist.

MedTrak's rules-based system allows building rules for *evidence-based medicine*. In this example, the physician's answer to the question about the need for an over-read automatically drives another order for the clinical staff to prepare the x-ray to be sent out for the over-read.

After entering the answers, the physician clicks the *Submit Answers* button or presses the *ENTER* key. Because the physician wants to go to the expanded answer screen for the **Initial Impression** question, the next screen to appear is the Expanded Answer screen (shown below).

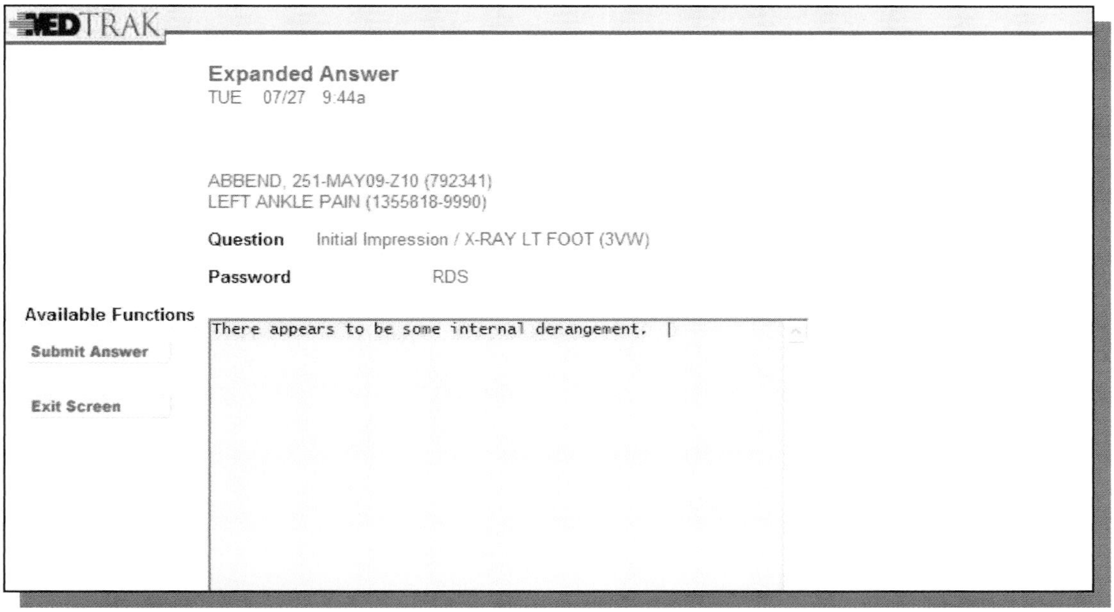

```
MEDTRAK
            Expanded Answer
            TUE   07/27  9:44a



            ABBEND, 251-MAY09-Z10 {792341}
            LEFT ANKLE PAIN (1355818-9990)

            Question   Initial Impression / X-RAY LT FOOT (3VW)

            Password        RDS
Available Functions
            There appears to be some internal derangement.  |
Submit Answer

Exit Screen
```

The physician answered all of the questions on the <u>Open Orders</u> processing screen; therefore, MedTrak automatically returns to the <u>Clinic Status</u> screen (shown below). Because the physician ordered the over-read for the x-ray, the word Open is still in the **ORDER** column, indicating to the clinical staff that they have something to do for the patient.

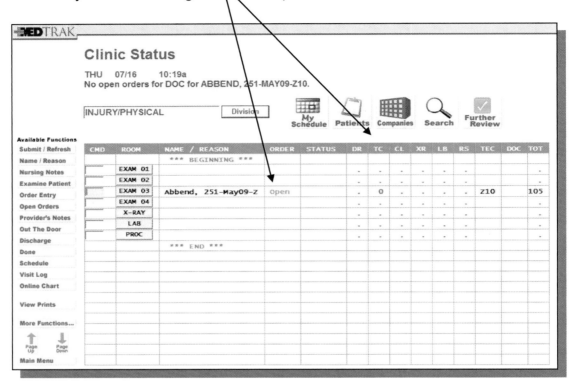

---

**Do This** ▶ **11.09** - Place the cursor next to your patient

**11.10** - Click the *Open Orders* button

**11.11** - Answer the *DOC* questions for the **X-RAY LT ANKLE (3VW)** order
  Type an **x** in the **Initial Impression** question entry field
  Type your employee initials in the **Completed By** entry field
  Type a **y** in the **Over-read Needed** question entry field

**11.12** - Click the *Submit Answers* button
  (you should be on the **Initial Impression** expanded answer)

**11.13** - Type the following in the expanded answer entry field
  "There appears to be some internal derangement."

**11.14** - Click the *Submit Answer* button
  (you should be on the <u>Clinic Status</u> screen)

The clinical staff places the cursor next to the patient and clicks the *Open Order* button.

The next screen to appear is the Open Orders processing screen (shown below). The clinical staff prepares the x-ray for an over-read and then documents the type of x-ray, the x-ray number, where the x-ray is being sent, and who prepared it for sending. After answering the questions, the clinical staff clicks the *Submit Answers* button. The red asterisk * to the right of the data input field indicates that the question must be answered. It is optional to answer the question if there is no red asterisk.

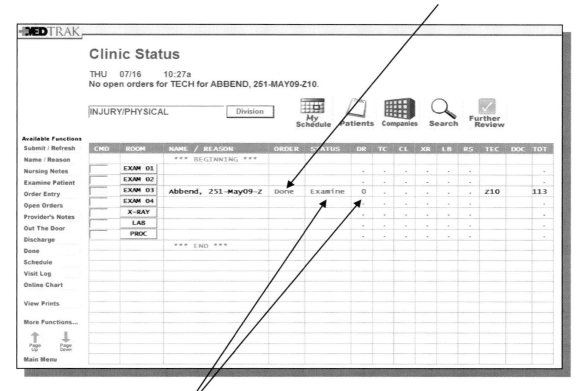

MedTrak automatically returns to the Clinic Status screen. The word **Done** is now in the **ORDER** column to indicate that there were open orders, and they are now *completed orders*.

In addition, MedTrak reset the time counter for the physician's waiting time column (**DR**) and changed the **STATUS** column back to Examine. MedTrak automatically sets the workflow status to Examine whenever all open orders are completed after the physician has picked up the patient's chart and placed orders for the patient.

With all open orders complete, the responsibility for determining the next step in the patient's care is passed back to the physician, and the Examine workflow status indicates the physician needs to place additional orders for the patient or finish with the patient and discharge him or her from this visit.

---

**Do This ▶**   **11.15** - Place the cursor next to your patient

**11.16** - Click the *Open Orders* button

**11.17** - Answer the **TECH** questions for the **X-RAY OVERREAD** order
   Type **Acme Xray** in the **X-ray sent to** entry field
   Type your employee initials in the **X-ray prepared by** entry field

**11.18** - Click the *Submit Answers* button
   (you should be on the Clinic Status screen)
   (your patient's workflow status should now be **Examine**)

---

# CHAPTER

# 12

# Out the Door - Overview

**Estimated time needed to complete this chapter  -  15** minutes

## What you need to know before doing this chapter

- ♦ How to log into MedTrak
- ♦ How to register a patient
- ♦ How to access <u>Clinic Status</u> off the <u>Main Menu</u>
- ♦ How to move a patient to a room and answer nursing notes
- ♦ How to place orders for a patient
- ♦ How to answer open orders

## Learning outcomes gained from this chapter

- ♦ An understanding of the <u>Visit Documentation</u> screen

## Key concepts in this chapter

*subjective*

*objective*

*assessment*

*plan*

*SOAP notes*

*right information to the right person at the right time*

*targeted information*

*blink speed*

*visit documentation*

*out the door*

## Out the Door - Overview

### Major Categories of Clinical Workflow

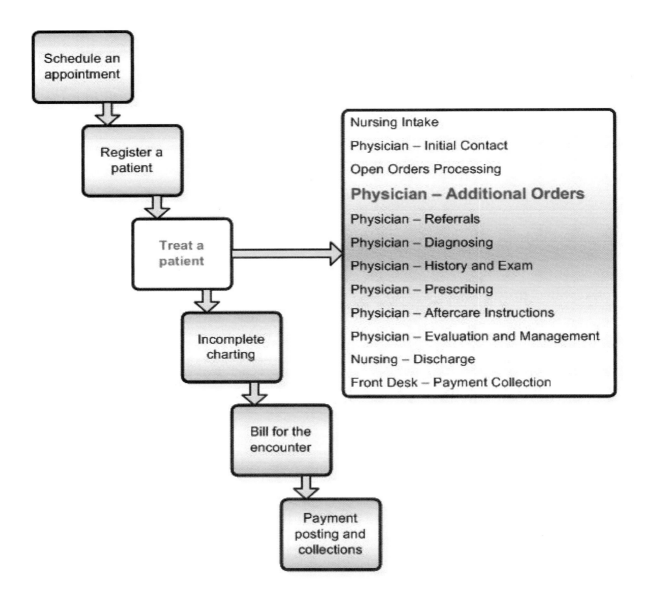

## Out the Door - Overview

Efficient medical clinic workflow minimizes the time that it takes physicians to document their *subjective* and *objective* findings based on the physical exam, their *assessment* of the patient's condition, and their *plan* for treatment. Together these components comprise the physician's *SOAP notes*.

One of MedTrak's goals is to present the *right information* to the *right person* at the *right time*. We do this by presenting only the information needed at the time to make a decision when requested. This saves on clutter on the screen so that the clinicians can focus on the *targeted information*. Additionally, the weight of each screen (amount of data on a screen) is minimal to enable *blink speed* screen changes.

As you learned in **Chapter 10 - Physician - Initial Contact**, MedTrak streamlined the order entry process by problem-focusing the order selection screens to present the most-likely orders that the physician would need for the presenting problem(s) with minimal clicks of the mouse (or touches on a touch-screen). To place the two orders (left ankle x-ray and ice treatment) for the example in this book, the physician needed to do eight clicks or touches. Two of those were to return to the Clinic Status screen from the Order Entry screen.

In keeping with our goal of targeted information, MedTrak developed a processor for physicians to use for *visit documentation* that includes the following sections of functionality and information:

- ◆ Additional orders needed for the patient's care
- ◆ Referrals to specialists
- ◆ Diagnosing
- ◆ Documenting the history and exam (subjective and objective findings)
- ◆ Ordering medications - both dispensed and prescribed
- ◆ Aftercare instructions for the patients to take with them
- ◆ Evaluation and management - level of service

To access the Visit Documentation screen (shown on the next page), the physician places the cursor next to the patient and clicks the *Out the Door* button.

The **Out the Door** term originated when MedTrak was being developed to run the emergency department of a hospital. During our visits to the emergency room, we would hear the physicians telling the ward clerk that they were done with the patient and wanted them "*out the door.*"

While doing time studies of the physicians using this processor, MedTrak started calling the **Out the Door** process the "two minute drill." Our goal is to have the physicians place additional orders, order a referral, diagnose the patient, prescribe the patient, provide the patient with aftercare instructions, and select the patient's level of service in two minutes or less.

The average length of time for a physician to use MedTrak's Visit Documentation screen is **less than two minutes**, without documenting the history and exam portions. The history and exam are the only two parts of the patient's visit that do not have to be documented before the patient leaves the medical facility. There are no charges directly related to the history and exam. The thoroughness of the history and the exam are documented in the level of the evaluation and management code selected by the physician.

## *Visit Documentation Screen*

The <u>Visit Documentation</u> screen enables physicians to document the patient's visit by working their way down the topics on the screen. As the physician documents, this screen refreshes to show the work.

The top of the screen displays the date of service for the visit, the clinical staff's answer to the medication allergies question, the patient's name and the chief complaint.

In this example, the physician previously placed orders for the x-ray and ice for the left ankle. Then, by way of answering positively to the question about whether the physician wanted an overread of the x-ray, the physician placed the order for the x-ray overread.

The following provides a description of the different areas on the <u>Visit Documentation</u> screen.

## Orders

The top portion on the screen is for **patient orders** and enables the physician to:

◆ Place additional orders using the problem-focused order entry method

◆ Place additional orders using order codes that can be entered directly on this screen

◆ Cancel an order

◆ Access the open orders processor to complete an order

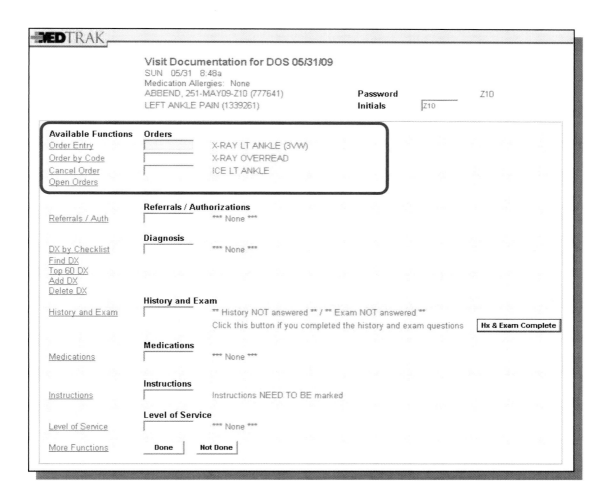

## *Referrals/Authorizations*

The next section is for **referrals/authorizations** and enables the physician to:

- ◆ Place an order for the patient to see a specialist (orthopedic surgeon, dermatologist, etc.)

- ◆ Place an order for physical therapy, occupational therapy, chiropractic care

- ◆ Place an order for an MRI, CT scan, EMG, or other scheduled testing

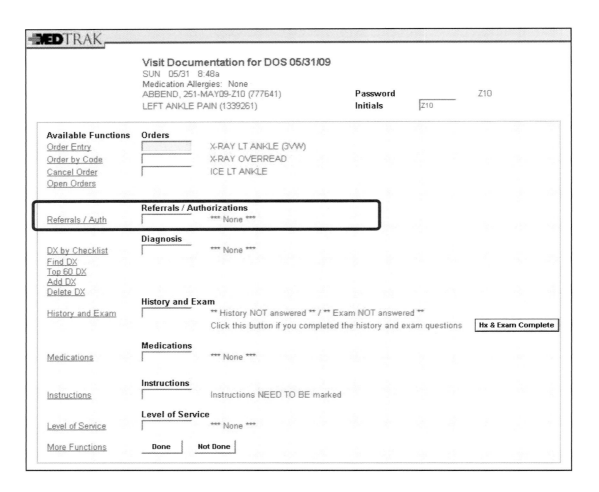

## *Diagnosis*

The next section on the screen is for the provider to choose and maintain the **diagnosis:**

- ◆ Using the problem-focused diagnoses tree based on the physician's checklist

- ◆ Using the **Find DX** process that provides seven different ways to locate the diagnosis

- ◆ Using the **Top 60 DX** process that displays the most common diagnoses on one screen

- ◆ Using the **Add DX** process that starts at the top of the diagnoses tree

- ◆ Using the **Delete DX** process to remove a diagnosis

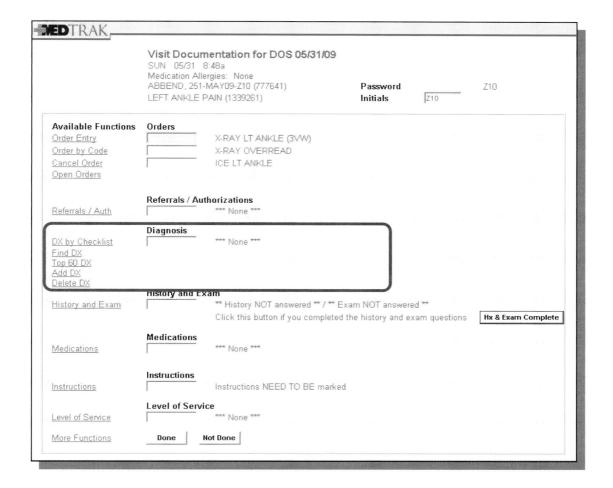

## *History and Exam*

The next section on the screen is for the physician to document the **History and Exam**:

- ◆ History and exam questions are based on the diagnoses.
- ◆ Physicians can use the check-box process with a touch-screen tablet.
- ◆ Physicians can use voice recognition software.
- ◆ Physicians can dictate the history and exam to a transcriptionist.
- ◆ Physicians can type their answers using a keyboard and the stored response processor.

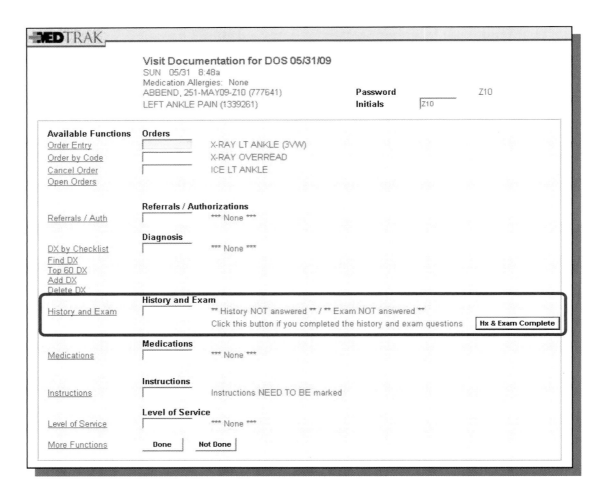

## *Medications*

The next section is for the physician to order both dispensed and prescription **medications**:

- ◆ Using the problem-focused order entry process

- ◆ Using the order codes process

- ◆ This section can also be used by a physician to cancel a medication order.

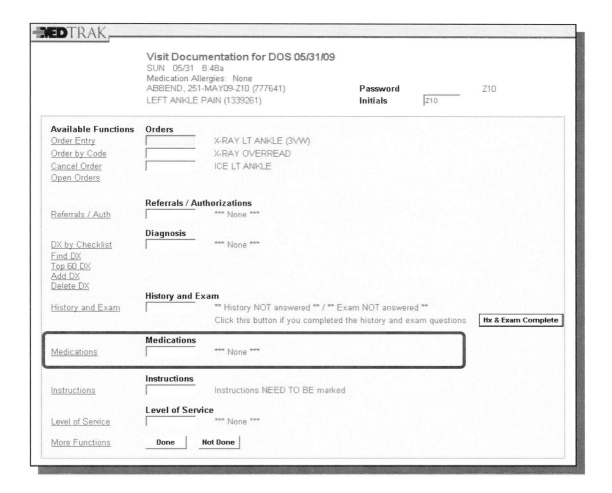

## Instructions  (For the Patients After They Leave the Clinic)

The next section is for the physician to select the patient's aftercare **instructions**:

- ◆ Instructions are problem-focused based on the diagnoses.

- ◆ Physicians can instruct the patient as to what to do at home.

- ◆ Physicians can instruct the patient as to what to do at work.

- ◆ Physicians can document their plan of care.

- ◆ Physicians schedule the patient's next appointment with minimal effort.

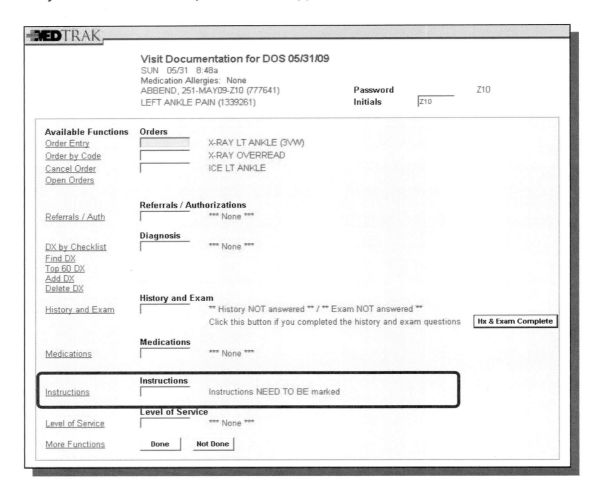

## Level of Service (Evaluation & Management)

The next section is for the physician to select the **level of service** for the visit:

- ◆ Based on the complexity of the history, exam, and decision making for primary care

- ◆ Based on the type of visit for orthopedics

- ◆ Provides for first aid designation for workers' compensation visits

- ◆ Provides for consultation visits

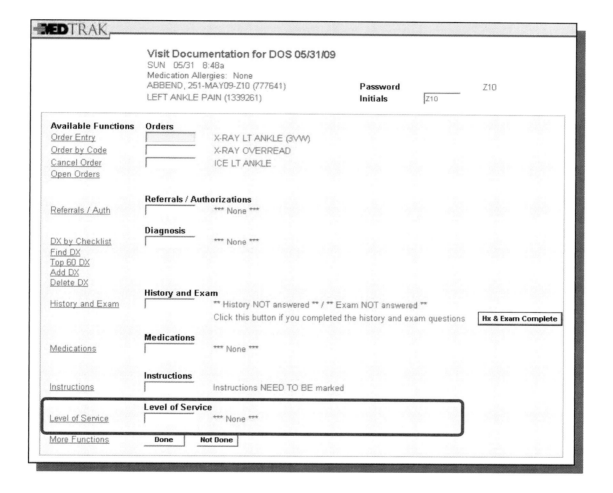

## *Done or Not Done*

The next section is for the physician to determine whether the visit documentation is **done** or **not done**:

    ♦    If the physician is done, he or she clicks the *Done* button.

    ♦    If the physician is not done, he or she clicks the *Not Done* button.

Sometimes physicians are interrupted with phone calls from patients or questions from the clinical staff and cannot finish the documentation of the visit at that time. That is the purpose of the *Not Done* button. Physicians can return to this screen at their convenience.

However, the patient will not be able to be discharged from the <u>Clinic Status</u> screen until the physician indicates that he or she is **Done** with the patient and wants them "**out the door**."

As you work through the next few chapters of the book, you will process your patient through each of the sections on the <u>Visit Documentation</u> screen.

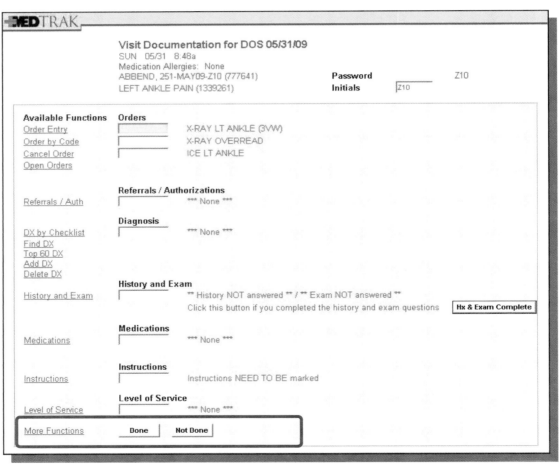

# CHAPTER

# 13

# Physician - Additional Orders

**Estimated time needed to complete this chapter - 15** minutes

## What you need to know before doing this chapter

- ◆ How to log into MedTrak
- ◆ How to register a patient
- ◆ How to access <u>Clinic Status</u> off the <u>Main Menu</u>
- ◆ How to move a patient to a room and answer nursing notes
- ◆ How to access the <u>Visit Documentation</u> processor (Out the Door)

## Learning outcomes gained from this chapter

- ◆ How to place additional orders using order codes

## *Physician - Additional Orders*

### Major Categories of Clinical Workflow

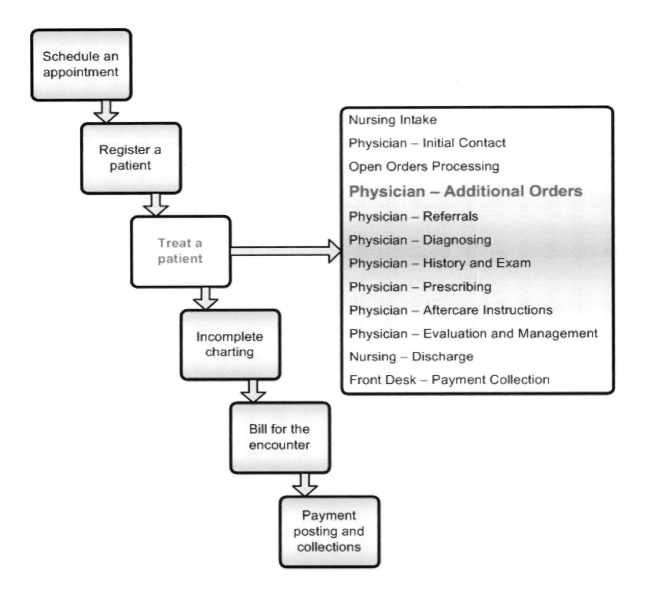

Schedule an appointment

Register a patient

Treat a patient

Incomplete charting

Bill for the encounter

Payment posting and collections

Nursing Intake

Physician – Initial Contact

Open Orders Processing

**Physician – Additional Orders**

Physician – Referrals

Physician – Diagnosing

Physician – History and Exam

Physician – Prescribing

Physician – Aftercare Instructions

Physician – Evaluation and Management

Nursing – Discharge

Front Desk – Payment Collection

If you are already on the <u>Visit Documentation</u> screen (shown below), then skip the next **Do This** section. If you are not on the <u>Visit Documentation</u> screen, then do the next steps.

---

**Do This** ▶ **13.01** - Place the cursor next to your patient

(you should be on the <u>Clinic Status</u> screen)

**13.02** - Click the ***Out the Door*** button

(you should be on the <u>Visit Documentation</u> screen)

---

In this example, the physician ordered the left ankle x-ray and the ice treatment after the initial contact with the patient. Then the physician ordered an x-ray over-read based on the initial impression of the x-ray.

After reviewing the x-ray and determining that the ankle has some internal derangement, the physician is going to provide a brace to the patient to help stabilize the ankle. The physician will place an order for the ankle brace.

In addition to the order entry process using the problem-focused <u>Visit Orders</u> screen, MedTrak also allows the placing of orders using ***order codes***. Physicians like to use order codes because it is faster than locating the desired order in the order entry screens.

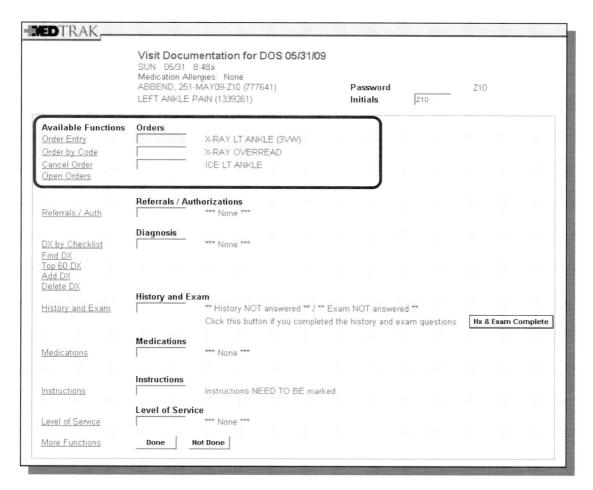

## Using Order Codes for Placing Orders

Order codes are names created by physicians for some of their *common orders* — orders placed on a frequent basis. The order code names (order codes) can be up to 10 characters in length. The only restriction on the order code is that it is unique. Each physician can create custom order codes. For example: Physician A could name an x-ray order for the right index finger **rtindexxr** and Physician B could name the same order **xrindexrt**. Both of these order codes refer to the same order, but the naming is specific to the individual physician.

In this example, the physician is placing an order for a left ankle appliance (brace). The order code created by the physician for the left ankle appliance is **lankappl** (as shown on the screen below). After entering the order code in the data entry field, the physician presses the *ENTER* key to place the order.

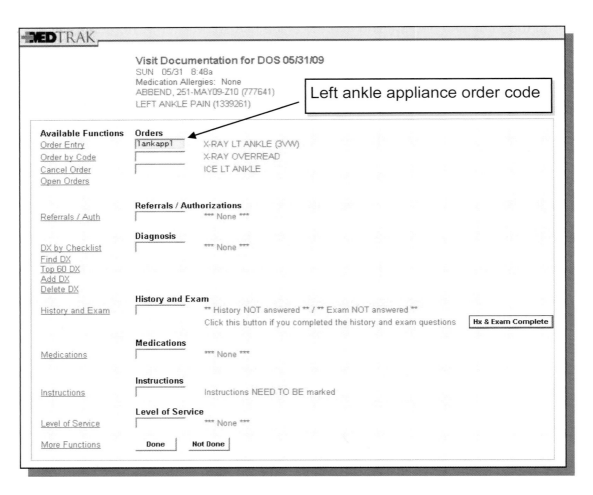

The next screen to appear is the <u>Order by Code</u> screen (shown below) with the left ankle appliance order automatically entered. To confirm the order, the physician clicks the *Submit* button.

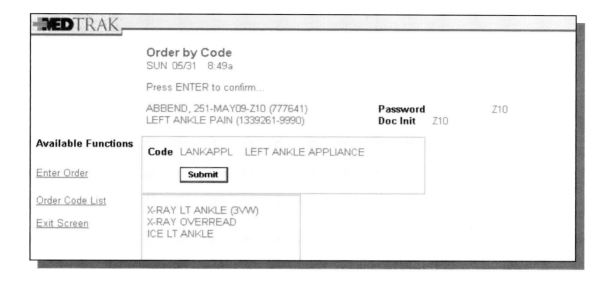

The physician clicks the *Submit* button to confirm that this is the right order.

If it is not the right order or the physician wants to place another order and does not know the order code, the physician can view all of the order codes by clicking the *Order Code List* button to select the order from the <u>Order Code: Select</u> screen (sample screen shown below). The *order code list* contains all of the order codes created by the users for that entity.

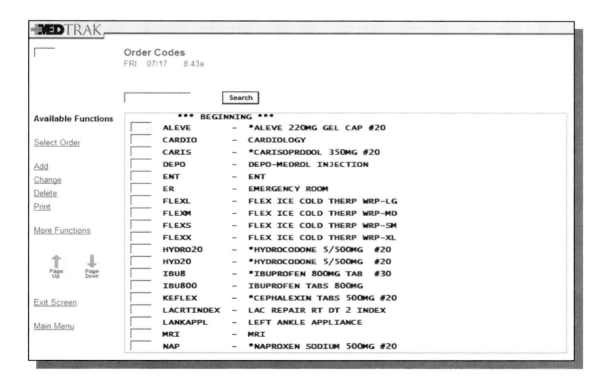

The Order by Code screen (shown below) refreshes, displaying the **Left Ankle Appliance** order underneath the **Ice LT Ankle** order. The physician can continue to stay on this screen and enter additional order codes or select them from the Order Code List screen as previously described.

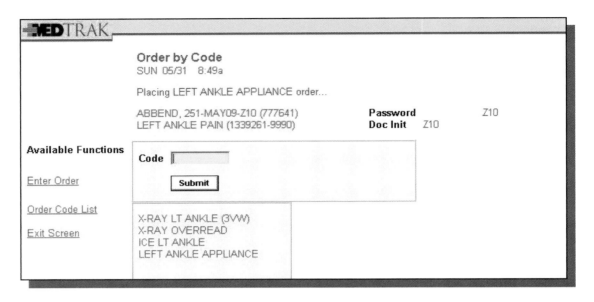

After placing the **Left Ankle Appliance** order, the physician clicks the *Exit Screen* button to return to the Visit Documentation screen (shown below). The **Left Ankle Appliance** order is an open order and will need to be completed by the clinical staff before discharging the patient from the medical facility.

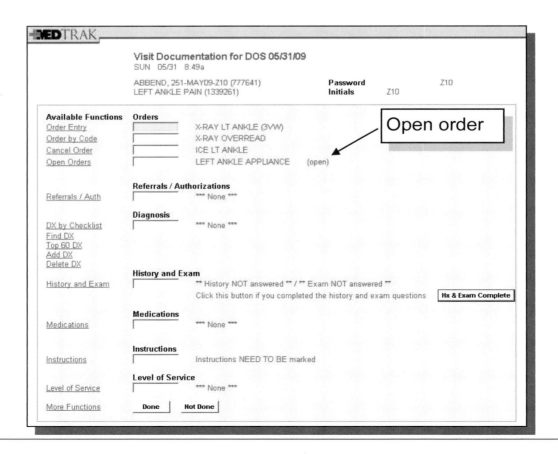

**Do This** ▶ **13.03** - Place the cursor in the top field of the Orders category

(you should be on the <u>Visit Documentation</u> screen)

**13.04** - Type **lankappl** in the data entry field

**13.05** - Press the *ENTER* key

**13.06** - Review the <u>Order by Code</u> screen to be sure of the right order

**13.07** - Press the *ENTER* key again to confirm the order

**13.08** - Press the *Order Code List* button to view other order codes

**13.09** - Click the *Exit Screen* button to return to the <u>Order by Code</u> screen

**13.10** - Click the *Exit Screen* button

(you should be on the <u>Visit Documentation</u> screen)

**If you are continuing with the next exercise (Physician - Referrals)**

**right now, skip the next Do This section.**

If you are not continuing on with the next chapter, do the next steps to sign out of MedTrak.

**Do This** ▶ **13.11** - Click the *Not Done* button

(you should be on the <u>Clinic Status</u> screen)

**13.12** - Click the *Exit Screen* or *Main Menu* button

(you should be on the MedTrak <u>Main Menu</u>)

**13.13** - Click the *Log Off* button to exit MedTrak

# CHAPTER

# 14

# Physician - Referrals

**Estimated time needed to complete this chapter  -  15** minutes

## What you need to know before doing this chapter

- ♦ How to log into MedTrak
- ♦ How to register a patient
- ♦ How to access <u>Clinic Status</u> off the <u>Main Menu</u>
- ♦ How to move a patient to a room and answer nursing notes
- ♦ How to access the <u>Visit Documentation</u> processor (Out the Door)

## Learning outcomes gained from this chapter

- ♦ How to place an order for a referral to a specialist

## Key concepts in this chapter

*referral*
*specialist*
*treatments*
*scheduled testing*
*tracking a referral*
*status of a referral*

## *Physician - Referrals*

## Major Categories of Clinical Workflow

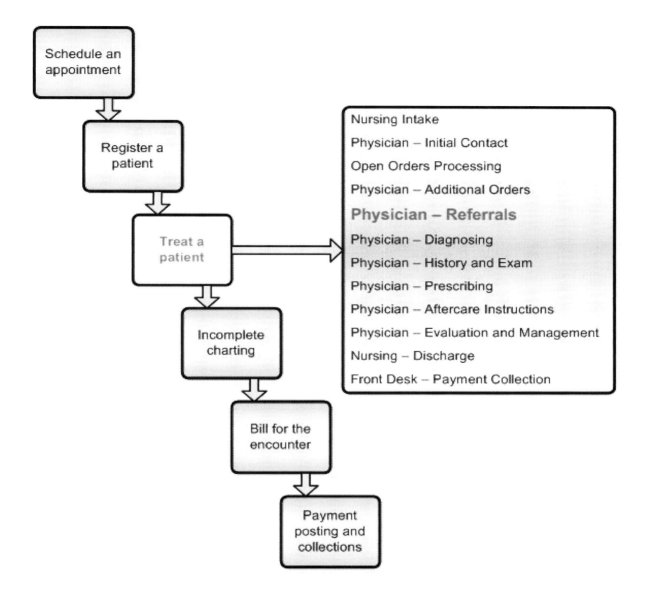

## *Physician - Referrals*

Many times patients present with problems that require medical skills and knowledge beyond the scope of abilities of the treating physician. In these situations, the treating physician will refer the patient to a specialist for further evaluation and/or treatment. When the treating physician makes this determination, an order for a *referral* will be placed.

These types of referrals are to see a *specialist*:

- Allergist
- Cardiologist
- Endocrinologist
- Gynecologist
- Hematologist
- Internal medicine doctor
- Oncologist
- Ophthalmologist
- Orthopedic surgeon
- Physiatrist
- Plastic surgeon
- Psychiatrist
- Rheumatologist
- Urologist

These types of referrals are for *treatments*:

- Physical therapist
- Chiropractor
- Acupuncturist

These types of referrals are for *scheduled testing*:

- MRI - magnetic resonance imaging
- CT scan - computed tomography scan
- EMG - electromyography

The treating physician provides the specialist with the following information about the referral:

- Body part(s) involved or systemic reason for the referral
- Scheduling priority - immediately, as soon as possible, or at their convenience
- Scheduling purpose - evaluate only, evaluate and treat, or assume care
- Special notes about the reason for the referral
- Chart for the most recent patient visit

*Tracking a referral* is an important function in clinical workflow. The medical facility needs to know the *status of a referral* at all times and be able to provide that status to the patient and everyone else who needs to know.

Once a physician orders a referral, the clinical staff will:

◆ Obtain authorization for the referral from the patient's payer

◆ Coordinate with the patient and the specialist's office to schedule the first appointment

◆ Receive the specialist's report after the patient's appointment and place it in the chart

◆ Alert the treating physician that the specialist's report is back and ready for review

If you are already on the Visit Documentation screen (shown below), then skip the next **Do This** section. If you are not on the Visit Documentation screen, then do the next steps.

---

**Do This** ▶ **14.01** - Place the cursor next to your patient on the Clinic Status screen

**14.02** - Click the *Out the Door* button

(you should be on the Visit Documentation screen)

---

In this example, based on the results of the x-ray, the treating physician determined that the patient needs an orthopedic consultation. To place the order for the orthopedic consultation, the physician decides to use the Order Entry screen by clicking the *Referrals/Auth* button on the Visit Documentation screen (shown below).

Because MedTrak is a problem-focused system, the Visit Orders screen for **Referrals/Authorizations** appears (shown on the next page), displaying the most likely referrals for the left ankle problem. To save the physician time, MedTrak immediately set the Visit Orders screen to the referral category.

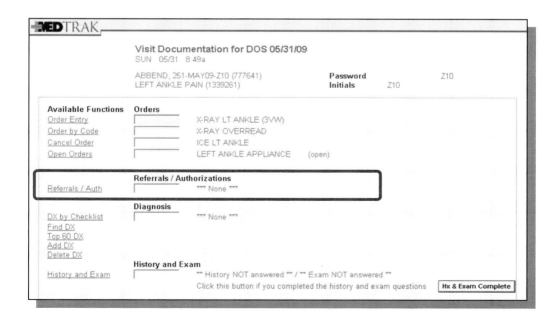

To place an order for an orthopedic evaluation and/or treatment for the left ankle injury, the physician clicks the green ⊠ button next to the **Orthopedic Consultation** order.

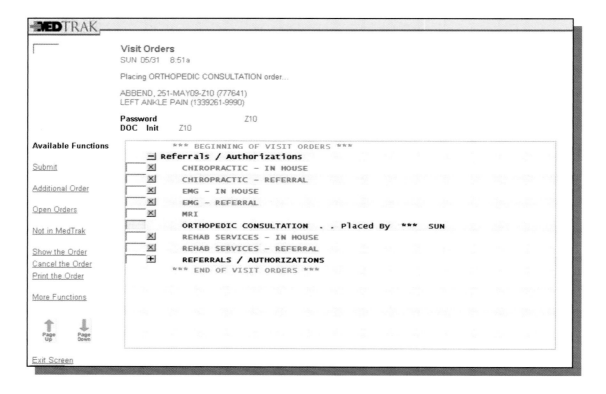

The Visit Orders screen for the **Referrals/Authorizations** category (shown below) refreshes, indicating that the physician placed an order for the **Orthopedic Consultation**.

After placing the **Orthopedic Consultation** order, the physician clicks the *Exit Screen* button to return to the <u>Visit Documentation</u> screen (shown below).

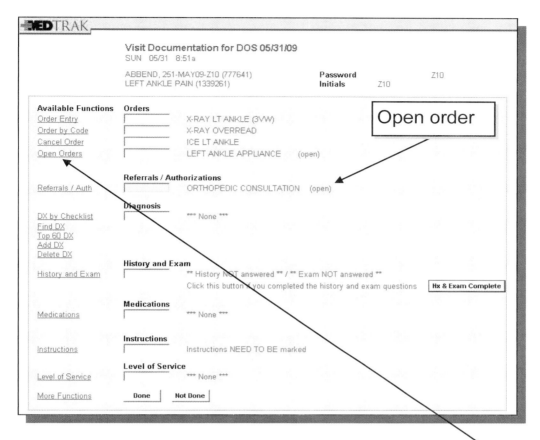

The clinical workflow calls for the physician to complete the first few questions of the **Orthopedic Consultation** open order. To answer open orders, the physician clicks the *Open Orders* button (as shown above). The <u>Open Orders</u> screen (shown below) appears with questions about the referral for the physician to answer. After filling in the answers (shown below), the physician clicks the *Submit Answers* button.

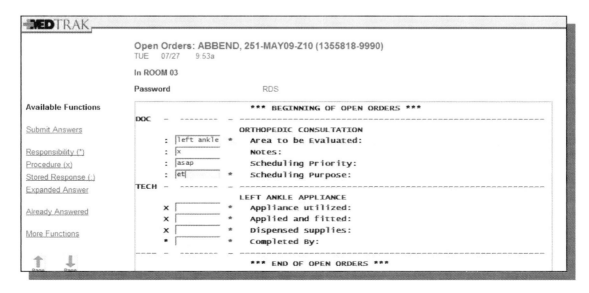

After filling in answers to all four questions about the referral, the physician clicks the *Submit Answers* button.

Because the provider entered an "**x**" in the **Notes** question data entry field to indicate that he or she wanted to go to the expanded answer screen to enter more than 1a 0 character answer, MedTrak displays the Expanded Answer screen (shown below). On this screen, the physician types "**Observed some internal derangement**" to provide some additional information to the specialist.

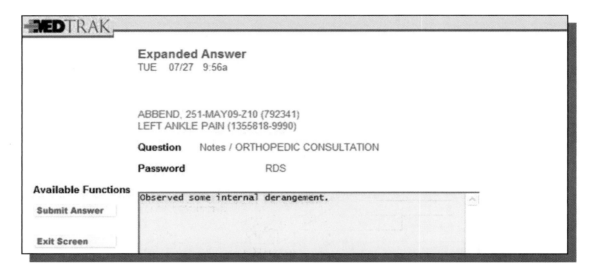

After entering the expanded answer, the physician clicks the *Submit Answer* button. MedTrak finishes processing the rest of the questions on the open order. To save time, the physician entered triggers to answer the remaining two questions on the open order.

Because the physician entered the trigger of **asap** in the **Scheduling Priority** question, MedTrak retrieved the stored response of **As soon as possible** and placed it in the answer field.

Because the physician entered the trigger of **et** in the **Scheduling Purpose** question, MedTrak retrieved the stored response of **Evaluate and treat as indicated - please send report** and placed it in the answer field.

The Visit Documentation screen (shown on the next page) reappears with the **(open)** designation on the referral for the **Orthopedic Consultation** removed.

The referral is now on the Referral Dashboard, which is an option off the Pending menu. The referral coordinator for the medical facility uses the Referral Dashboard to keep track of the open referrals. Each stage of the workflow for the referral is processed using this dashboard.

You can view your referral on this dashboard by going to the Pending menu off the MedTrak Main Menu and then clicking the *Referral Dashboard* button. The processing of referrals is not covered in this book.

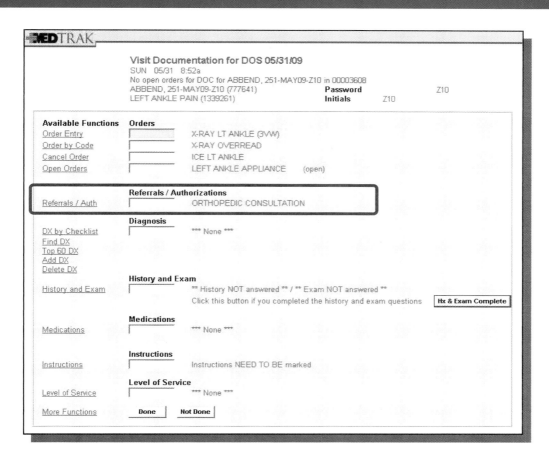

**Do This** ▶ **14.03** - Click the *Referrals/Auth* button

**14.04** - Click the *Orthopedic Consultation* order selection button ☒

**14.05** - Click the *Exit Screen* button

(you should be on the Visit Documentation screen)

**14.06** - Click the *Open Orders* button

**14.07** - Answer the *DOC* questions for the **Orthopedic Consultation** order

Type **left ankle** in the **Area to be evaluated** question

Type an **x** in the **Notes** question

Type **asap** in the **Scheduling Priority** question

Type **et** in the **Scheduling Purpose** question

**14.08** - Click the *Submit Answers* button

**14.09** - Answer the **Notes** question with the following:

**Observed some internal derangement.**

**14.10** - Click the *Submit Answer* button

(you should be on the Visit Documentation screen)

**If you are continuing with the next exercise (Physician - Diagnosing)**
**right now, skip the next Do This section.**

If you are not continuing on with the next chapter, do the next steps to sign out of MedTrak.

**Do This** ▶ **14.11** - Click the *Not Done* button
(you should be on the Clinic Status screen)

**14.12** - Click the *Exit Screen* or *Main Menu* button
(you should be on the MedTrak Main Menu)

**14.13** - Click the *Log Off* button to exit MedTrak

# CHAPTER

# 15

# Physician - Diagnosing

**Estimated time needed to complete this chapter - 15** minutes

**What you need to know before doing this chapter**

- ♦ How to log into MedTrak
- ♦ How to register a patient
- ♦ How to access <u>Clinic Status</u> off the <u>Main Menu</u>
- ♦ How to move a patient to a room and answer nursing notes
- ♦ How to access the <u>Visit Documentation</u> processor (Out the Door)

**Learning outcomes gained from this chapter**

- ♦ How to add diagnoses to a patient

## *Physician - Diagnosing*

### Major Categories of Clinical Workflow

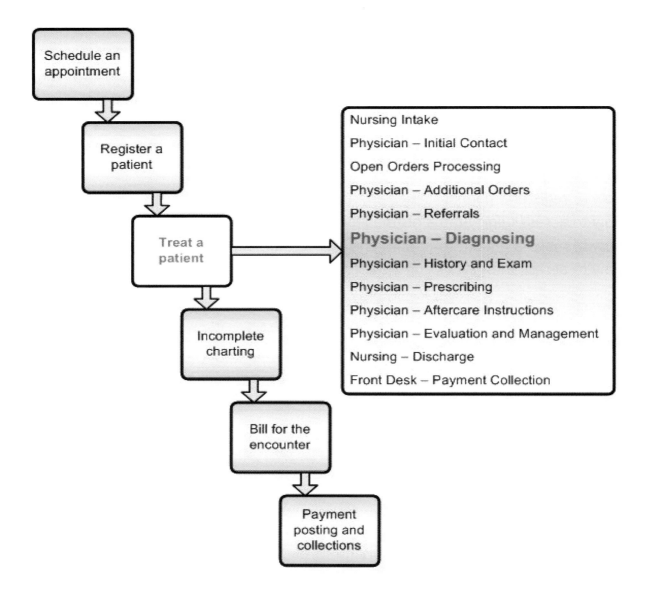

Identifying the condition or symptom that is the reason for the patient's visit is a key responsibility of the physician. The physician must diagnose the patient, and the *diagnosis* must be converted to an *ICD-9 code* to be submitted to the payer for payment of services. ICD-9 codes are provided by the World Health Organization's 9th Revision, International Classification of Diseases (ICD-9).

MedTrak enables physicians to select the diagnoses for the patient in multiple ways:

- By **Description** - entering the words describing the diagnosis in any order
- By **ICD-9** code - entering the ICD-9 code, if they know it
- By the **Top 60** diagnoses seen by clinics for musculoskeletal problems
- Based on **Checklists** - based on the presenting problems selected at the front desk
- By **Tree** structure – starting at the top of the diagnosis tree
- By **Problem** - based on the presenting problem
- By **Body Part** - based on the body part involved

Once the physician examines the patient, he or she will decide what the patient's diagnoses are. These diagnoses might not coincide with what the patient indicated to the front desk person or the clinical staff. MedTrak has the physician select the diagnoses right after placing any additional orders for the patient because the diagnoses determine what history and exam questions and patient aftercare instructions the physician needs to use for documenting the patient's visit. The alignment of the history and exam questions and aftercare instructions are another part of MedTrak's problem-focused functionality.

If you are already on the Visit Documentation screen (shown on the next page), then skip the next Do This section. If you are not on the Visit Documentation screen, then do the next steps.

---

**Do This ▶** **15.01** - Place the cursor next to your patient on the Clinic Status screen

**15.02** - Click the *Out the Door* button

(you should be on the Visit Documentation screen)

---

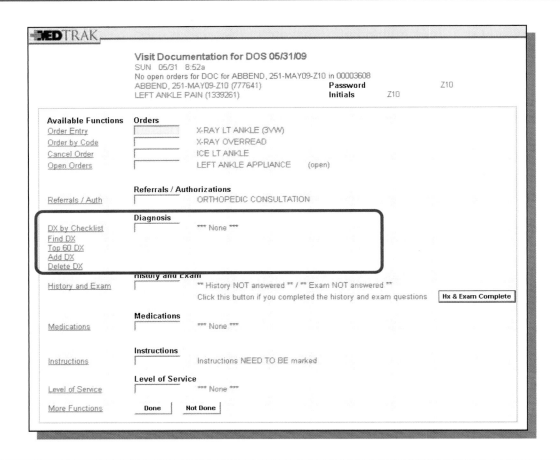

## Selecting a Diagnosis Based on the Presenting Problem(s)

In this example, the presenting problem entered by the front desk is **left ankle pain**. The physician clicks the *DX by Checklist* button to display the Add Diagnosis screen (shown on the next page) starting at **Muscles/Joints/Bones Left Ankle**, because this was the presenting problem category. At the top of the screen, a note identifying the presenting problem appears in red  -  **Note: Left Ankle Muscles/Joints/Bones**. The most common diagnoses for this problem appear on the screen for the physician to make selection(s).

The Add Diagnosis screen functions just like the Order Entry screen does. The yellow plus sign buttons indicate that there are more selections available by clicking the button. The green buttons indicate that these are selectable diagnoses. The yellow minus sign button on the top line indicates that there are more diagnoses by going up the diagnosis tree.

To select the **Derangement, Unspecified** diagnosis, the physician clicks the green ⊠ button to the left of the diagnosis.

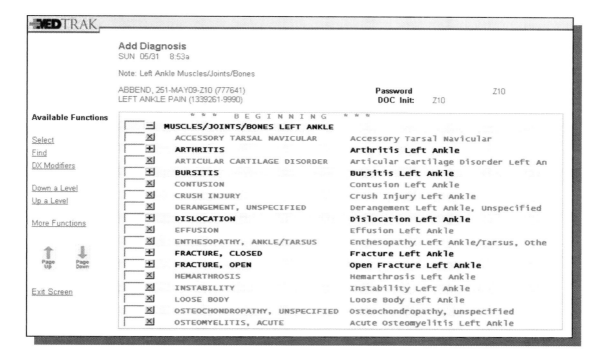

The Add Diagnosis screen (shown below) refreshes with the message "**Adding: Derangement Left Ankle, Unspecified**" in red at the top of the screen.

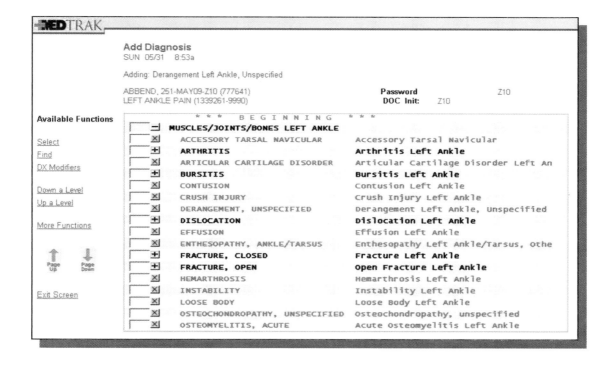

After selecting the diagnosis, the physician clicks the *Exit Screen* button to return to the Visit Documentation screen (shown below). The **Unspecified Left Ankle Derangement** displays with the ICD-9 code of **718.97**.

The physician selected the diagnosis by using the MedTrak Diagnosis Tree. MedTrak attached the ICD-9 codes to the diagnosis descriptions. Therefore, when a physician selects a diagnosis, the ICD-9 code is automatically loaded for documentation and billing purposes.

There could be multiple diagnoses needed for the patient's encounter. In a like manner, the physician can select all of the appropriate diagnoses.

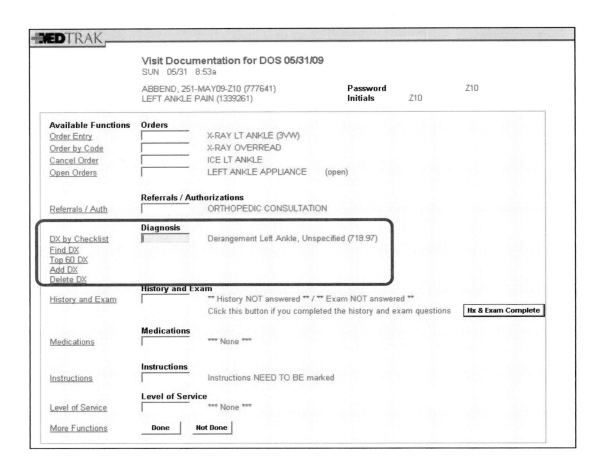

## Selecting a Diagnosis Based on the Description

Another diagnosis search function that the providers like to use is the **Find Dx by Description**. To access this processor, the physician clicks on the *Find Dx* button. The next screen to appear is the Diagnosis: Find screen (shown on the next page).

The physician types "**left ankle derangement**" in the data input field for the description and clicks the *Submit* button.

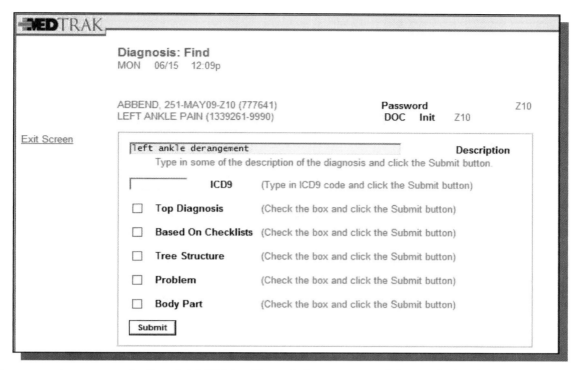

The next screen to appear is the Add DX by Description screen (shown below). The physician clicks the green ☒ button to the left of the **Left Ankle Derangement Unspecified** diagnosis to select it. The physician can type the diagnosis description words in any order. For example, typing **Ankle Unspecified Derangement Left** would also find the correct diagnosis. The order of the words does not matter.

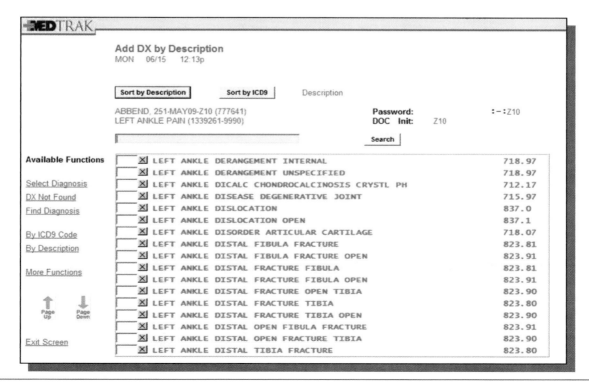

MedTrak refreshes the screen with a message at the top that the diagnosis was added. If the physician needs to select another diagnosis, the next description can be typed in the **Search** field and clicking the *Search* button. When done selecting diagnoses, the physician clicks the *Exit Screen* button to return to the <u>Visit Documentation</u> screen (shown below).

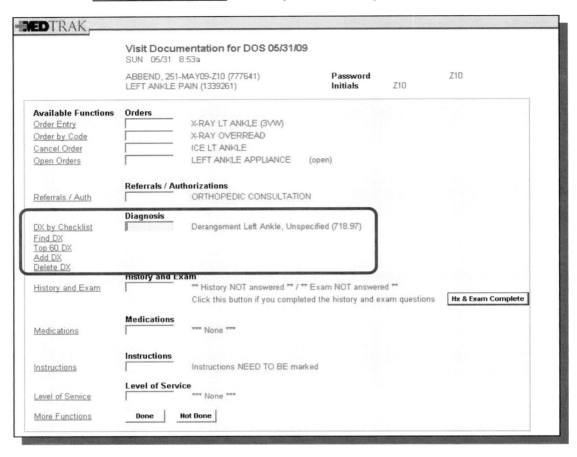

The <u>Visit Documentation</u> screen (shown above) lists the selected diagnoses in the **Diagnosis** section. To delete a diagnosis, the physician places the cursor next to the diagnosis that needs deleting and clicks the *Delete Dx* button.

**Do This** ▶ **15.03** - Click the *Find Dx* button

**15.04** - Type the following diagnosis in the description field:

      **left ankle derangement**

**15.05** - Click the *Submit* button

**15.06** - Click the **left ankle derangement unspecified** diagnosis button ⊠

**15.07** - Click the *Exit Screen* button again

      (you should be on the <u>Visit Documentation</u> screen)

      (your diagnosis should appear in the **Diagnoses** section)

**If you are continuing with the next exercise (Physician - Patient History and Physical Exam) right now, skip the next Do This section.**

If you are not continuing with the next chapter, do the next steps to sign out of MedTrak.

---

**Do This** ▶ **15.08** - Click the **Not Done** button
(you should be on the <u>Clinic Status</u> screen)

**15.09** - Click the **Exit Screen** or **Main Menu** button
(you should be on the MedTrak <u>Main Menu</u>)

**15.10** - Click the **Log Off** button to exit MedTrak

---

# CHAPTER 16

# Physician - Patient History and Physical Exam

**Estimated time needed to complete this chapter - 30** minutes

## What you need to know before doing this chapter

- ♦ How to log into MedTrak
- ♦ How to register a patient
- ♦ How to access Clinic Status off the Main Menu
- ♦ How to move a patient to a room and answer nursing notes
- ♦ How to access the Visit Documentation processor (Out the Door)

## Learning outcomes gained from this chapter

- ♦ How to document the physician's history and exam of the patient

## Physician - Patient History and Physical Exam

### Major Categories of Clinical Workflow

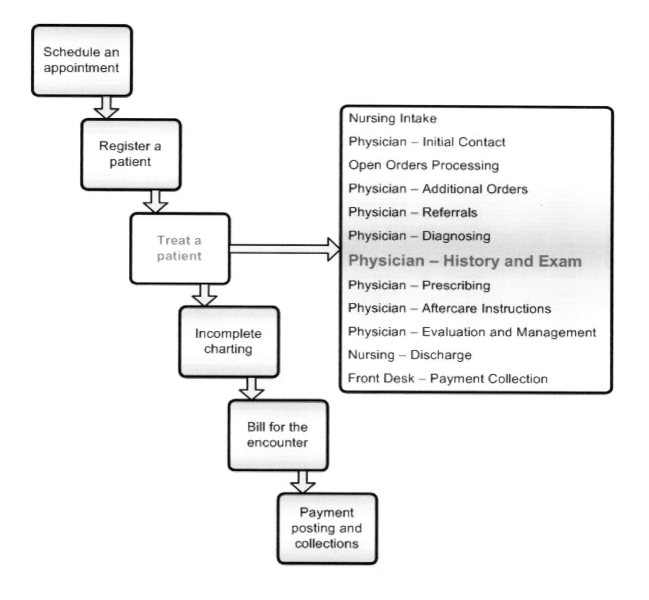

The next section on the Visit Documentation screen (shown below) is for the physician to document the *patient's history and physical examination*. This is the only section that does not need to be completed before discharging the patient from this visit to the medical facility. All of the other sections must be done. The history and exam questions are based (problem-focused) on the diagnoses selected by the physician. If there are *multiple diagnoses*, then MedTrak prepares a blended checklist of history and exam questions from head to toe. Questions that are common to each diagnosis of a multiple-diagnoses patient visit only appear once in the checklist.

If you are already on the Visit Documentation screen, then skip the next Do This section. If you are not on the Visit Documentation screen, then do the next steps.

---

**Do This** ▶ **16.01** - Place the cursor next to your patient on the Clinic Status screen

**16.02** - Click the *Out the Door* button

(you should be on the Visit Documentation screen)

---

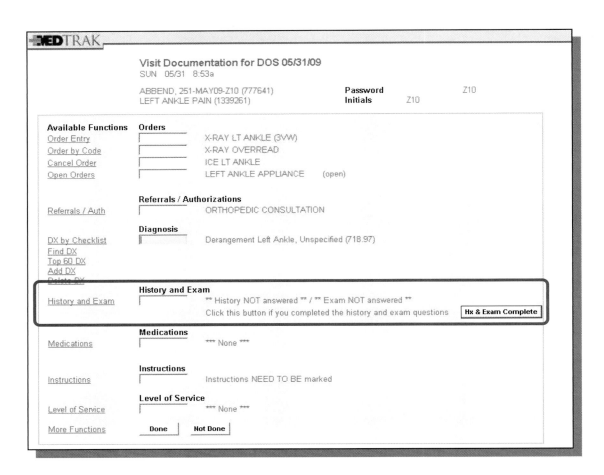

In this example, the physician diagnosed the patient with an unspecified derangement of the left ankle. Therefore, the questions in the **History and Exam** section are specific to a musculoskeletal problem of the left ankle.

The physician clicks the *History and Exam* button to display the <u>Doctor Checklist Processor</u> screen (shown below). This screen displays the names of the doctor's checklists that correspond to the diagnoses selected by the physician.

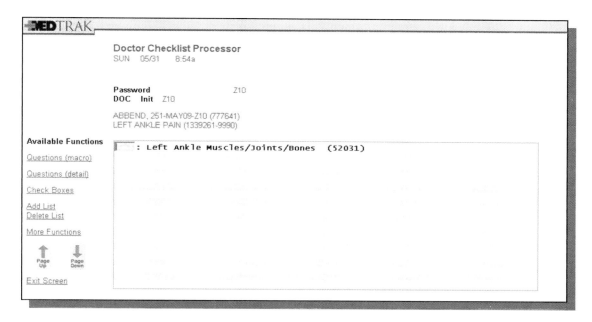

MedTrak allows three ways for the physician to answer the history and exam questions:

- ◆ By **Dictation Topic** - for physicians who dictate their history and exam questions at a macro level using voice recognition (or with the help of a transcriptionist).

- ◆ By **Detailed Questions** - for physicians who use the keyboard to type their answers using a detailed checklist of questions.

- ◆ By **Check Boxes** - for physicians who take a wireless tablet computer into the exam room and check off answers on the touch screen while examining the patient.

---

**Do This** ▶ **16.03** - Click the *History and Exam* button
(you should be on the <u>Doctor Checklist Processor</u> screen)

---

## Answering Questions Using the Macro Method

If the physician clicks the *Questions (macro)* button, the Doctor's Checklist screen (shown below) appears.

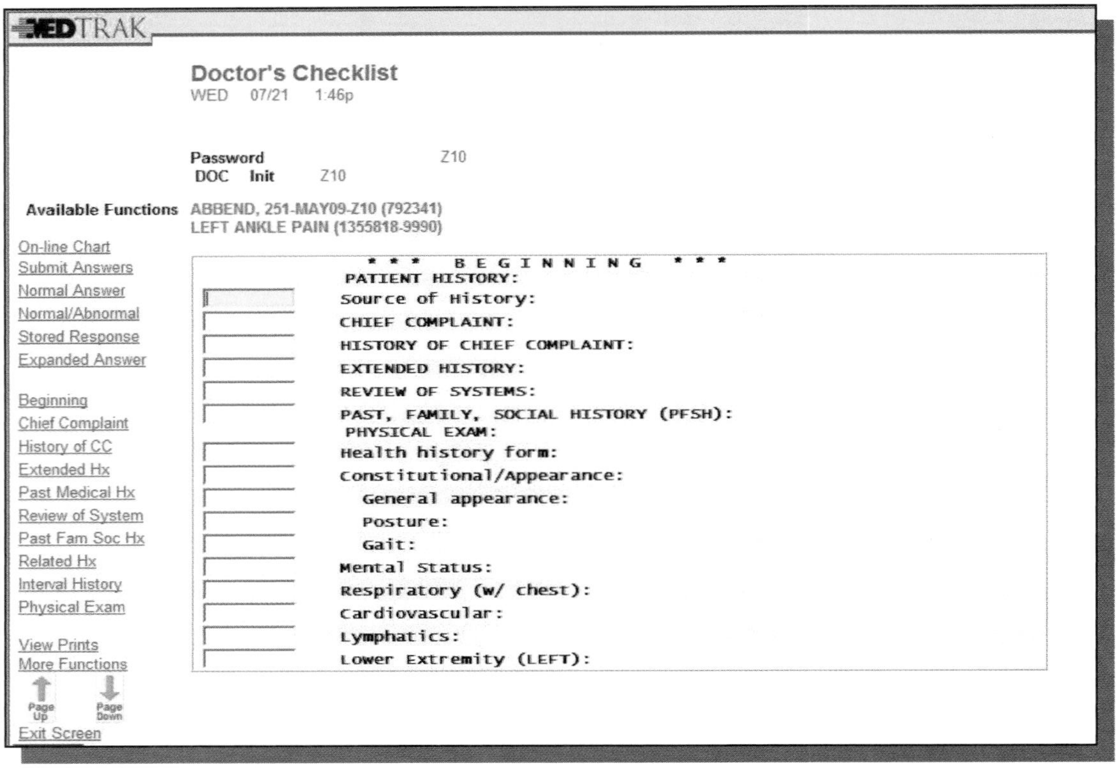

```
MEDTRAK

            Doctor's Checklist
            WED   07/21   1:46p


            Password                        Z10
            DOC   Init      Z10

Available Functions   ABBEND, 251-MAY09-Z10 (792341)
                      LEFT ANKLE PAIN (1355818-9990)
On-line Chart
Submit Answers               * * *   B E G I N N I N G   * * *
Normal Answer                PATIENT HISTORY:
Normal/Abnormal        [   ]  Source of History:
Stored Response        [   ]  CHIEF COMPLAINT:
Expanded Answer        [   ]  HISTORY OF CHIEF COMPLAINT:
                       [   ]  EXTENDED HISTORY:
Beginning              [   ]  REVIEW OF SYSTEMS:
Chief Complaint        [   ]  PAST, FAMILY, SOCIAL HISTORY (PFSH):
History of CC                 PHYSICAL EXAM:
Extended Hx            [   ]  Health history form:
Past Medical Hx       [   ]  Constitutional/Appearance:
Review of System      [   ]    General appearance:
Past Fam Soc Hx       [   ]    Posture:
Related Hx            [   ]    Gait:
Interval History      [   ]  Mental Status:
Physical Exam         [   ]  Respiratory (w/ chest):
                       [   ]  Cardiovascular:
View Prints           [   ]  Lymphatics:
More Functions        [   ]  Lower Extremity (LEFT):
  ↑        ↓
 Page    Page
 Up      Down
Exit Screen
```

The questions (especially for the history) are at a macro level. Physicians who like to dictate their chart typically use this processor to either transcribe their answers or enter their answers using voice recognition software.

The top section of buttons on the left side of the screen is for reviewing the on-line chart and answering the questions. The lower section of the buttons is for navigating the list of questions.

---

**Do This ▶**  **16.04** - Click the *Questions (macro)* button
(from the Doctor Checklist Processor screen)

**16.05** - Read the questions on the Doctor's Checklist screen and review the buttons

**16.06** - Click the *Exit Screen* button
(you should be on the Visit Documentation screen)

**16.07** - Click the *History and Exam* button
(you should be on the Doctor Checklist Processor screen)

---

## Answering Questions Using the Detail Method

If the physician clicks the *Questions (detail)* button, the Doctor's Checklist screen (shown below) appears.

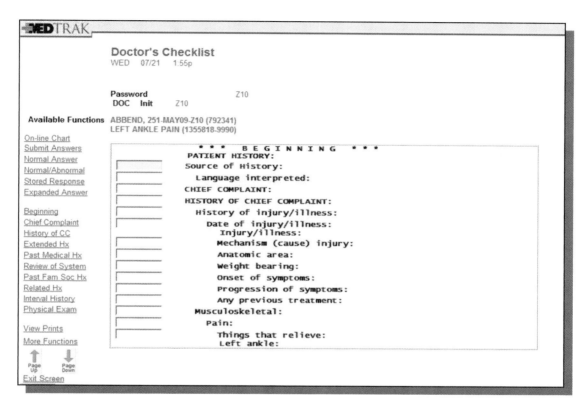

The questions are at a detail level. For example, the **History of Chief Complaint** question is now exploded to show all of its detailed questions. Physicians who like to use the keyboard to type their answers typically use this processor.

The top section of buttons is for reviewing the on-line chart and answering the questions. The lower section of the buttons is for navigating the list of questions.

---

**Do This ►**  **16.08** - Click the *Questions (detail)* button
(from the Doctor Checklist Processor screen)

**16.09** - Read the questions on the Doctor's Checklist and review the buttons

**16.10** - Click the *Exit Screen* button
(you should be on the Visit Documentation screen)

**16.11** - Click the *History and Exam* button
(you should be on the Doctor Checklist Processor screen)

---

## Answering Questions Using the Check Boxes Method

If the physician clicks the *Check Boxes* button, the Doctor's Checklist screen (shown below) appears.

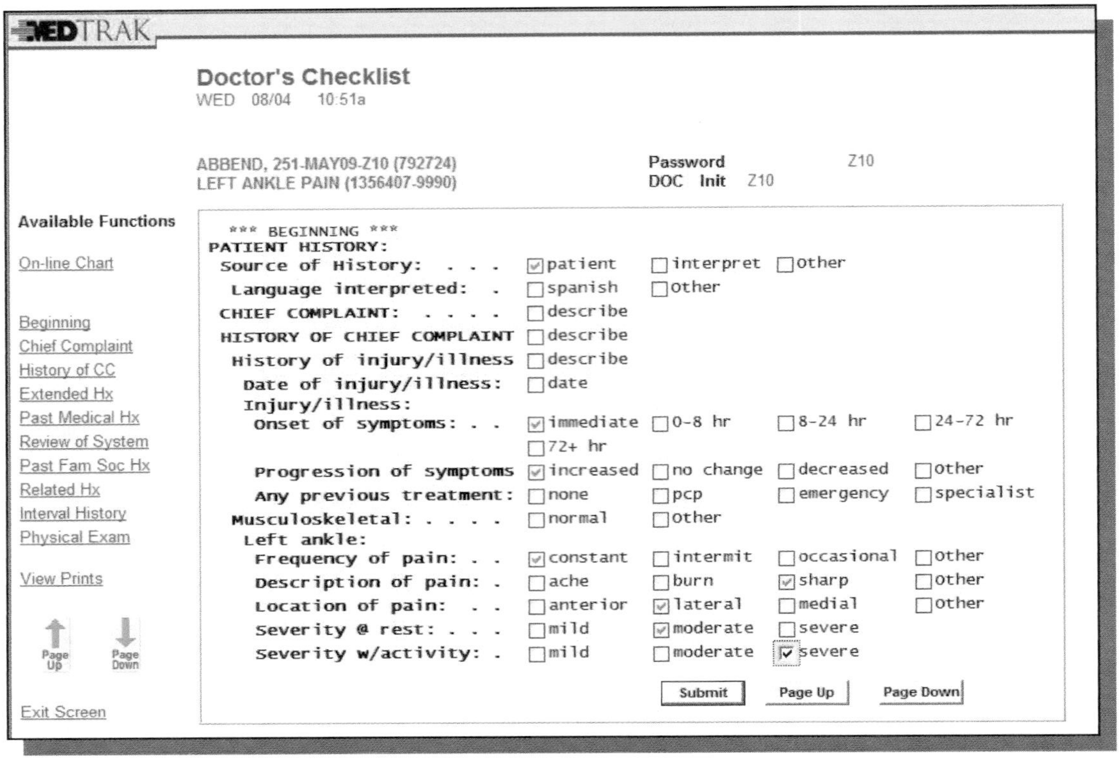

MedTrak builds the screen with the triggers to the questions appearing to the right of the questions with check boxes in front of the triggers for selection purposes. By checking the trigger check boxes, the physician answers the questions. Some questions are answered simply by checking one or more trigger check boxes, whereas other questions may require going to the Expanded Answer screen to enter a more specific answer.

In this example, the physician answers some of the history questions on this screen by checking the following trigger check boxes.

       **Source of History** - patient

       **Onset of symptoms** - immediate

       **Progression of symptoms** - increased

       **Any previous treatment** - none

       **Frequency of pain** - constant

       **Description of pain** - sharp

       **Location of pain** - lateral

       **Severity @ rest** - mod

       **Severity w/activity** - severe

**NOTE**: Normally, the physician would click the *describe* check boxes to answer the **Chief Complaint** and the **History of the Chief Complaint** using the Expanded Answer screen, but not for this example.

The physician clicks the *Submit* button to record the selections and stay on the same screen, or clicks the *Page Down* button to record the changes and move down the checklist to the next set of questions on the following screen.

To review the answers using the on-line chart (shown below), the physician clicks the *On-line Chart* button on the Doctor's Checklist screen.

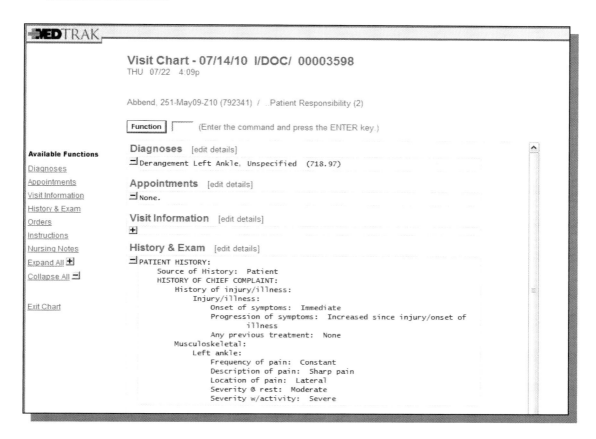

The On-line Chart has navigation buttons to reset to a specific section of the chart and yellow plus  and minus  signs to use for expanding and collapsing the sections of the chart. After reviewing the on-line chart, the physician clicks the *Exit Chart* button to return to the Doctor's Checklist check box processor.

---

**Do This** ▶  **16.12** - Click the *Check Boxes* button

**16.13** - Click the patient history *check boxes* as listed on the previous page

**16.14** - Click the *Submit* button

**16.15** - Click the *On-line Chart* button
(review your answers on the on-line chart)

**16.16** - Click the *Exit Chart* button
(you should be on the check box processor)

**16.17** - Click the *Page Down* button to go to the next screen

---

In this example, the physician continues to answer patient history questions by clicking the *Page Down* button to display the next screen (shown below).

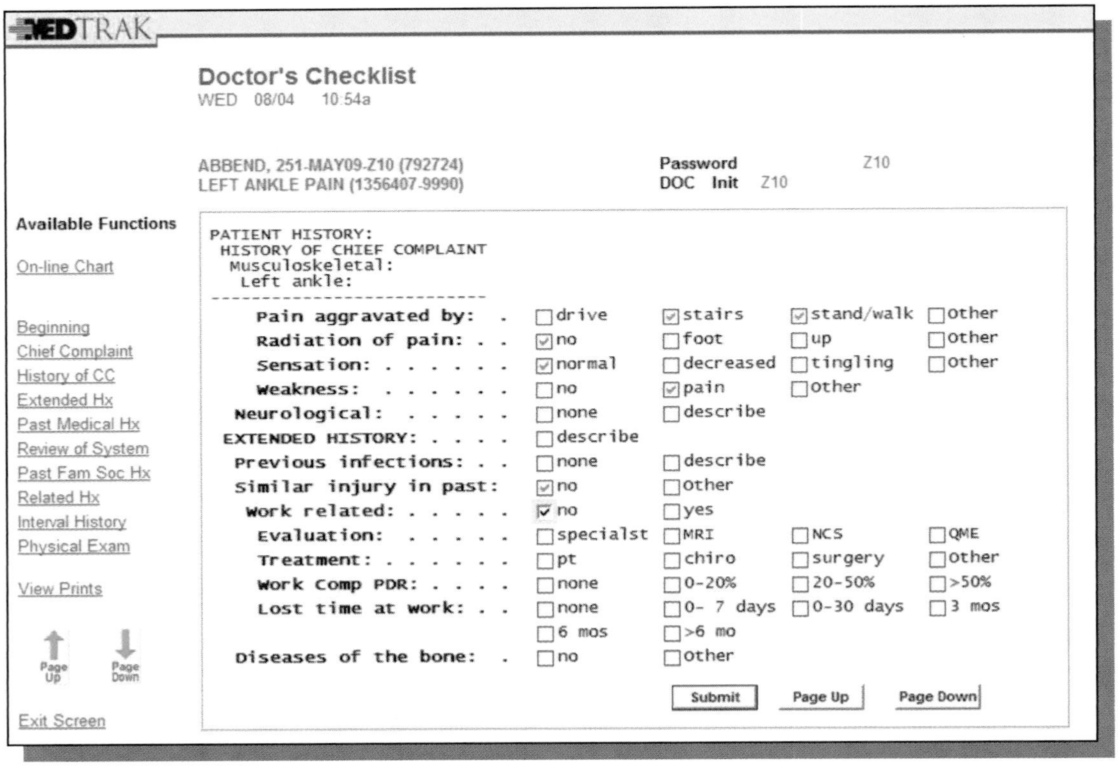

On this screen, the physician answers more of the history questions by checking the following trigger check boxes:

**Pain aggravated by** - stairs, stand/walk  (two triggers selected)

**Radiation of pain** - no

**Sensation** - normal

**Weakness** - pain

**Similar injury in the past** - no

**Work related** - no

The physician continues to answer patient history questions by clicking the *Page Down* button to display the next screen (shown on the next page).

---

**Do This** ▶    **16.18** - Click the patient history *check boxes* as shown above

         **16.19** - Click the *Page Down* button

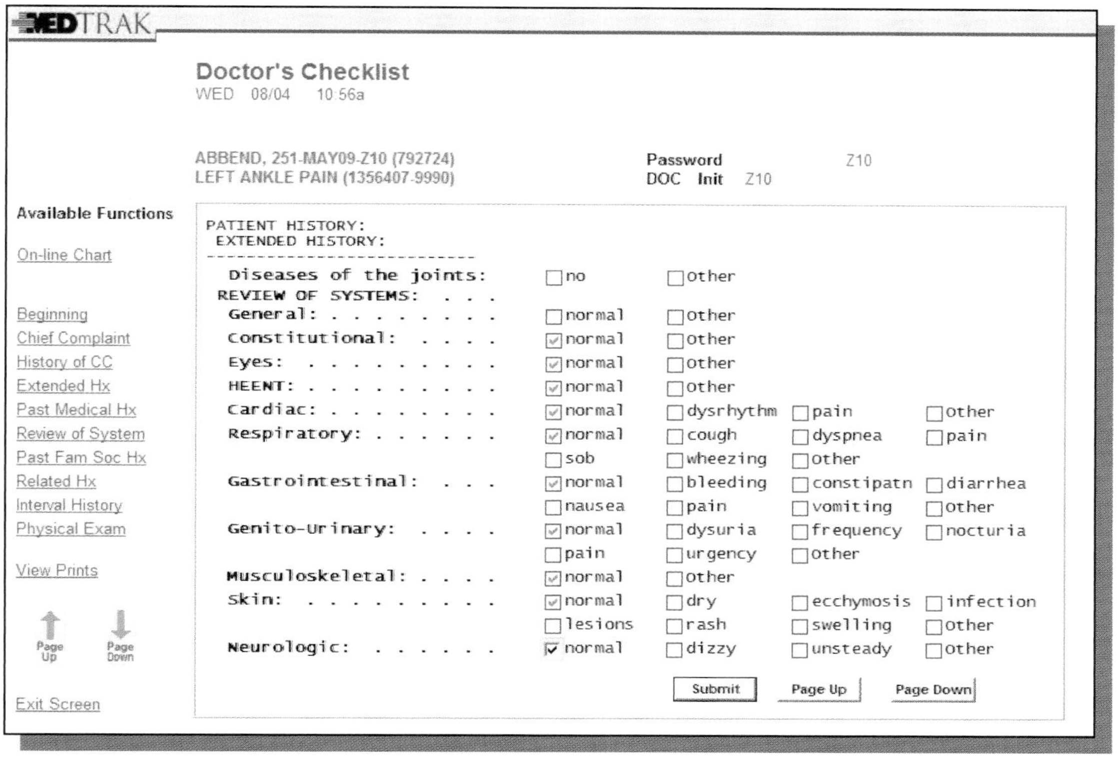

```
MEDTRAK

        Doctor's Checklist
        WED  08/04  10:56a


        ABBEND, 251-MAY09-Z10 (792724)          Password          Z10
        LEFT ANKLE PAIN (1356407-9990)          DOC  Init   Z10
```

**Available Functions**

On-line Chart

Beginning
Chief Complaint
History of CC
Extended Hx
Past Medical Hx
Review of System
Past Fam Soc Hx
Related Hx
Interval History
Physical Exam

View Prints

↑ Page Up    ↓ Page Down

Exit Screen

```
PATIENT HISTORY:
  EXTENDED HISTORY:
  ---------------------------
    Diseases of the joints:      ☐no        ☐other
  REVIEW OF SYSTEMS:  . . .
    General: . . . . . . . .     ☐normal    ☐other
    Constitutional:  . . . .     ☑normal    ☐other
    Eyes:  . . . . . . . . .     ☑normal    ☐other
    HEENT: . . . . . . . . .     ☑normal    ☐other
    Cardiac: . . . . . . . .     ☑normal    ☐dysrhythm  ☐pain        ☐other
    Respiratory: . . . . . .     ☑normal    ☐cough      ☐dyspnea     ☐pain
                                 ☐sob       ☐wheezing   ☐other
    Gastrointestinal:  . . .     ☑normal    ☐bleeding   ☐constipatn  ☐diarrhea
                                 ☐nausea    ☐pain       ☐vomiting    ☐other
    Genito-Urinary:  . . . .     ☑normal    ☐dysuria    ☐frequency   ☐nocturia
                                 ☐pain      ☐urgency    ☐other
    Musculoskeletal: . . . .     ☑normal    ☐other
    Skin: . . . . . . . . .      ☑normal    ☐dry        ☐ecchymosis  ☐infection
                                 ☐lesions   ☐rash       ☐swelling    ☐other
    Neurologic:  . . . . . .     ☑normal    ☐dizzy      ☐unsteady    ☐other

                                           [Submit]  [Page Up]  [Page Down]
```

On this screen, the physician answers the following history questions by checking the trigger check boxes:

**Constitutional** - normal

**Eyes** - normal

**HEENT** - normal

**Cardiac** - normal

**Respiratory** - normal

**Gastrointestinal** - normal

**Genito-Urinary** - normal

**Musculoskeletal** - normal

**Skin** - normal

**Neurologic** - normal

The physician continues to answer patient history questions by clicking the *Page Down* button to display the next screen (shown on the next page).

---

**Do This** ▶ **16.20** - Click the patient history *check boxes* as shown above

**16.21** - Click the *Page Down* button

---

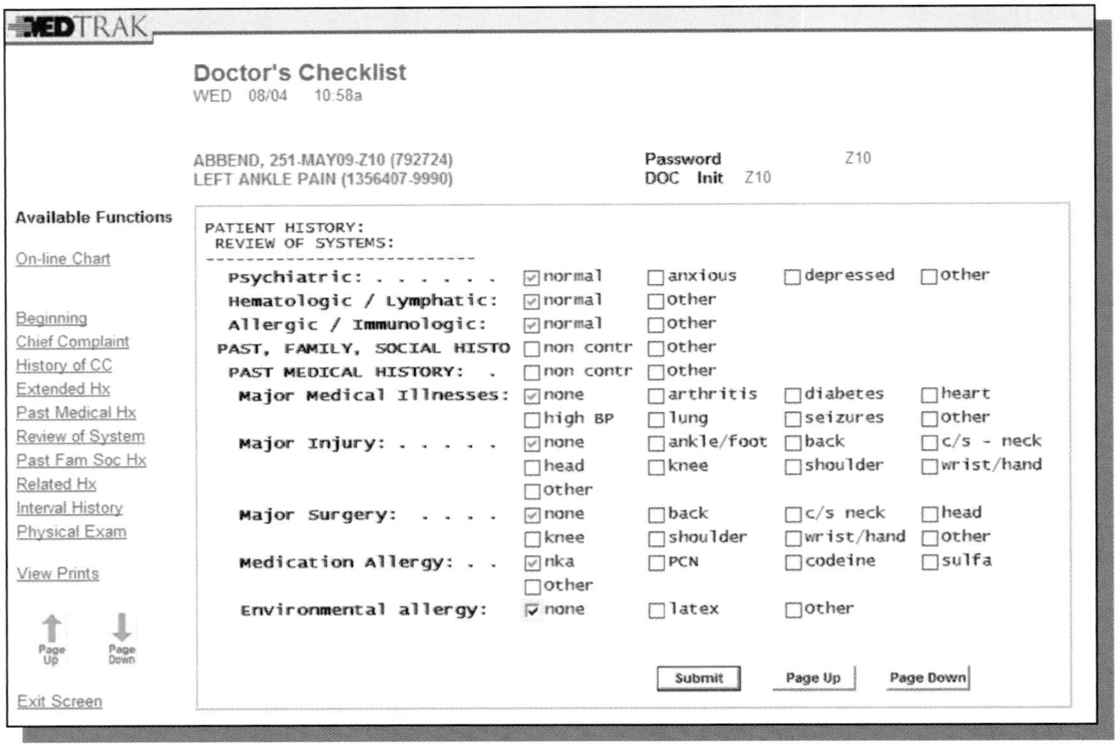

```
MEDTRAK

                    Doctor's Checklist
                    WED  08/04  10:58a


                    ABBEND, 251-MAY09-Z10 (792724)          Password            Z10
                    LEFT ANKLE PAIN (1356407-9990)          DOC  Init   Z10

Available Functions    PATIENT HISTORY:
                         REVIEW OF SYSTEMS:
On-line Chart          ---------------------------
                         Psychiatric: . . . . . .  ☑normal    ☐anxious     ☐depressed   ☐other
                         Hematologic / Lymphatic:  ☑normal    ☐other
Beginning                Allergic / Immunologic:   ☑normal    ☐other
Chief Complaint        PAST, FAMILY, SOCIAL HISTO  ☐non contr ☐other
History of CC          PAST MEDICAL HISTORY:  .    ☐non contr ☐other
Extended Hx              Major Medical Illnesses:  ☑none      ☐arthritis   ☐diabetes    ☐heart
Past Medical Hx                                    ☐high BP   ☐lung        ☐seizures    ☐other
Review of System         Major Injury: . . . . .   ☑none      ☐ankle/foot  ☐back        ☐c/s - neck
Past Fam Soc Hx                                     ☐head      ☐knee        ☐shoulder    ☐wrist/hand
Related Hx                                          ☐other
Interval History         Major Surgery:  . . . .   ☑none      ☐back        ☐c/s neck    ☐head
Physical Exam                                       ☐knee      ☐shoulder    ☐wrist/hand  ☐other
                         Medication Allergy: . .    ☑nka       ☐PCN         ☐codeine     ☐sulfa
View Prints                                         ☐other
                         Environmental allergy:    ☑none      ☐latex       ☐other
  ↑      ↓
 Page   Page
  Up    Down                                    [Submit]   [Page Up]  [Page Down]
Exit Screen
```

On this screen, the physician answers the following history questions by checking the trigger check boxes:

**Psychiatric** - normal
**Hematologic/Lymphatic** - normal
**Allergic/Immunologic** - normal
**Major Medical Illnesses** - none
**Major Injury** - none
**Major Surgery** - none
**Medication Allergy** - nka (which is the trigger for no known allergies)
**Environmental Allergy** - none

The physician continues to answer patient history questions by clicking the *Page Down* button to display the next screen (shown on the next page).

**Do This** ▶ 16.22 - Click the patient history *check boxes* as shown above

16.23 - Click the *Page Down* button

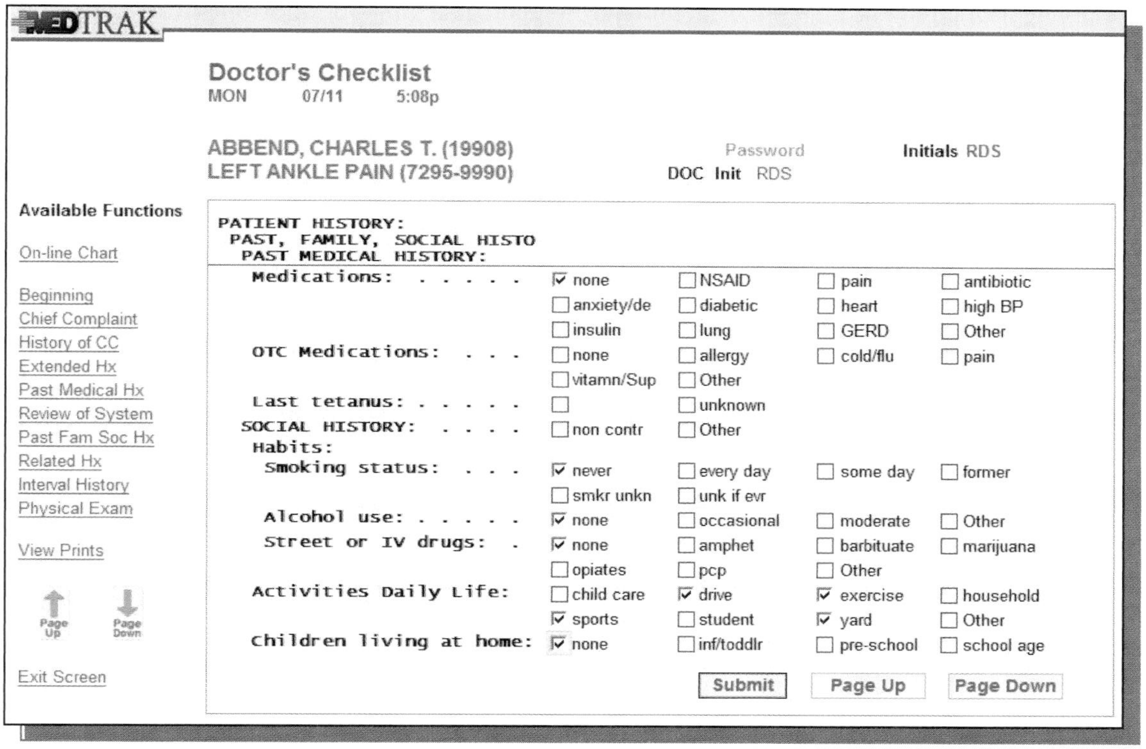

**MEDTRAK**

**Doctor's Checklist**
MON    07/11    5:08p

ABBEND, CHARLES T. (19908)      Password      Initials RDS
LEFT ANKLE PAIN (7295-9990)      DOC Init   RDS

**Available Functions**

On-line Chart

Beginning
Chief Complaint
History of CC
Extended Hx
Past Medical Hx
Review of System
Past Fam Soc Hx
Related Hx
Interval History
Physical Exam

View Prints

↑ Page Up    ↓ Page Down

Exit Screen

```
PATIENT HISTORY:
  PAST, FAMILY, SOCIAL HISTO
  PAST MEDICAL HISTORY:
    Medications:  . . . . .    ☑ none      ☐ NSAID       ☐ pain       ☐ antibiotic
                               ☐ anxiety/de ☐ diabetic    ☐ heart      ☐ high BP
                               ☐ insulin    ☐ lung        ☐ GERD       ☐ Other
    OTC Medications:  . . .    ☐ none       ☐ allergy     ☐ cold/flu   ☐ pain
                               ☐ vitamn/Sup ☐ Other
    Last tetanus: . . . . .    ☐            ☐ unknown
  SOCIAL HISTORY:  . . . .     ☐ non contr  ☐ Other
  Habits:
    Smoking status:  . . .     ☑ never      ☐ every day   ☐ some day   ☐ former
                               ☐ smkr unkn  ☐ unk if evr
    Alcohol use: . . . . .     ☑ none       ☐ occasional  ☐ moderate   ☐ Other
    Street or IV drugs:  .     ☑ none       ☐ amphet      ☐ barbituate ☐ marijuana
                               ☐ opiates    ☐ pcp         ☐ Other
    Activities Daily Life:     ☐ child care ☑ drive       ☑ exercise   ☐ household
                               ☑ sports     ☐ student     ☑ yard       ☐ Other
    Children living at home:   ☑ none       ☐ inf/toddlr  ☐ pre-school ☐ school age
```

[ Submit ]   [ Page Up ]   [ Page Down ]

On this screen, the physician answers the following history questions by checking the trigger check boxes:

> **Medications** - none
>
> **Tobacco** - never
>
> **Alcohol use** - none
>
> **Street or IV drugs** - none
>
> **Activities Daily Life** - drive, exercise, sports, yard (four triggers selected)
>
> **Children living at home** - none

This was the last full screen of history questions. When the physician clicks the *Page Down* button to display the next screen, the first screen displaying some of the physical examination questions appears (not shown in this example).

---

**Do This** ►    **16.24** - Click the patient history *check boxes* as shown above

             **16.25** - Click the *Page Down* button

To reset to the top of the first screen of the physical examination questions for the <u>Doctor's Checklist</u> (shown below), the physician clicks the *Physical Exam* navigation button.

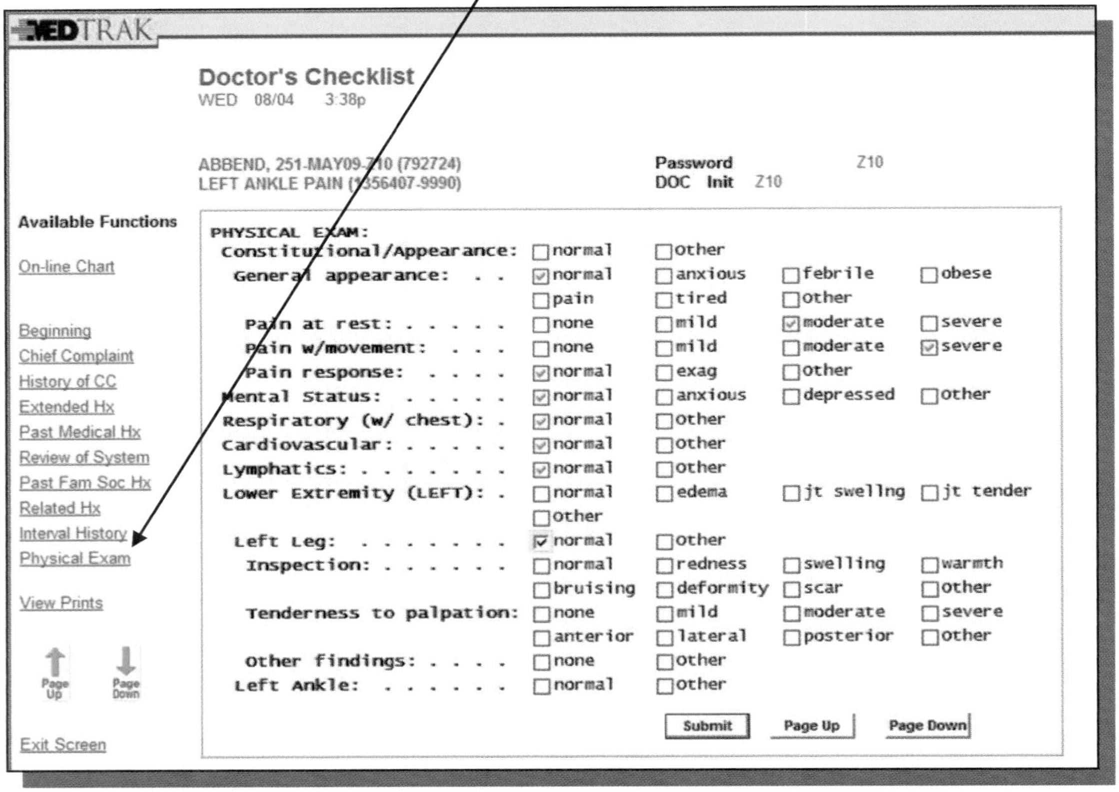

The physician answers some of the physical examination questions on this screen by checking the following trigger check boxes:

> **General appearance** - normal
> **Pain at rest** - moderate
> **Pain w/ movement** - severe
> **Pain response** - normal
> **Mental Status** - normal
> **Respiratory (w/ chest)** - normal
> **Cardiovascular** - normal
> **Lymphatics** - normal
> **Left Leg** - normal

The physician clicks the *Page Down* button to record the selections and moves down the checklist to the next set of physical examination questions (shown on the next page).

---

**Do This** ▶  **16.26** - Click the *Physical Exam* navigation button

**16.27** - Click the physical exam *check boxes* as shown above

**16.28** - Click the *Page Down* button

---

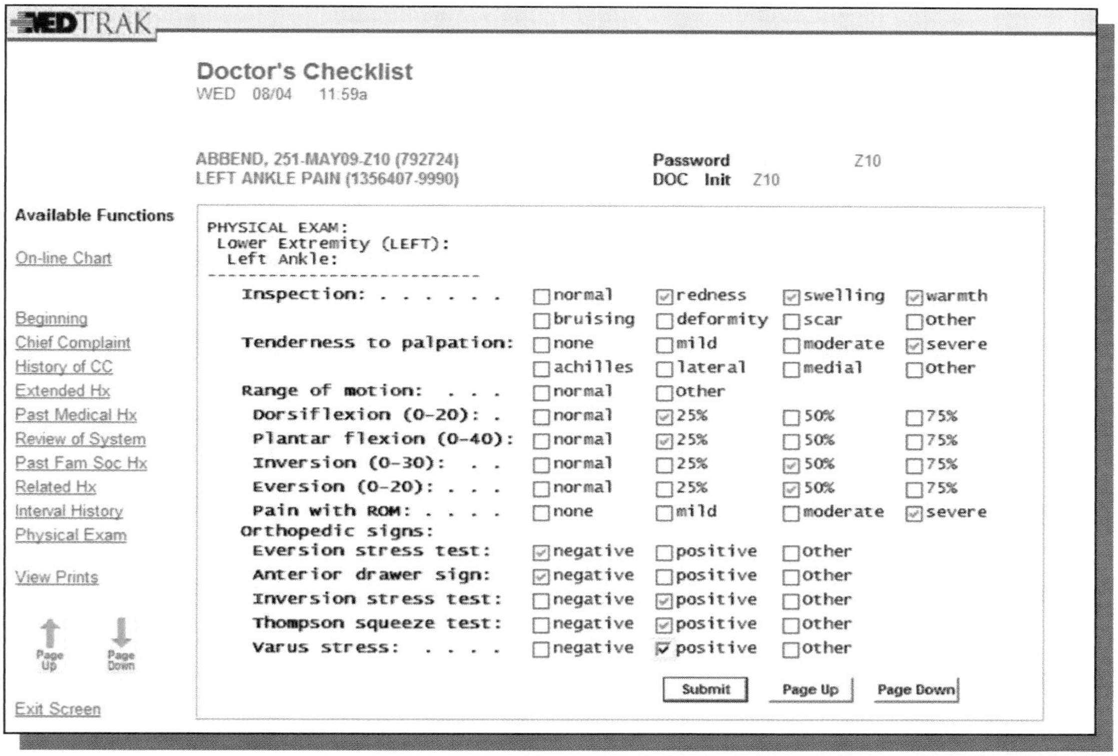

## Doctor's Checklist
WED 08/04 11:59a

ABBEND, 251-MAY09-Z10 (792724)          Password          Z10
LEFT ANKLE PAIN (1356407-9990)          DOC Init   Z10

**Available Functions**

On-line Chart

Beginning
Chief Complaint
History of CC
Extended Hx
Past Medical Hx
Review of System
Past Fam Soc Hx
Related Hx
Interval History
Physical Exam

View Prints

↑ Page Up     ↓ Page Down

Exit Screen

```
PHYSICAL EXAM:
  Lower Extremity (LEFT):
   Left Ankle:
  ------------------------
    Inspection: . . . . . .   □normal    ☑redness    ☑swelling   ☑warmth
                              □bruising  □deformity  □scar       □other
    Tenderness to palpation:  □none      □mild       □moderate   ☑severe
                              □achilles  □lateral    □medial     □other
    Range of motion: . . .    □normal    □other
    Dorsiflexion (0-20): .    □normal    ☑25%        □50%        □75%
    Plantar flexion (0-40):   □normal    ☑25%        □50%        □75%
    Inversion (0-30): . .     □normal    □25%        ☑50%        □75%
    Eversion (0-20): . . .    □normal    □25%        ☑50%        □75%
    Pain with ROM: . . . .    □none      □mild       □moderate   ☑severe
  Orthopedic signs:
    Eversion stress test:     ☑negative  □positive   □other
    Anterior drawer sign:     ☑negative  □positive   □other
    Inversion stress test:    □negative  ☑positive   □other
    Thompson squeeze test:    □negative  ☑positive   □other
    Varus stress: . . . .     □negative  ☑positive   □other
```

Submit    Page Up    Page Down

In this example, the physician answers some of the physical examination questions on this screen by checking the following trigger check boxes:

**Inspection** - redness, swelling, warmth  (three triggers selected)

**Tenderness to palpation** - severe

**Dorsiflexion (0-20)** - 25%

**Plantar flexion (0-40)** - 25%

**Inversion (0-30)** - 50%

**Eversion (0-20)** - 50%

**Pain with ROM** - severe

**Eversion stress test** - negative

**Anterior drawer sign** - negative

**Inversion stress test** - positive

**Thompson squeeze test** - positive

**Varus stress** - positive

The physician clicks the *Page Down* button to record the selections and move down the checklist to the next set of physical examination questions (shown on the next page).

---

**Do This** ▶  **16.29** - Click the physical examination *check boxes* as shown above

**16.30** - Click the *Page Down* button

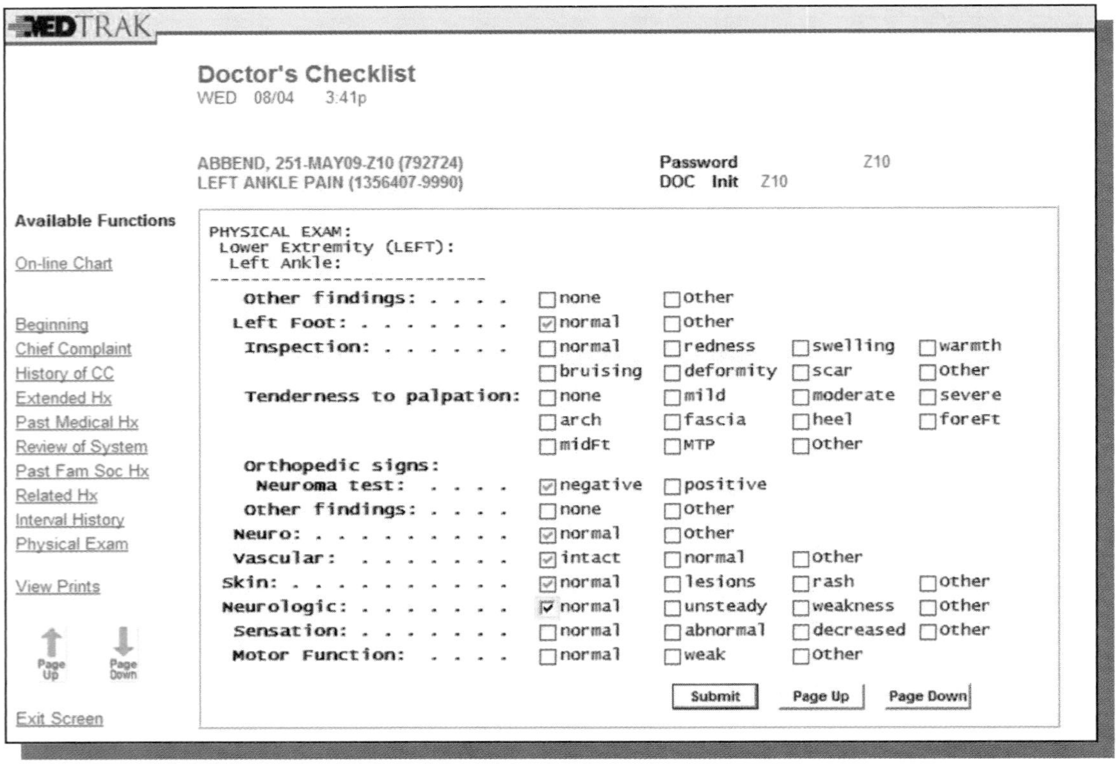

```
MEDTRAK

        Doctor's Checklist
        WED  08/04   3:41p


        ABBEND, 251-MAY09-Z10 (792724)          Password          Z10
        LEFT ANKLE PAIN (1356407-9990)          DOC  Init   Z10

Available Functions   PHYSICAL EXAM:
                       Lower Extremity (LEFT):
On-line Chart           Left Ankle:
                       ---------------------------
                         Other findings: . . . .  ☐none      ☐other
Beginning                Left Foot: . . . . . . .  ☑normal    ☐other
Chief Complaint            Inspection: . . . . .   ☐normal    ☐redness    ☐swelling   ☐warmth
History of CC                                      ☐bruising  ☐deformity  ☐scar       ☐other
Extended Hx                Tenderness to palpation: ☐none     ☐mild       ☐moderate   ☐severe
Past Medical Hx                                    ☐arch      ☐fascia     ☐heel       ☐foreFt
Review of System                                   ☐midFt     ☐MTP        ☐other
Past Fam Soc Hx          Orthopedic signs:
Related Hx                 Neuroma test: . . . .   ☑negative  ☐positive
Interval History         Other findings: . . . .  ☐none      ☐other
Physical Exam            Neuro: . . . . . . . . .  ☑normal    ☐other
                         vascular: . . . . . . .   ☑intact    ☐normal     ☐other
View Prints            Skin: . . . . . . . . . .   ☑normal    ☐lesions    ☐rash       ☐other
                       Neurologic: . . . . . . .   ☑normal    ☐unsteady   ☐weakness   ☐other
  ↑      ↓             Sensation: . . . . . . .    ☐normal    ☐abnormal   ☐decreased  ☐other
 Page   Page           Motor Function:  . . . .    ☐normal    ☐weak       ☐other
 Up     Down
                                                    [ Submit ]  [ Page Up ]  [ Page Down ]
Exit Screen
```

In this example, the physician answers some of the remaining physical examination questions on this screen by checking the following trigger check boxes:

> **Left Foot** - normal
> **Neuroma test** - negative
> **Neuro** - normal
> **Vascular** - intact
> **Skin** - normal
> **Neurologic** - normal

The physician clicks the *Submit* button to record the remaining physical examination answers.

The physician clicks the *Exit Screen* button to return to the <u>Visit Documentation</u> screen (shown on the next page).

**Do This** ▶   **16.31** - Click the physical examination *check boxes* as shown above

                    **16.32** - Click the *Submit* button

                    **16.33** - Click the *Exit Screen* button

                           (you should be on the <u>Visit Documentation</u> screen)

The **History and Exam** section now reads Some History answered/Some Exam answered. This message is updated to remind the physician that he has answered some of the patient's history questions and some of the physical examination questions.

If the physician is done answering the history and exam questions, he clicks the *Hx & Exam Complete* button to alert the clinical staff and billing department that this part of the patient's record is complete for this encounter.

```
MEDTRAK

        Visit Documentation for DOS 05/31/09
        SUN   05/31   9:00a

        ABBEND, 251-MAY09-Z10 (777641)          Password              Z10
        LEFT ANKLE PAIN (1339261)               Initials     Z10

Available Functions  Orders
Order Entry          [     ]     X-RAY LT ANKLE (3VW)
Order by Code        [     ]     X-RAY OVERREAD
Cancel Order         [     ]     ICE LT ANKLE
Open Orders          [     ]     LEFT ANKLE APPLIANCE      (open)

                     Referrals / Authorizations
Referrals / Auth     [     ]     ORTHOPEDIC CONSULTATION

                     Diagnosis
DX by Checklist      [     ]     Derangement Left Ankle, Unspecified (718.97)
Find DX
Top 60 DX
Add DX
Delete DX

                     History and Exam
History and Exam     [     ]     Some History answered / Some Exam answered
                                 Click this button if you completed the history and exam questions  [ Hx & Exam Complete ]

                     Medications
Medications          [     ]     *** None ***

                     Instructions
Instructions         [     ]     Instructions NEED TO BE marked

                     Level of Service
Level of Service     [     ]     *** None ***

More Functions       [ Done ]   [ Not Done ]
```

**If you are continuing with the next chapter (Physician - Prescribing)**

**right now, skip the next Do This section.**

If you are not continuing with the next chapter, do the next steps to sign out of MedTrak.

**Do This** ▶ **16.34** - Click the *Not Done* button
(you should be on the Clinic Status screen)

**16.35** - Click the *Exit Screen* or *Main Menu* button
(you should be on the MedTrak Main Menu)

**16.36** - Click the *Log Off* button to exit MedTrak

# CHAPTER

# 17

# Physician - Prescribing

**Estimated time needed to complete this chapter  -  15** minutes

## What you need to know before doing this chapter

- ♦ How to log into MedTrak
- ♦ How to register a patient
- ♦ How to access Clinic Status off the Main Menu
- ♦ How to move a patient to a room and answer nursing notes
- ♦ How to access the Visit Documentation processor (Out the Door)

## Learning outcomes gained from this chapter

- ♦ How to prescribe dispensed and prescription medications

## *Physician - Prescribing*

### Major Categories of Clinical Workflow

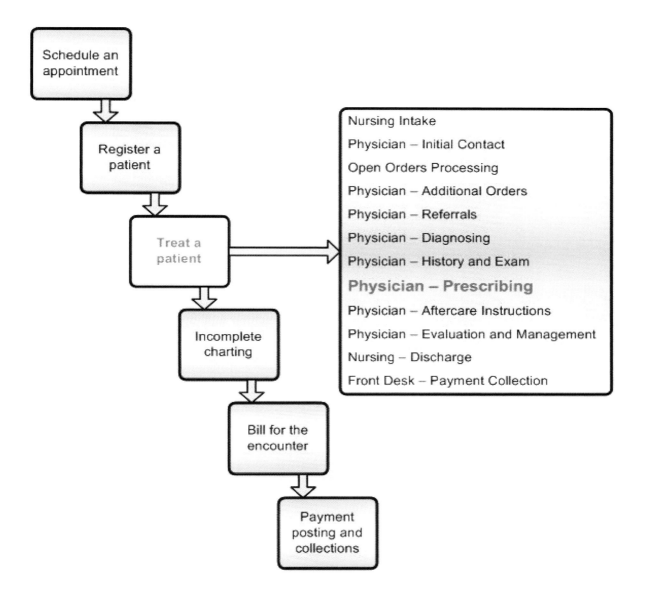

The next section on the Visit Documentation screen (shown below) is used to place orders for dispensed and prescription medications. Dispensed medications are those that the medical facility has on hand to provide to the patient. Prescription medications are those that the patient needs to have filled at a pharmacy.

If you are already on the Visit Documentation screen, then skip the next **Do This** section. If you are not on the Visit Documentation screen, then do the next steps.

**Do This** ► **17.01** - Place the cursor next to your patient on the Clinic Status screen

**17.02** - Click the *Out the Door* button

(you should be on the Visit Documentation screen)

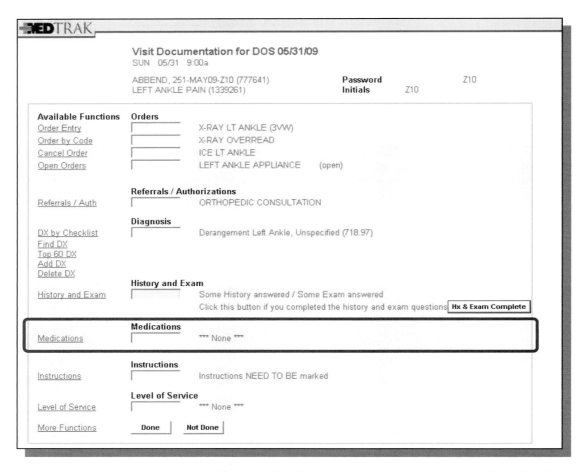

The two ways for the physician to prescribe medications are the same two ways the physician uses to place orders for x-rays or treatments as described in the **Physician - Initial Contact** chapter.

## Ordering Medications Using the Problem-Focused Method

To use the problem-focused <u>Visit Orders</u> screen (shown below) to prescribe medications, the physician clicks the **Medications** button.

```
MEDTRAK

                    Visit Orders
                    SAT  07/18  1:17p

                    Medication Allergies:  None

                    ABBEND, 251-JUN09-Z10 (778929)
                    LEFT ANKLE PAIN (1340757-9990)

                    Password                        Z10
                    DOC  Init      Z10

Available Functions         *** BEGINNING OF VISIT ORDERS ***
                        ⊟ Medications (Disp OR Rx)
Submit                  ⊞    .MEDS - DISPENSED
                        ⊞    .MEDS - PRESCRIBED
Additional Order            Musculoskeletal Disorders
                        ⊞    MUSCLE RELAXANTS
Open Orders                 Pain & Pyrexia
                        ⊞    NSAID
Not in MedTrak          ⊞    NARCOTIC
                        ⊞  MEDICATIONS
Show the Order              *** END OF VISIT ORDERS ***
Cancel the Order
Print the Order

More Functions

    ↑         ↓
  Page      Page
   Up       Down

Exit Screen
```

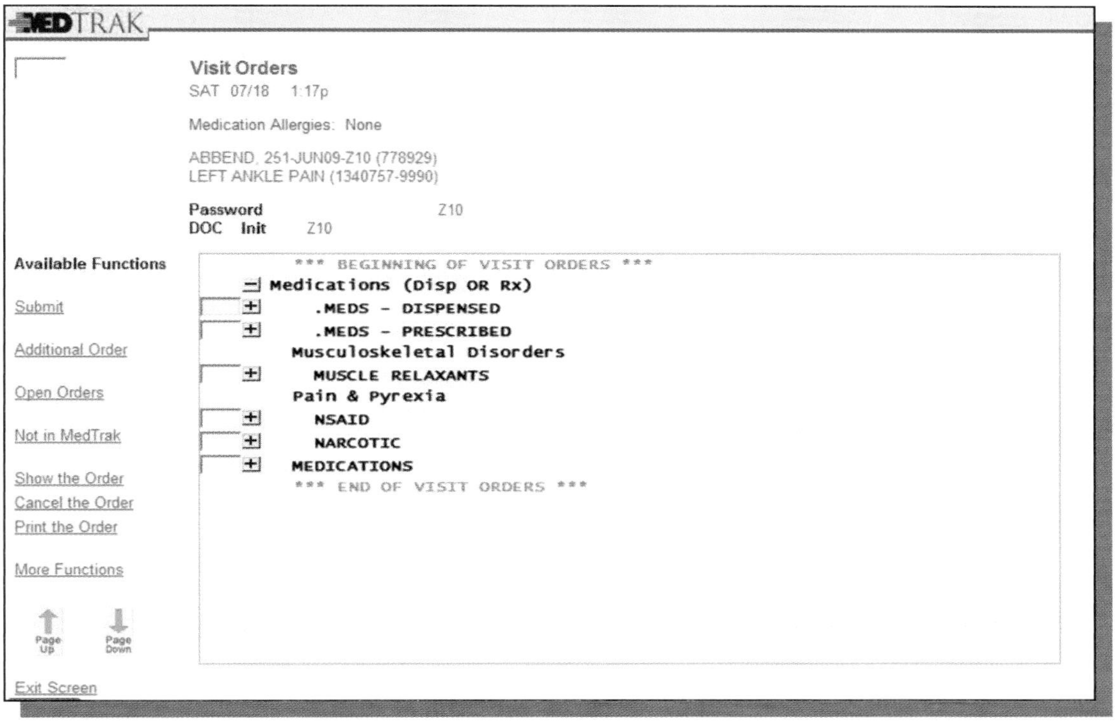

The provider uses the yellow plus ⊞ and minus ⊟ buttons to navigate to the right medication, then clicks the green ⊠ button to select the medication.

---

**Do This ▶**   **17.03** - Click the **Medications** button

**17.04** - Using the yellow plus ⊞ and minus ⊟ signs navigate around
(do not place an order for a medication - just look at them)

**17.05** - Click the **Exit Screen** button
(you should be on the <u>Visit Documentation</u> screen)

---

## Ordering Medications Using the Order Code Method

The second way for the physician to place an order for a medication is to use the order code. The order code can be entered directly into the **Medication** data entry field on the <u>Visit Documentation</u> screen (shown below).

In this example, the physician wants the patient to take **Ibuprofen** to help with the swelling and pain in his left ankle. To order the prescription, the physician types "**ibu800**" in the **Medication** field and presses the *ENTER* key. This is faster because the physician just has to type the name of the medication on the <u>Visit Documentation</u> screen rather than locate the medication in the medication tree.

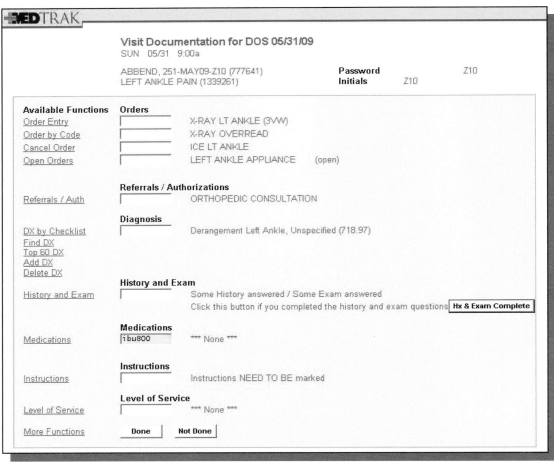

The next screen to appear is the <u>Order by Code</u> screen (shown on the next page). Based on the order code entered on the <u>Visit Documentation</u> screen, the <u>Order by Code</u> processor reads the code and displays the related order.

The provider clicks the *Submit* button to confirm that this is the right medication order.

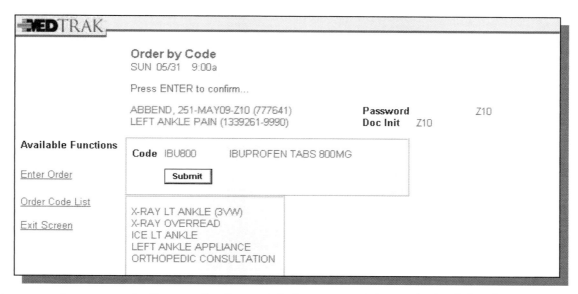

The next screen to appear is the medications details screen (shown below) for the **Ibuprofen Tabs 800 mg** medication, displaying the number to dispense and the directions for taking the medication.

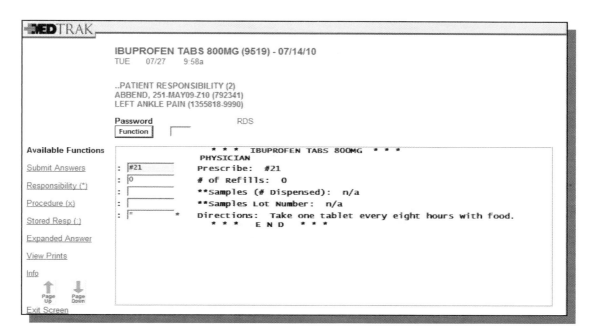

To save the physician time, MedTrak fills in the normal way the physician writes the prescription, because physicians typically write prescriptions the same way each time. The medication normals can be by medical facility and individual physician.

In the example above, the prescribed number of tablets is **21**, the number of refills is **zero**, and the directions are to "**Take one tablet every eight hours with food.**" If the physician wanted the patient to take the medication for 10 days rather than the standard seven, he or she would type over the prescribe amount with the number **30**. This screen has the same functionality as the open orders screen.

For prescription medications, MedTrak includes two questions about samples:

- ◆ How many samples did the physician dispense?

- ◆ What is the lot number of the sample medication?

If for some reason there was a recall on the sample medication given to the patient, the medical facility could run a report to see which patients received the lot number for the sample medication and notify the patients about the recall.

To finish ordering this medication, the physician clicks the *Submit Answers* button. MedTrak refreshes the Order by Code screen (shown below), displaying the addition of the **Ibuprofen Tabs 800 mg** prescription.

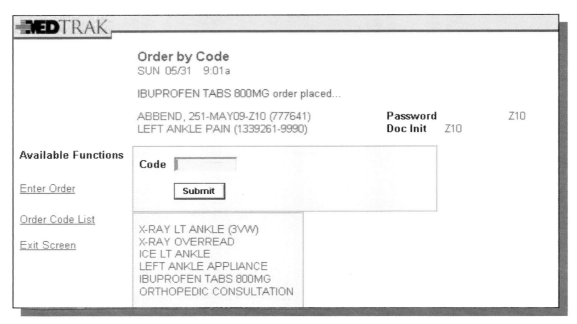

If the physician needs to order another medication, he or she could enter the order code or select the order code from the **Order Code List**.

In this example, the physician only wants to order the **Ibuprofen**, so he or she clicks the *Exit Screen* button to return to the Visit Documentation screen (shown on the next page).

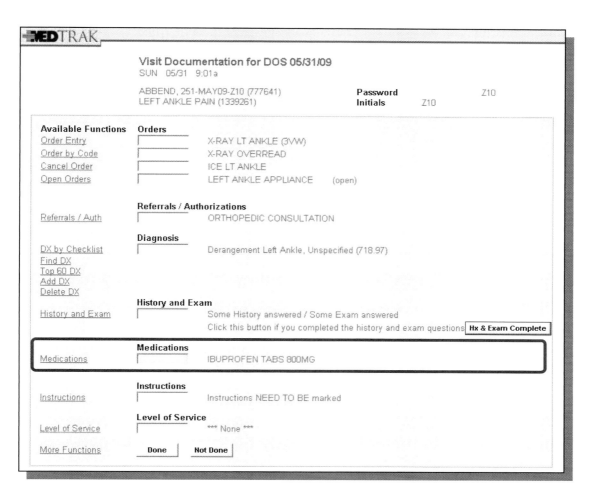

The **Ibuprofen Tabs 800 mg** medication order displays to the right of the medication data entry field. If the physician placed the wrong medication order, he or she would cancel it by placing the cursor in the data entry field next to the medication and clicking the *Cancel Order* button located in the **Orders** section.

**Do This** ▶ **17.06** - Type the order code **ibu800** in the **Medications** data entry field

**17.07** - Press the *ENTER* key to place the order
(you should be on the Order by Code screen)

**17.08** - Press the *Submit* button to confirm the order

**17.09** - Press the *Submit Answers* button to confirm the med directions
(you should be on the Ibuprofen directions screen)

**17.10** - Click the *Exit Screen* button on the Order by Code screen
(you should be on the Visit Documentation screen)

**If you are continuing with the next exercise (Physician - Aftercare Instructions) right now, skip the next Do This section.**

If you are not continuing with the next chapter, do the next steps to sign out of MedTrak.

---

**Do This** ▶  **17.11** - Click the *Not Done* button
(you should be on the <u>Clinic Status</u> screen)

**17.12** - Click the *Exit Screen* or *Main Menu* button
(you should be on the MedTrak <u>Main Menu</u>)

**17.13** - Click the *Log Off* button to exit MedTrak

---

CHAPTER

18

# Physician - Aftercare Instructions

**Estimated time needed to complete this chapter - 30** minutes

## What you need to know before doing this chapter

- ◆ How to log into MedTrak
- ◆ How to register a patient
- ◆ How to access Clinic Status off the Main Menu
- ◆ How to move a patient to a room and answer nursing notes
- ◆ How to access the Visit Documentation processor (Out the Door)

## Learning outcomes gained from this chapter

- ◆ How to select, modify and create patient aftercare instructions

## Key terms used in this chapter

*aftercare instructions*
*important points to remember*
*what to be concerned about*
*medications*
*work status*
*work restrictions*
*follow-up*
*assessment and plan of care*
*summation*
*case closed*
*standard instructions*
*modifiable instructions*
*specific instructions*

## Physician - Aftercare Instructions

### Major Categories of Clinical Workflow

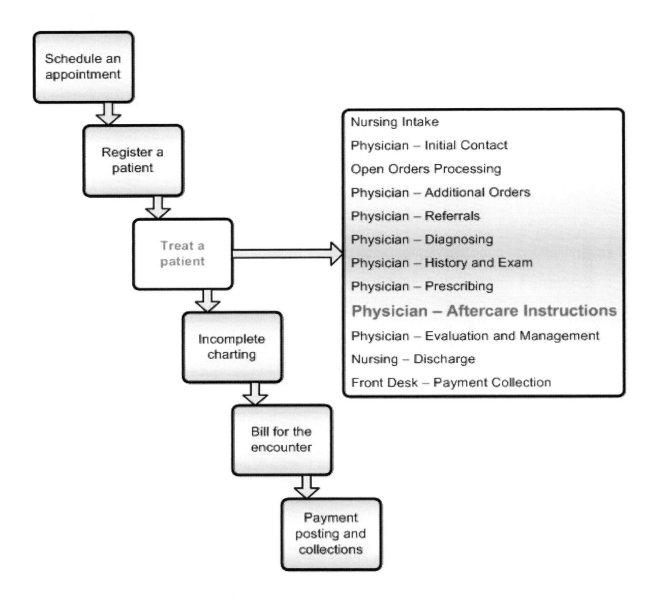

Once the physician finishes placing orders, diagnosing, and answering the history and exam, the next step in the workflow is to select the *aftercare instructions* for the patients to take with them when they leave the medical facility. MedTrak's instruction processor is problem-focused based on the diagnoses selected by the physician. The physician chooses from instructions that are directly related to the patient's condition. This saves the physician time searching for the appropriate aftercare instructions to provide the patient.

The aftercare instructions inform the patients as to what they can do for self care after they leave the medical facility, and what they should limit doing or not do. The aftercare instructions also inform the patient as to how to self-treat, how to take the prescribed medications, and when to return to the medical facility.

For workers' compensation patients, the physician also specifies whether the patient can work without restrictions, needs to work with the restrictions specified by the provider, or is incapable of working at this time. Based on these work-related instructions, MedTrak sends emails and faxes to the employers with the work status so that the employer knows the employee's condition as soon as the patient leaves the medical facility.

The main sections of the patient aftercare instructions are as follows:

*Important Points to Remember* - instructions about what the patients should and should not do to self treat their injury or illness

*What to be Concerned About* - instructions to inform the patients about what they should do if their condition should worsen

*Medications* - instructions about whether the patients should continue taking or stop taking medications that they were already taking before they came to the medical facility

*Work Status* - contains the physician's recommendation about whether the patients should go back to work, and if so, any restrictions about what they can or cannot do while at work

*Work Restrictions* - instructions about what the patient is encouraged to do, should limit doing, or should not do while at work

*Follow-up* - instructions about when the patient should return to the medical facility

*Assessment and Plan of Care* - contains the physician's detailed plan for treating the patient's condition

*Summation* - contains the physician's opinion of the patient's present condition

*Case Closed* - the physician uses this section to close workers' compensation cases

MedTrak has three types of instructions that the physician can use:

*Standard instructions* - where the wording for the instruction is from the MedTrak library of instructions. For example, the **Reduce Activity** instruction is a standard instruction.

*Modifiable instructions* - where a specific word or words (marked with brackets < > on either side of them) in the instruction can be changed.

*Specific instructions* - where the provider types in (or uses voice recognition) to create instructions that are specific to the patient.

If you are already on the <u>Visit Documentation</u> screen, then skip the next **Do This** section. If you are not on the <u>Visit Documentation</u> screen, then do the next steps.

**Do This** ▶ **18.01** - Place the cursor next to your patient on the <u>Clinic Status</u> screen

           **18.02** - Click the ***Out the Door*** button

                    (you should be on the <u>Visit Documentation</u> screen)

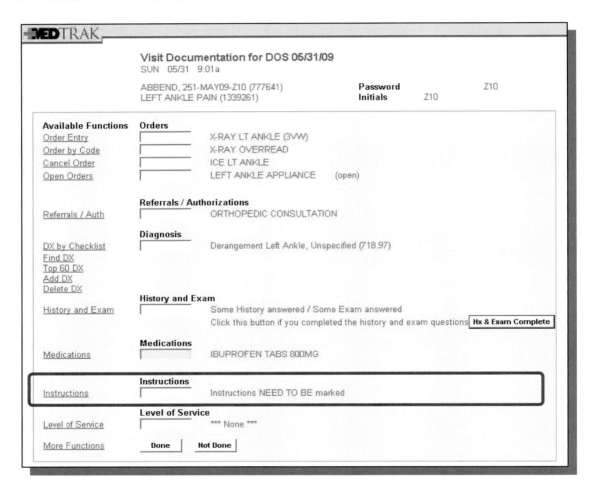

In this example, the provider clicks the ***Instructions*** button to access the first screen of patient <u>Instructions</u> (shown on the next page).

## *Important Points to Remember*

```
═MEDTRAK
                Instructions
                SUN  05/31   9:02a


                ABBEND, 251-MAY09-Z10 (777641)
                LEFT ANKLE PAIN (1339261-9990)

                Password        Z10

Available Functions      Important Points to Remember
                           Activity:
Submit Selections    □         Normal Activity.
                     ☑         Reduce activity.
More Functions       □         Rest and Relax.
                     □         Resume activity when feeling better.
                     □         <Specific Activity Instruction>.        □▭
                     ☑         Let pain be the guide.
   Page    Page      □         <Specific Instruction>                  □▭
   Up      Down                Rest and Don't Use
                     ☑            Ankle.
Exit Screen                    Rest and Limit Use
                     □            Ankle.
```

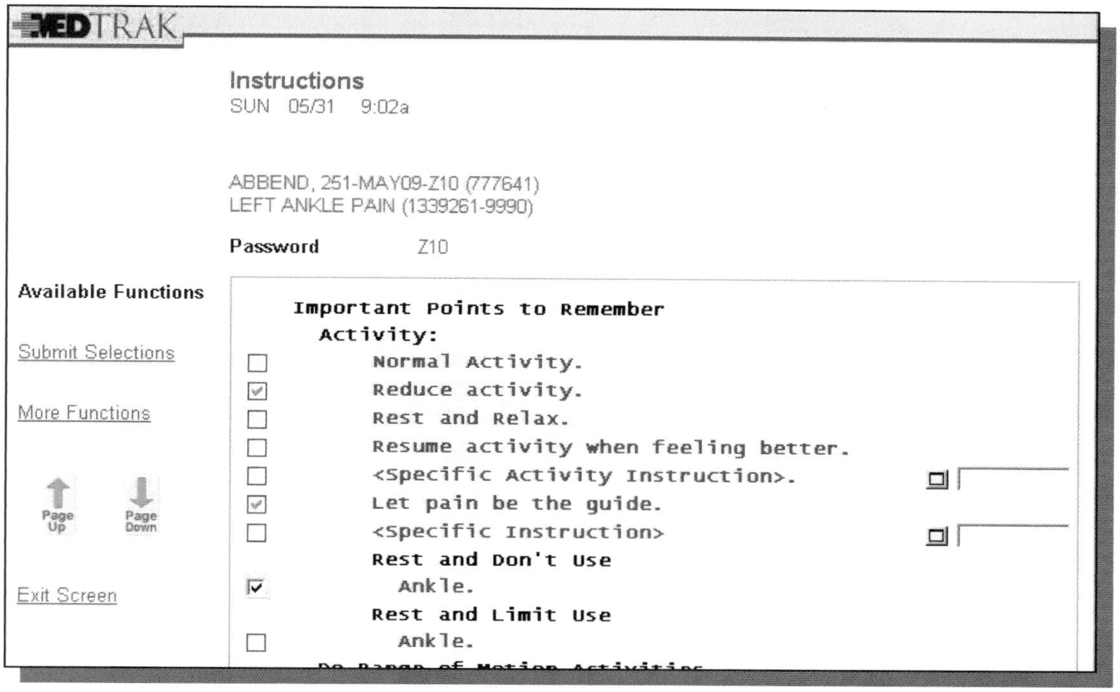

On this screen the physician selects the following MedTrak standard instructions by clicking the *check boxes*:

- **Reduce Activity.**
- **Let pain be the guide.**
- **Rest and Don't Use** - Ankle

Then the physician clicks the *Submit Selections* button to accept the selections. The screen refreshes with the selected instructions in blue and bold. The physician clicks the *Submit Selections* button again to advance to the next screen of instructions (shown on the next page).

MedTrak automatically moves to the next screen within the same main section of instructions. Since the Important Points to Remember section is comprised of several screens of instruction choices, MedTrak moves to the next screen of instructions in this section.

---

**Do This** ▶ **18.03** - Click the *Instructions* button

(the Instructions list processor will appear)

**18.04** - Click the same check boxes as on the above screen

**18.05** - Click the *Submit Selections* button

(the first Important Points to Remember screen refreshes)

**18.06** - Click the *Submit Selections* button again

(the second Important Points to Remember screen appears)

---

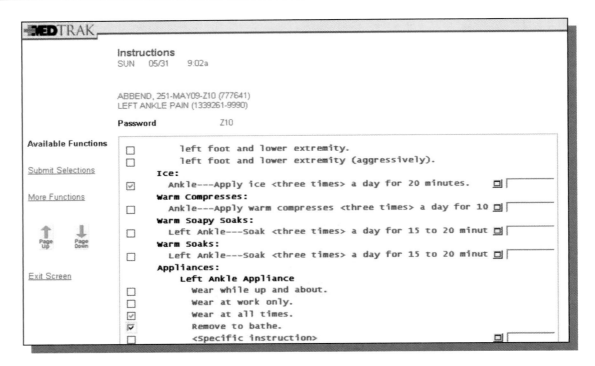

On this screen, the physician selects the following instructions by clicking the *check boxes*:

- **Ice -** Ankle - Apply ice <three times> a day for 20 minutes (modifiable instruction)
- **Appliances - Left Ankle Appliance -** Wear at all times and

  Remove to bathe (both standard instructions)

Then the physician clicks the *Submit Selections* button to accept the selections. The screen refreshes with the selected instructions in black. The physician clicks the *Submit Selections* button again to advance to the <u>Medications</u> instructions (shown below).

**Do This** ► **18.07** - Click the same check boxes as on the previous screen

**18.08** - Click the **Submit Selections** button
(the second Important Points to Remember screen refreshes)

**18.09** - Click the **Submit Selections** button again
(the Medications screen appears)

## Medications

Since the patient is not currently taking any medications, the physician is not selecting any of the Medications instructions, so he or she clicks the **Submit Selections** button to advance to the Work Status instructions (shown on the next page).

If the patient was already taking prescription or over-the-counter medications, the physician would need to instruct the patient as to whether he should continue taking his current medications given his present condition. This is especially important if the physician is prescribing any additional medications for the patient.

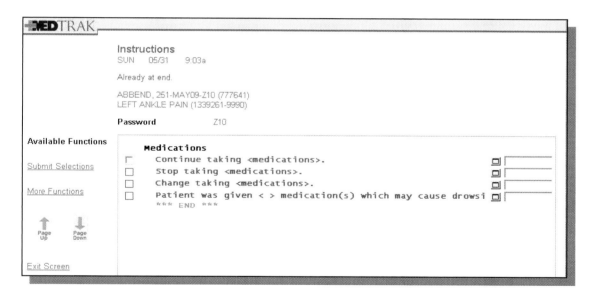

**Do This** ► **18.10** - Click the **Submit Selections** button
(the Work Status screen appears)

## *Work Status*

On this screen the physician selects the following instruction by clicking the *check box*:

### Return to modified work duties <today>

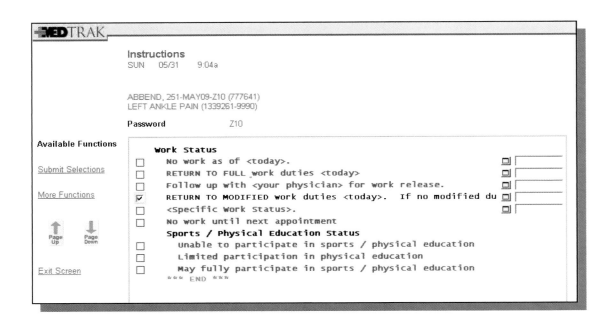

Then the physician clicks the *Submit Selections* button to accept the selection. Since this is the only screen of <u>Work Status</u> instructions, the screen refreshes with the checked instruction in **black** to indicate its selection.

The physician clicks the *Submit Selections* button again to advance to the <u>Work Restrictions</u> instructions (shown below).

**Do This** ▶  **18.11** - Click the check box for the return to modified duty

**18.12** - Click the *Submit Selections* button
(the <u>Work Status</u> screen refreshes)

**18.13** - Click the *Submit Selections* button again
(the <u>Work Restrictions</u> screen appears)

## *Work Restrictions*

The physician clicks the *check box* for the specific instruction in the encourage area of <u>Work Restrictions</u> and clicks the *specific instruction screen icon* ▯ to the right of the instruction.

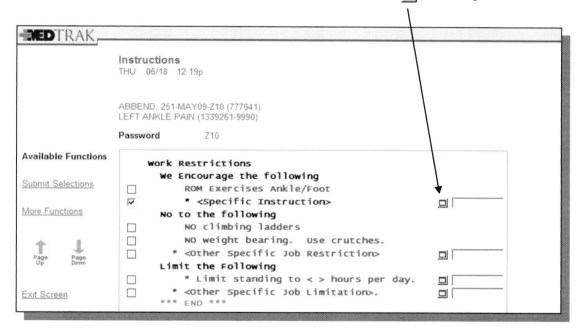

The next screen to appear is the specific instruction screen for the Encourage section of <u>Work Restrictions</u> (shown on the next page). The physician either types into the entry field or turns on voice recognition and dictates directly into the field.

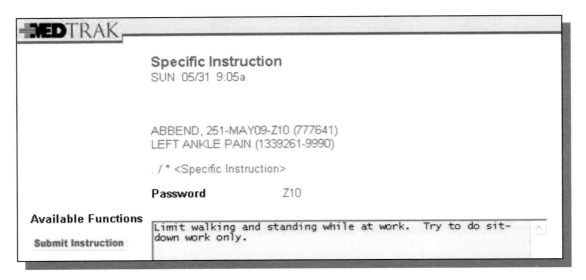

After entering the specific instruction, the physician clicks the **Submit Instruction** button. MedTrak automatically refreshes the Instructions screen (shown below) with the specific instruction now appearing under the instruction.

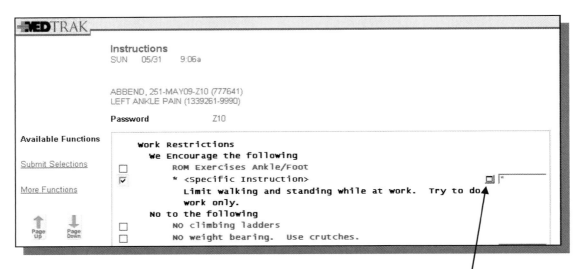

The physician clicks the **Submit Selections** button again to advance to the Follow-Up instructions (shown on the next page).

**Do This ▶**   **18.14** - Click the check box for the encourage specific instruction

**18.15** - Click the *specific instruction screen icon* 🖥

**18.16** - Enter the specific instruction as shown above

**18.17** - Click the *Submit Instruction* button
(the Work Restrictions screen refreshes)

**18.18** - Click the *Submit Selections* button again
(the Follow-Up screen appears)

## Follow Up

The physician checks the *check box* for the specific instruction of return for next visit in the Follow-Up section and clicks the *specific instruction screen icon* ▢ to the right of the instruction.

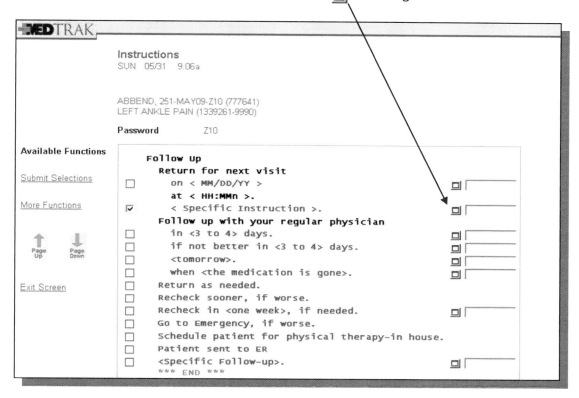

The next screen to appear is the Specific Instruction screen for return for next visit (shown below). The physician either types into the entry field or turns on voice recognition and dictates directly into the field.

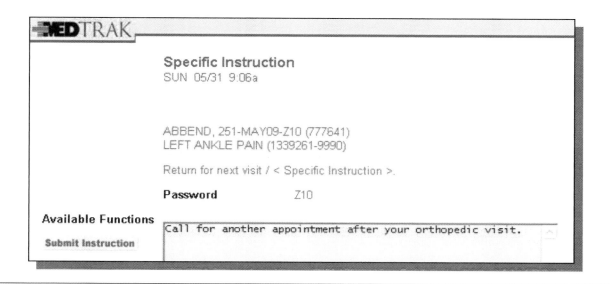

The physician clicks the *Submit Instruction* button, and MedTrak automatically returns to the <u>Follow Up</u> section of the <u>Instructions</u> screen with the specific instruction now appearing under the instruction.

The physician clicks the *Submit Selections* button again to advance to the <u>Assessment and Plan of Care</u> instructions (shown below).

---

**Do This** ▶    **18.19** - Click the *check box* for the return for next visit specific instruction

         **18.20** - Click the *specific instruction screen icon* ▢
                (the <u>Specific Instruction</u> screen appears)

         **18.21** - Enter the specific instruction as shown on the previous screen

         **18.22** - Click the *Submit Instruction* button
                (the <u>Follow Up</u> screen refreshes with the specific instruction)

         **18.23** - Click the *Submit Selections* button again
                (the <u>Assessment and Plan of Care</u> screen appears)

---

## Assessment and Plan of Care

The physician checks the *check box* for the modifiable instruction of **Discussion of treatment options/contingencies** in the **Additional Comments for Plan** section and clicks the *specific instruction screen icon* ▢ to the right of the instruction.

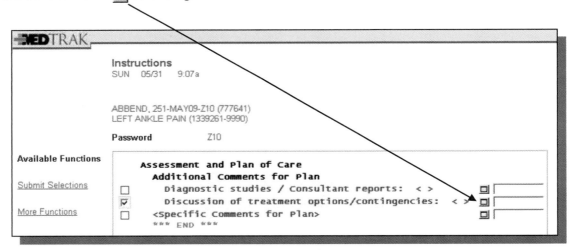

The next screen to appear is the specific instruction screen for <u>Assessment and Plan of Care</u> (shown on the next page). The physician either types into the entry field or turns on voice recognition and dictates directly into the field.

After entering the specific instruction, the physician clicks the *Submit Instruction* button to record the instruction.

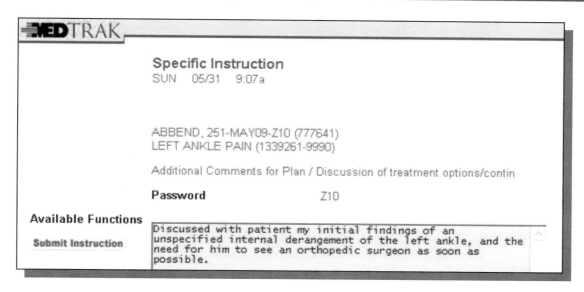

The physician clicks the *Submit Selections* button again to advance to the <u>Summation</u> instructions (shown on the next page).

**Do This ▶** **18.24** - Click the check box for **Discussion of Treatment** specific instruction

**18.25** - Click the *specific instruction screen icon* □|
(the <u>Specific Instruction</u> screen appears)

**18.26** - Enter the specific instruction as shown above

**18.27** - Click the *Submit Instruction* button
(the <u>Assessment and Plan of Care</u> screen refreshes)

**18.28** - Click the *Submit Selections* button again
(the <u>Summation</u> screen appears)

## *Summation*

The physician clicks the *check box* for the condition on discharge in the <u>Summation</u>, types the word **fair** in the data input field to the right of the instruction, and clicks the *Submit Selections* button. When there is an input field to the right of the instruction, the brackets on either side of a word (or group of words) designate the modifiable part of the instruction. If the physician needs more than 10 characters for the modifier of the instruction, he or she will click the expanded instruction screen icon □| to the right of the instruction.

In this example, the physician is indicating that the patient's condition on discharge is **fair**. The standard answer for the patient's condition is **good**. The bracketed instruction field allows the physician to modify the instruction to indicate whatever the physician feels is the patient's current condition. Whatever the physician types in the input field or in the expanded instruction field replaces the word or words inside the brackets.

The Summation section of the Instructions screen (shown below) refreshes with the word **fair** under the instruction. When MedTrak prints the aftercare instructions, the condition on discharge will read as **fair**.

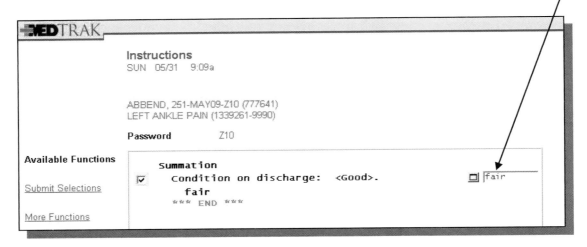

After finishing selecting, modifying, and creating specific patient aftercare instructions, the physician clicks the *Submit Selections* button again to display the patient aftercare instructions Summary screen (shown on the next page).

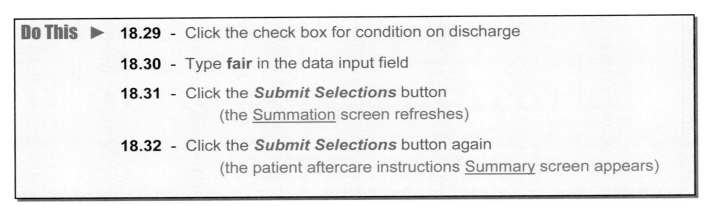

**Do This** ▶   **18.29** - Click the check box for condition on discharge

**18.30** - Type **fair** in the data input field

**18.31** - Click the *Submit Selections* button
(the Summation screen refreshes)

**18.32** - Click the *Submit Selections* button again
(the patient aftercare instructions Summary screen appears)

## Aftercare Instructions Summary Screens

The summary screens of the <u>Instructions</u> (shown below) display selected instructions in **black**. If upon review, the physician decides to add, change, or remove instructions in a section, he or she clicks the green ☒ button to the left of the section name to access the selection screen for that section of aftercare instructions.

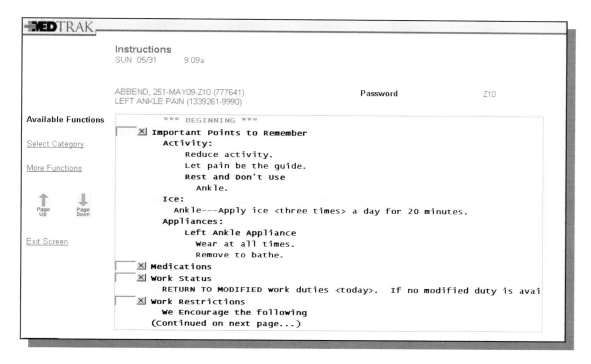

By clicking the *Page Down* button, the physician scrolls down to see the next summary screen of instructions (shown below).

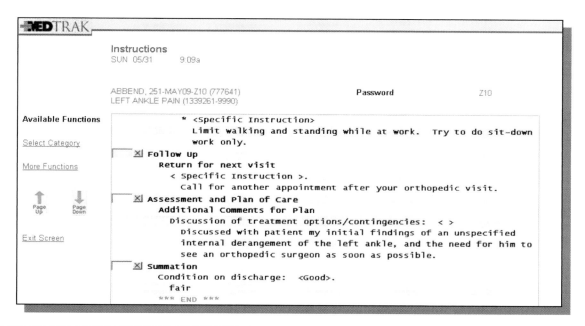

After reviewing the summary screens of instructions, the physician clicks the *Exit Screen* button to return to the <u>Visit Documentation</u> screen (shown below). The **Instructions** section displays a message that "**Instructions have been marked**."

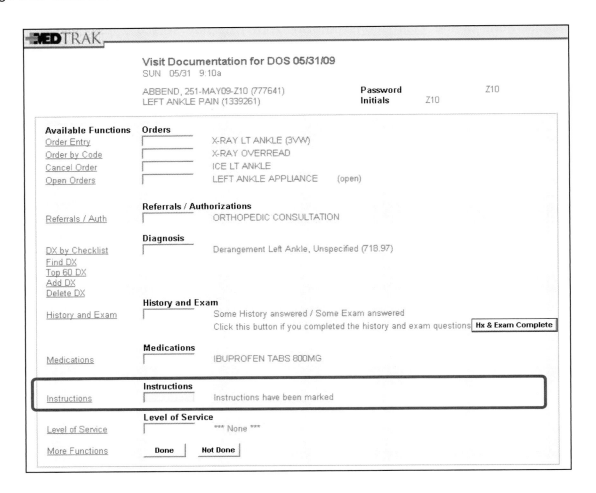

---

**Do This** ► **18.33** - Review the instructions on the first <u>Instructions</u> summary screen

**18.34** - Click the *Page Down* button
(you should be on the second <u>Instructions</u> summary screen)

**18.35** - Review the instructions on the second <u>Instructions</u> summary screen

**18.36** - Click the *Exit Screen* button
(you should be on the <u>Visit Documentation</u> screen)

**If you are continuing with the next exercise (Physician - Evaluation & Management) right now, skip the next Do This section.**

If you are not continuing with the next chapter, do the next steps to sign out of MedTrak.

**Do This** ▶ **18.37** - Click the *Not Done* button
(you should be on the <u>Clinic Status</u> screen)

**18.38** - Click the *Exit Screen* or *Main Menu* button
(you should be on the MedTrak <u>Main Menu</u>)

**18.39** - Click the *Log Off* button to exit MedTrak

# CHAPTER 19

# Physician - Evaluation and Management

**Estimated time needed to complete this chapter  -  15** minutes

## What you need to know before doing this chapter

- ◆ How to log into MedTrak
- ◆ How to register a patient
- ◆ How to access Clinic Status off the Main Menu
- ◆ How to move a patient to a room and answer nursing notes
- ◆ How to access the Visit Documentation processor  (Out the Door)

## Learning outcomes gained from this chapter

- ◆ How to select the evaluation and management level of service

## Key terms used in this chapter

*professional services*
*evaluation and management services*
*levels of service*
*key components*
*contributory factors*
*history*
*exam*
*decision making*

## Physician - Evaluation and Management

### Major Categories of Clinical Workflow

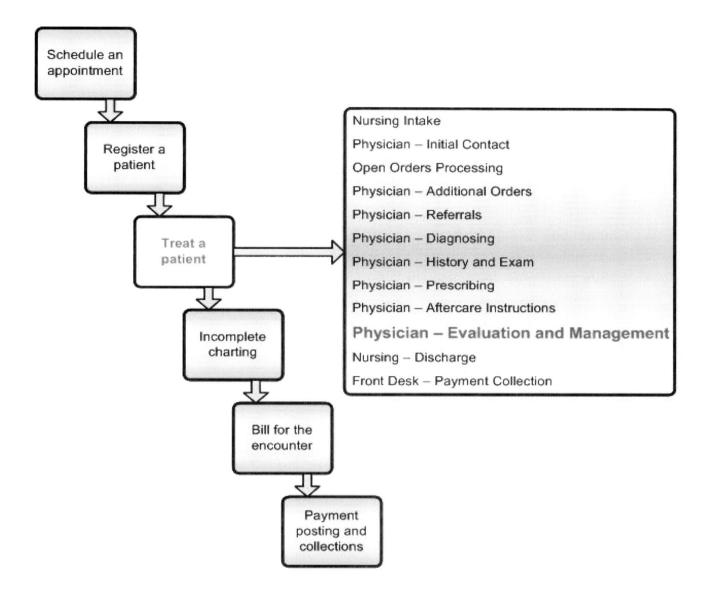

The face-to-face time spent by the physician with a patient obtaining history, doing examinations, evaluating, treating, conferring with, and suggesting preventive health measures constitutes *professional services*. Physicians charge for these professional services called evaluation and management (E/M) services with specific CPT codes.

The *evaluation and management services* (also called *levels of service*) differ depending on:

+ Place of service
+ Type of service
+ Content of the service
+ Nature of the presenting problem
+ Time typically required to provide the service

For reporting purposes there are up to five levels of E/M services available, defined by six different components:

+ History
+ Examination
+ Medical decision making
+ Counseling
+ Coordination of care
+ Nature of the presenting problem

The *key components* in deciding the level of E/M services are the first three. The last three components are *contributory factors* and are not required to be provided during each patient encounter.

In this example, the physician:

+ questions the patients about their history
+ examines their major systems
+ specifically examines the left ankle
+ orders a diagnostic x-ray
+ orders an overread of the x-ray
+ orders an ice treatment
+ orders an ankle support
+ refers the patient to see an orthopedic surgeon
+ prescribes a medication
+ diagnoses the patient with an internal derangement of the left ankle

All of these actions constitute the key components of the E/M services.

The level of service CPT codes also vary depending on the type of visit. Primary care, urgent care, and workers' compensation visits to a primary care physician use the same series of CPT codes. Orthopedic medicine and rehab services have their own sets of CPT codes.

If you are already on the Visit Documentation screen, then skip the next **Do This** section. If you are not on the Visit Documentation screen, then do the next steps.

---

**Do This** ▶ **19.01** - Place the cursor next to your patient on the Clinic Status screen

**19.02** - Click the **Out the Door** button

(you should be on the Visit Documentation screen)

---

**MEDTRAK**

**Visit Documentation for DOS 05/31/09**
SUN 05/31 9:01a

ABBEND, 251-MAY09-Z10 (777641)          Password          Z10
LEFT ANKLE PAIN (1339261)               Initials     Z10

**Available Functions**   **Orders**
Order Entry            |____|  X-RAY LT ANKLE (3VW)
Order by Code          |____|  X-RAY OVERREAD
Cancel Order           |____|  ICE LT ANKLE
Open Orders            |____|  LEFT ANKLE APPLIANCE      (open)

                      **Referrals / Authorizations**
Referrals / Auth       |____|  ORTHOPEDIC CONSULTATION

                      **Diagnosis**
DX by Checklist        |____|  Derangement Left Ankle, Unspecified (718.97)
Find DX
Top 60 DX
Add DX
Delete DX

                      **History and Exam**
History and Exam       |____|  Some History answered / Some Exam answered
                               Click this button if you completed the history and exam questions [ **Hx & Exam Complete** ]

                      **Medications**
Medications            |____|  IBUPROFEN TABS 800MG

                      **Instructions**
Instructions           |____|  Instructions NEED TO BE marked

                      **Level of Service**
Level of Service       |____|  *** None ***

More Functions      [ **Done** ]  [ **Not Done** ]

In this example, the physician clicks the **Level of Service** button to access the Level of Service screen (shown on the next page).

On the <u>Level of Service</u> screen (shown below), the physician clicks the following check boxes for the key components of the E/M level of service code:

♦ *History* - **CC, HPI(>3), P or F or S, ROS Prob Sys and Mult Other Sys**

This means that the physician reviewed the chief complaint (**CC**) with the patient, asked him about the history of the present illness/injury (**HPI**), reviewed either his past history of any similar injuries (**P**), reviewed the history of his problem system (**Prob Sys**) and multiple other systems (**Mult Other Sys**).

♦ *Exam* - **Limited Exam of Affected Body Area and Other Related Sys**

This means that the physician examined the left ankle and joints on either side of the ankle.

♦ *Decision Making* - **Low 1-2 Diff DX, Limited Data Review, Low Risk of Complications**

This means that the physician selected one diagnosis for the patient's condition and reviewed the left ankle x-ray and felt that there was a low risk of long-term complications with this injury.

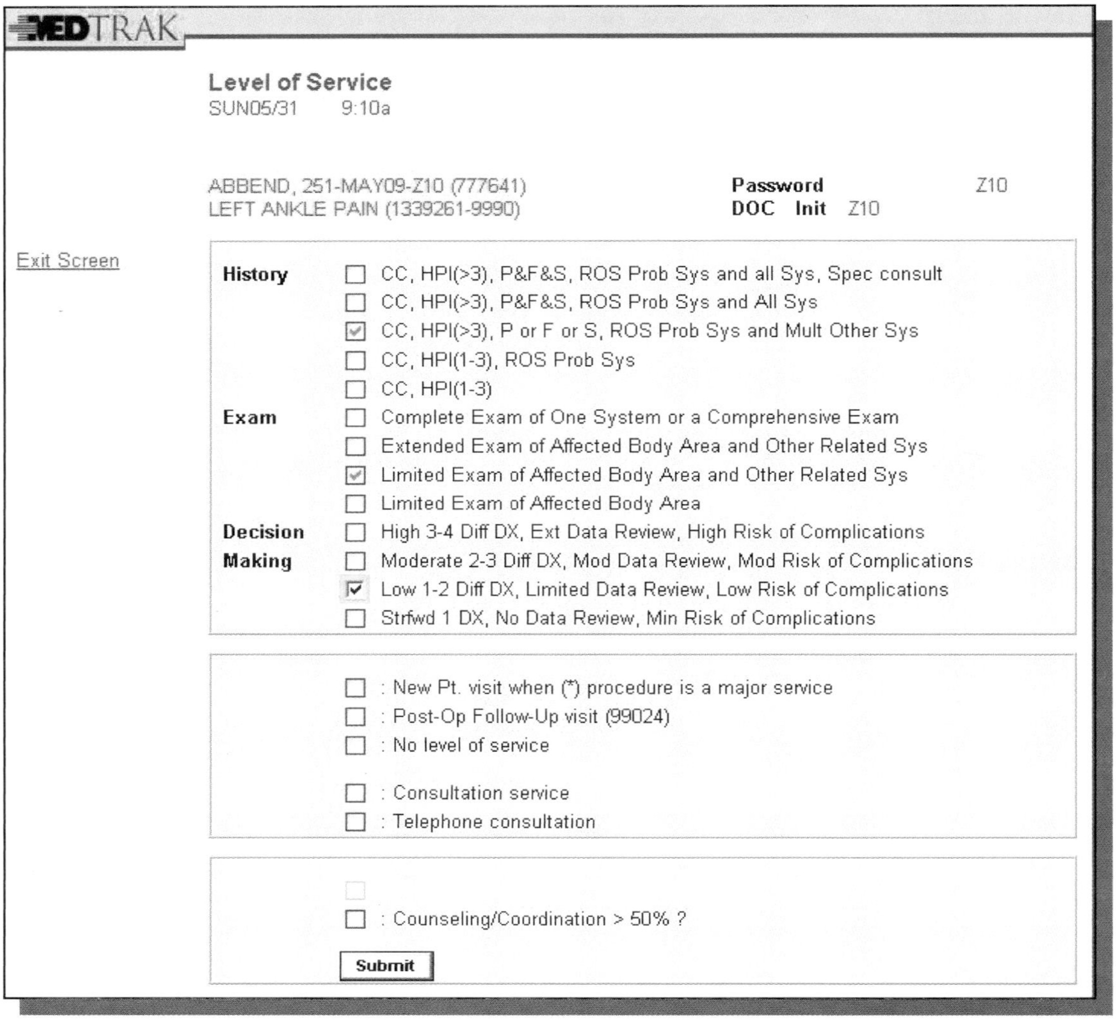

**MED**TRAK

**Level of Service**
SUN05/31   9:10a

ABBEND, 251-MAY09-Z10 (777641)      **Password**        Z10
LEFT ANKLE PAIN (1339261-9990)       **DOC Init**  Z10

Exit Screen

**History**
- ☐ CC, HPI(>3), P&F&S, ROS Prob Sys and all Sys, Spec consult
- ☐ CC, HPI(>3), P&F&S, ROS Prob Sys and All Sys
- ☑ CC, HPI(>3), P or F or S, ROS Prob Sys and Mult Other Sys
- ☐ CC, HPI(1-3), ROS Prob Sys
- ☐ CC, HPI(1-3)

**Exam**
- ☐ Complete Exam of One System or a Comprehensive Exam
- ☐ Extended Exam of Affected Body Area and Other Related Sys
- ☑ Limited Exam of Affected Body Area and Other Related Sys
- ☐ Limited Exam of Affected Body Area

**Decision Making**
- ☐ High 3-4 Diff DX, Ext Data Review, High Risk of Complications
- ☐ Moderate 2-3 Diff DX, Mod Data Review, Mod Risk of Complications
- ☑ Low 1-2 Diff DX, Limited Data Review, Low Risk of Complications
- ☐ Strfwd 1 DX, No Data Review, Min Risk of Complications

- ☐ : New Pt. visit when (*) procedure is a major service
- ☐ : Post-Op Follow-Up visit (99024)
- ☐ : No level of service

- ☐ : Consultation service
- ☐ : Telephone consultation

- ☐
- ☐ : Counseling/Coordination > 50% ?

**Submit**

After clicking the check boxes, the physician clicks the *Submit* button to accept the choices. The Level of Service screen (shown below) refreshes with the E/M level of service CPT code of **99203** displayed at the top of the screen.

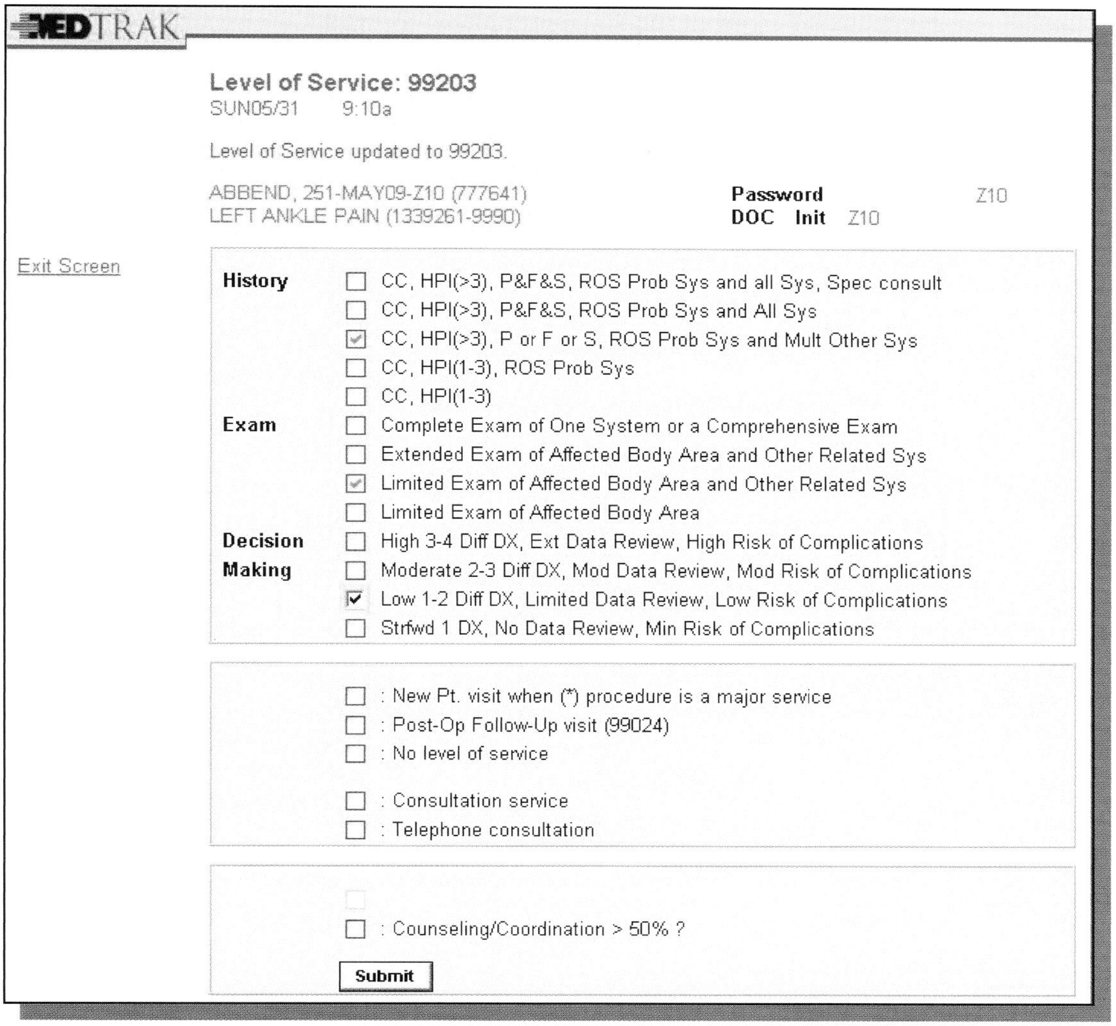

Many of the providers know the level of service CPT codes without the need to check the boxes for the history, exam, and decision making. The provider can type the level of service CPT code in the input field on the Visit Documentation screen and press the *ENTER* key. MedTrak will automatically check the appropriate boxes for history, exam, and decision making based on the CPT code entered by the provider. After reviewing the Level of Service screen, the provider clicks the *Submit* button to accept the code. The Level of Service screen (shown above) refreshes with the message **Level of service updated to 99203**.

Then the provider clicks the *Exit Screen* button to return to the Visit Documentation screen (shown below). The E/M level of service CPT code of **99203** appears next to the **Level of Service** data input field.

Your Visit Documentation screen should look similar to this one, with information about each of the sections selected displayed to the right of the data entry field for that section.

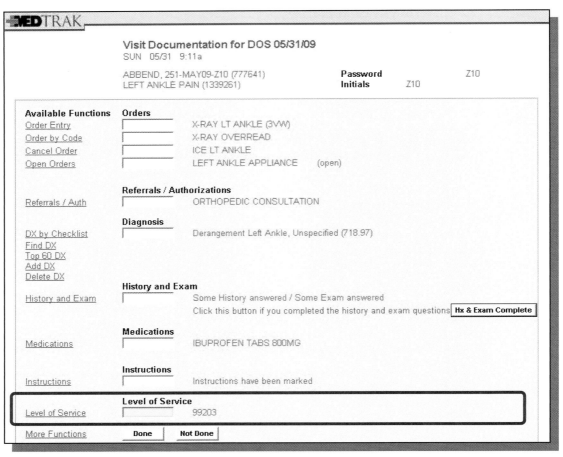

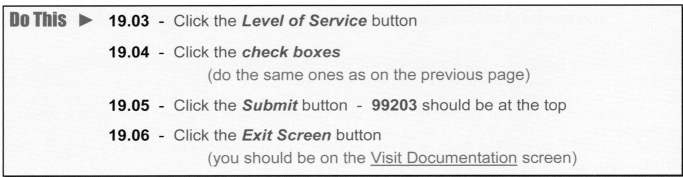

**Do This ▶   19.03** - Click the *Level of Service* button

**19.04** - Click the *check boxes*
(do the same ones as on the previous page)

**19.05** - Click the *Submit* button - **99203** should be at the top

**19.06** - Click the *Exit Screen* button
(you should be on the Visit Documentation screen)

The physician clicks the *Done* button to notify MedTrak that the **Out the Door** process is finished (visit documentation).

**Do This ▶   19.07** - Click the *Done* button
(you should be on the Clinic Status screen)

**Do This** ▶ **19.08** - Place the cursor next to your patient on the <u>Clinic Status</u> screen

**19.09** - Click the *Visit Log* button

(you should be on the <u>Visit Log</u> screen)

**19.10** - Place the cursor in the command field next to one of the log records

**19.11** - Type the command to print the patient's chart - **PRCH**

**19.12** - Press the *ENTER* key

(this will send the printed chart to your PDF print queue)

**19.13** - Click the *View Prints* button

(this will open another window displaying your PDF print queue)

(this screen is called <u>Available User Reports</u>)

**19.14** - Place the cursor in the command field next to the patient's chart

**19.15** - Click the *View Report* button

(this will open Adobe displaying the PDF of your chart)

**19.16** - Click the *diskette* icon at the top right of the PDF

**19.17** - Save this PDF to a folder for your class assignments

**19.18** - Attach the PDF to your assignment from this folder

**19.19** - Close the *Adobe* window displaying your chart

**19.20** - Close the <u>Available User Reports</u> window

**19.21** - Click the *Exit Screen* button

(you should be on the <u>Clinic Status</u> screen)

# CHAPTER

# 20 Nursing Discharge

**Estimated time needed to complete this chapter  -  15** minutes

## What you need to know before doing this chapter

- ◆ How to log into MedTrak
- ◆ How to register a patient
- ◆ How to access Clinic Status off the Main Menu
- ◆ How to move a patient to a room and answer nursing notes
- ◆ How to use the Visit Documentation processor  (Out the Door process)

## Learning outcomes gained from this chapter

- ◆ How to discharge a patient from the back examination area

# Nursing Discharge

## Major Categories of Clinical Workflow

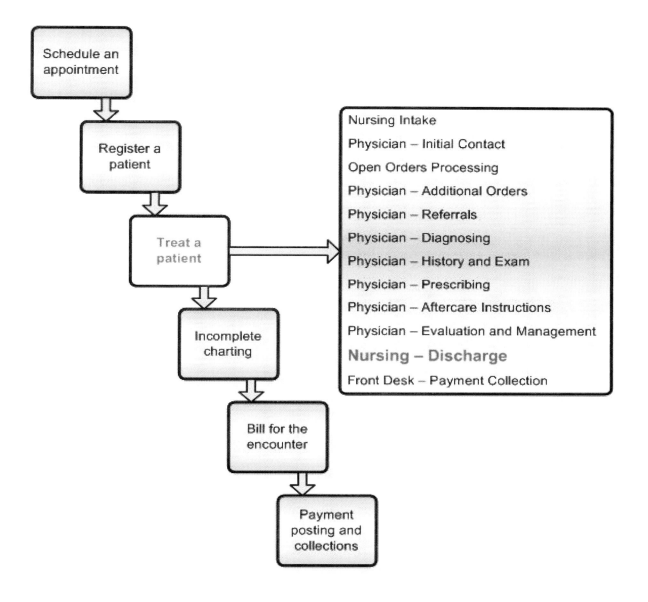

When the physician is done with the patient and finishes the **Out the Door** process, the physician might have placed orders that need completion (open orders) before the patient can be discharged with his or her paperwork from the medical facility. Even though the physician is now seeing another patient, there could still be open orders in MedTrak for the clinical staff to complete with this patient.

The *nursing discharge* workflow step is important for several reasons:

♦ The physician can focus on treating the other patients without having to worry about whether any orders are missed for this patient.

♦ The clinical staff does not need to wait for the physician to come out of an exam room to know what the physician wants them to do for the patient.

♦ Everyone in the medical facility knows that everything will be done for a patient before he or she is discharged from the medical facility.

The physician might have ordered a medication. If it was a dispensed medication, the clinical staff will need to take the medication off the shelf, record the lot number, and give it to the patient. If it was a prescription, the clinical staff might need to obtain the physician's signature on the prescription before giving it to the patient. If the patient was in the medical facility for an injury or an illness, the clinical staff will need to give the patient the aftercare instructions.

If you are already on the Clinic Status screen (shown below), then skip the next **Do This** section. If you are not on the Clinic Status screen, then do the next steps.

---

**Do This ▶**    **20.01** - Sign in to MedTrak

**20.02** - Click the *Clinic Status* button

---

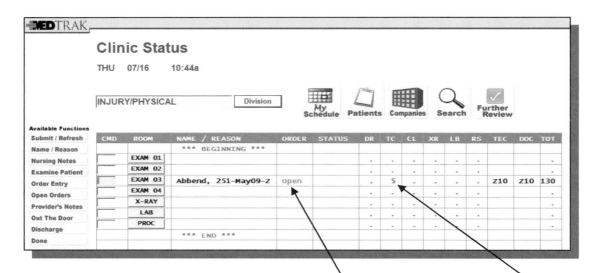

In this example, the physician placed an order for a left ankle appliance during the **Out the Door** process. That is why the **ORDER** column has the word Open in it with a time value of **5** minutes in the **TC** column on the Clinic Status screen (shown above).

The clinical staff places the cursor in the input field next to the patient and clicks the *Open Orders* button to see what orders need to be completed for the patient.

The Open Orders screen (shown below) appears, showing the clinical staff what needs to be done. In this example, the clinical staff needs to go to the procedure screens for the first three questions, so they enter an "**x**" in each of the data entry fields. Then the clinical staff enters the employee initials in the **Completed By** question. As you can see in this example, to save time the clinical staff answers each question before clicking the *Submit Answers* button.

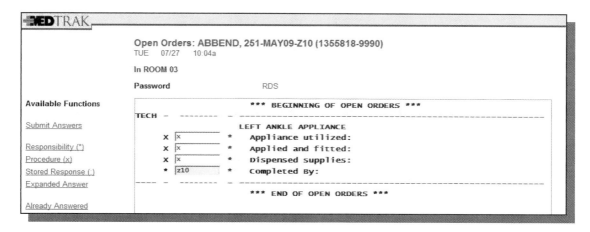

The next screen to appear is the procedure screen for the **Appliance Utilized** question (shown below). The clinical staff selects the **Md-Lace-up ankle brace** by typing an **x** in the data input field and clicking the *Submit* button.

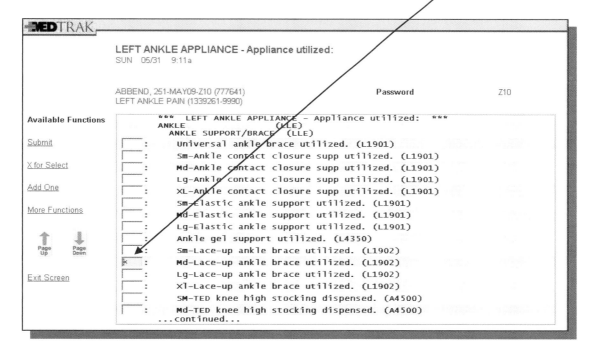

MedTrak records the selection of the brace and automatically advances to the next procedure selection screen for the Appliance Utilized because there are multiple screens of appliance choices.

The clinical staff clicks the *Exit Screen* button to go the **Applied and fitted** question (shown on the next page) in the workflow.

On this screen, the clinical staff selects the **Applied and fitted short leg appliance** option by typing an **x** in the data input field next to the option and clicking the *Submit* button.

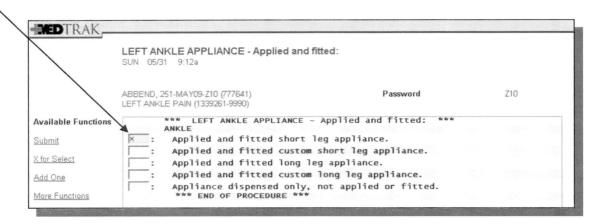

MedTrak records the selection of the **Applied and fitted** option and automatically advances to the procedure screen for the **Dispensed supplies** question (shown below).

On this screen, the clinical staff selects the **No other supplies dispensed** option by typing an **x** in the data input field next to the option and clicking the *Submit* button.

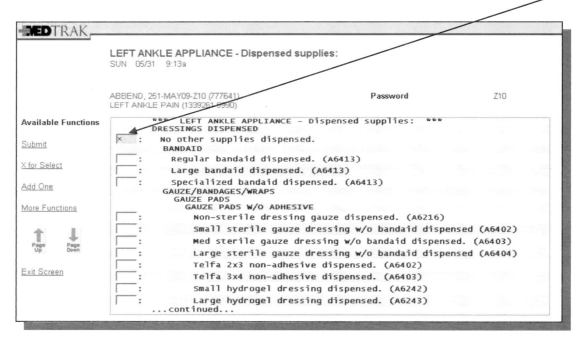

MedTrak records the selection of no dispensed supplies and automatically advances to the next procedure screen for the **Dispensed supplies**.

When the clinical staff clicks the *Exit Screen* button, MedTrak checks several conditions (rules) to see whether the patient is ready to be discharged from the clinic:

1. Has the physician finished the **Out the Door** process?
2. Are all open orders complete?

The **ORDER** column now has the word Done in it to indicate that there were open orders and they are now completed.

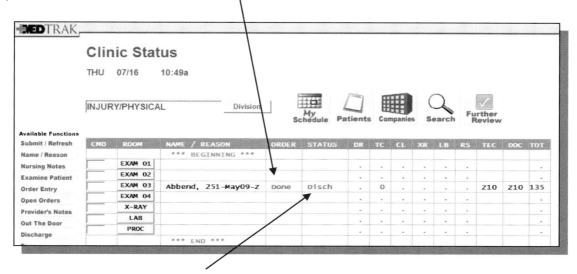

The workflow **STATUS** column has Disch in it to indicate to the clinical staff that the paperwork for this patient printed and is now ready to review with the patient and discharge the patient from the medical facility.

**Do This ▶**   **20.03** - Click the *Open Orders* button

**20.04** - Type in the following answers to the **Left ankle appliance** questions:

**Appliance utilized** - type an x

**Applied and fitted** - type an x

**Dispensed supplies** - type an x

**Completed by** - type your employee initials

**20.05** - Click the *Submit Answers* button

(you should be on the Appliance utilized procedure screen)

**20.06** - Type an x in the **Md-Lace-up ankle brace utilized** option

**20.07** - Click the *Submit* button

**20.08** - Click the *Exit Screen* button

(you should be on the Applied and fitted procedure screen)

**20.09** - Type an x in the **Applied and fitted short leg appliance** option

**20.10** - Click the *Submit* button

(you should be on the Dispensed supplies procedure screen)

**(go to the Do This box on the next page)**

**Do This** ▶ **20.11** - Type an **x** in the **No other supplies dispensed** option

**20.12** - Click the **Submit** button

**20.13** - Click the **Exit Screen** button
(you should be on the Clinic Status screen)

For their part in finishing the clinical portion of the workflow, it is the clinical staff's responsibility to:

♦ Retrieve the paperwork for the patient from the printer
♦ Retrieve dispensed medications from the cupboard (if ordered)
♦ Get the provider's signature on any prescription forms (if prescribed)
♦ Go back into the room to see the patient
♦ Review the aftercare instructions with the patient
♦ Review the medications (both prescription and dispensed) with the patient
♦ Review the charges with the patient (for patient responsibility visits only)
♦ Instruct the patient to stop back at the front desk for payment (for patient responsibility patients only)
♦ Discharge the patient from the Clinic Status screen

To discharge the patient from the Clinic Status screen, the clinical staff places the cursor in the entry field next to the patient and clicks the **Discharge** button to display the Discharging screen (shown below).

To discharge the patient, the clinical staff enters their password in the password entry field and clicks the **Submit** button. If the clinical staff has a global password, they just need to click the **Submit** button.

In this example, the employee has a **global password**, so the password and employee initials are automatically filled in. In the real clinical setting, the clinical staff typically shares Internet terminals that are in the common hallways, therefore the clinical staff will need to enter their employee password on this screen.

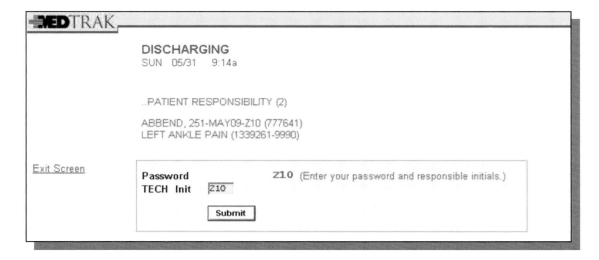

In this example, since this is a patient responsibility client, the Clinic Status screen (shown below) re-appears with the patient moved to the waiting room (front desk) for payment of services for the visit.

The workflow **STATUS** is now Done. This notifies the front desk person that the charges for the visit need to be reviewed with the patient, and reminds the front desk person to collect any monies due at this time.

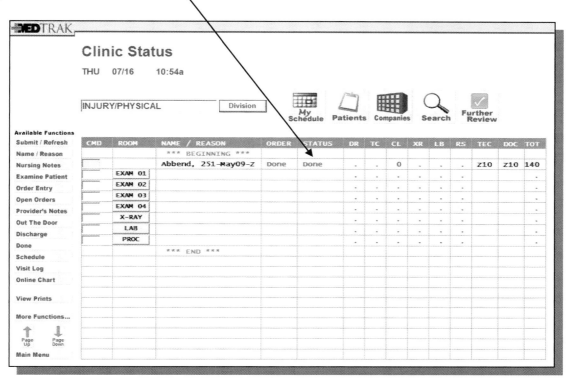

**Do This** ▶ **20.14** - Place the cursor next to your patient on the Clinic Status screen

**20.15** - Click the **Discharge** button

(you should be on the Discharging screen)

(you might need to enter your password and/or initials)

**20.16** - Click the **Submit** button

(you should be on the Clinic Status screen)

(your patient will be in the waiting room with a **STATUS** of Done)

# CHAPTER 21

# Front Desk - Payment Collection

**Estimated time needed to complete this chapter - 15** minutes

## What you need to know before doing this chapter

- How to log into MedTrak
- How to register a patient
- How to access Clinic Status off the Main Menu
- How to move a patient to a room and answer nursing notes
- How to use the Visit Documentation processor  (Out the Door)
- How to discharge the patient from the back examination area

## Learning outcomes gained from this chapter

- How to collect money at the front desk and finish the clinical part of the workflow

## Key terms used in this chapter

*occupational health reason*

*personal reason*

*co-payment*

*co-insurance*

*global billing period*

## Front Desk - Payment Collection

### Major Categories of Clinical Workflow

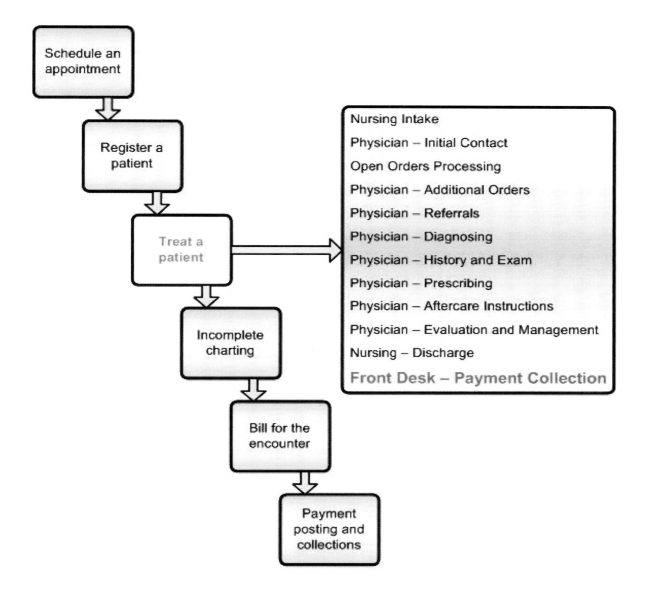

When the clinical staff finishes reviewing the paperwork with the patient, they discharge the patient from the back examination area. The physician scheduled the patient for his or her next appointment, and the clinical staff reviewed the patient's paperwork with him or her, so the only part of the patient's visit that remains is to collect any money due at this visit. The amount owed by the patient is known, since MedTrak accumulated the charges for the visit based on the clinical documentation by the physician and the clinical staff.

If the patient visited the medical facility for an *occupational health reason*, the bill for the visit will be sent to the employer or to the employer's insurance company. The patient, therefore, is not responsible for the charges for the visit and does not need to stop at the front desk.

If the patient visited the clinic for a *personal reason*, they are responsible for the charges for the visit (self pay), or the guarantor is responsible (the patient is under 18 years old), or the appropriate group health insurer will pay for the visit. All of the charges, some of the charges, or none of the charges for their patient responsibility visit will need to be paid when they leave the medical facility. The clinical staff provided these patients with a detailed listing of their charges and the amount that they are responsible to pay at this visit.

There are a variety of payment situations for patient responsibility patients:

♦ It is a self pay patient and they owe for all of the charges for the visit.

♦ The patient's insurance plan requires a *co-payment* for the physician's time.

♦ The patient's insurance plan requires that the patient pay for a percentage of the total cost for the visit, called a *co-insurance* amount.

♦ The patient owes both a co-payment and co-insurance amount.

♦ The patient does not owe anything (the group health insurer is billed for all charges).

♦ The visit is within a *global billing period* for a surgical procedure and there are no charges for this visit. Global billing periods are either 10 days or 90 days depending on the type of surgery. Any patient visits during the global billing period are included in the cost of the surgery unless the patient is diagnosed with another presenting problem that is not related to the surgery.

If you are already on the <u>Clinic Status</u> screen (shown below), then skip the next **Do This** section. If you are not on the <u>Clinic Status</u> screen, then do the next steps.

**Do This** ▶ **21.01** - Sign in to MedTrak

**21.02** - Click the *Clinic Status* button

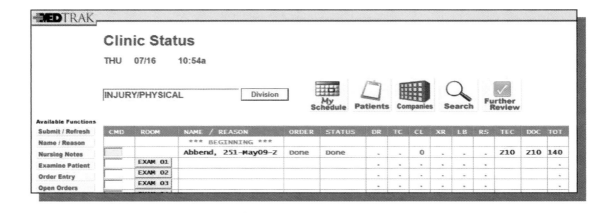

In this example, the front desk person places the cursor next to the patient and clicks the *Done* button.

The next screen to appear is the <u>Done</u> screen (shown below), displaying the total of the charges and the payment amount needed from the patient for the visit. This screen also has fields on it for the front desk to record the payment information.

If the patient does not make a payment and one is due, the front desk person will record why the patient did not pay anything in the **Payment Information Note** field.

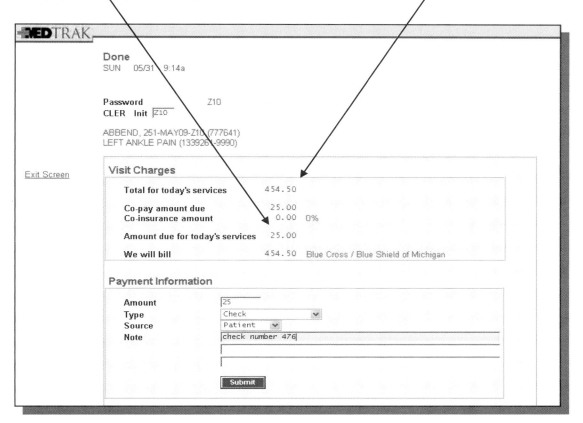

For this visit, the patient owes $25.00 for the co-payment of the level of service charge amount. Blue Cross/Blue Shield of Michigan will be billed for the full amount of the charges, but when the insurer pays, they will reduce their payment amount for the office visit by the co-payment amount due from the patient.

On this screen the front desk records the following payment information:

- ◆ **Amount** - $25.00 (this can be entered as 25 since the cents portion is zero)
- ◆ **Type** - Check
- ◆ **Source** - Patient
- ◆ **Note** - check number 476

Then the front desk clicks the *Submit* button to accept the payment information and automatically returns to the <u>Clinic Status</u> screen (shown on the next page).

The patient no longer appears on the screen because the clinical visit is done.

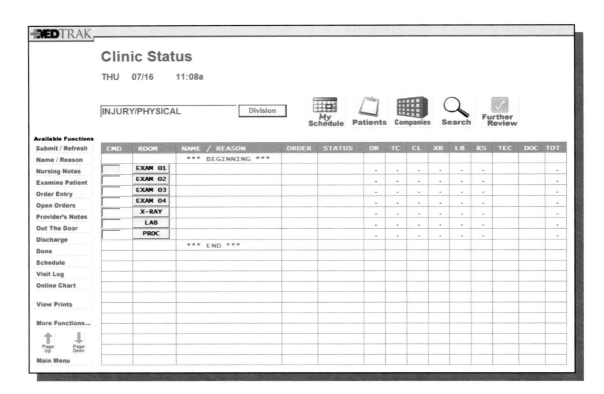

**Do This** ▶ **21.03** - Place the cursor next to your patient on the <u>Clinic Status</u> screen

**21.04** - Click the *Done* button

(you should be on the <u>Done</u> screen)

**21.05** - Enter the patient's co-payment information

(use the same information as shown on the previous page)

**21.06** - Click the *Submit* button

(you should be on the <u>Clinic Status</u> screen)

(your patient should not be on the screen)

# CHAPTER
# 22

# Pending Results

**Estimated time needed to complete this chapter  -  60** minutes

## What you need to know before doing this chapter

- How to log into MedTrak
- How to register a patient
- How to access Clinic Status off the Main Menu
- How to move a patient to a room and answer nursing notes
- How to use the Visit Documentation processor (Out the Door)
- How to discharge the patient from the back examination area
- How to collect the payment from the patient at the front desk

## Learning outcomes gained from this chapter

- How to process the incomplete charts using the **Pending** processors
- How to process a referral using the **Referral Dashboard**

## *Pending Results*

### Major Categories of Clinical Workflow

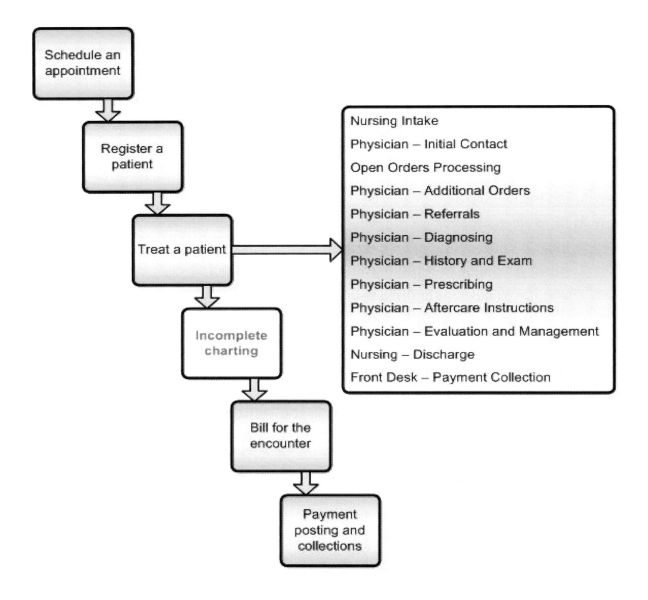

## *Pending Results*

When the patient leaves the healthcare facility, his or her clinical treatment for the visit is complete, but there could still be *results pending* for tests and treatments not provided at that facility. *Incomplete visits* are defined as patient encounters where results are pending for x-rays, laboratory tests, or treatments and opinions from referrals to specialists.

The importance of accurate and efficient tracking of results of outside testing and treatments cannot be overemphasized. If the physician does not review the results of an outside lab or an image or the opinion of a specialist in a timely fashion, the patient's health could be at risk. If the administrative staff enters the outside test results in the patient's chart and does not notify the physician that the results are back, the patient's treatment for a serious medical problem will be delayed. Every step in the patient's treatment could be perfect, but the simple misfiling of test results or the lack of notification to the physician that the test results are back could cancel all of the positive effects of the patient's care. Every step in the patient's care is important, right down to the simple process of filing and notification of test results.

MedTrak's **Pending** module also provides functionality to manage billing issues, track referrals, manage the authorization process for surgical procedures, and review company demographic changes.

To access the Pending Menu (shown below), the user signs into MedTrak and clicks the *Pending Menu* tab at the top of the screen.

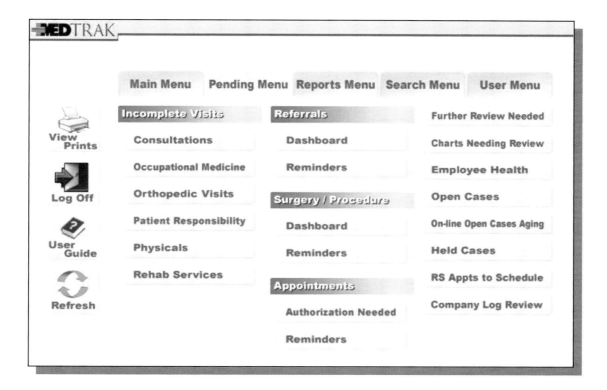

From the Pending Menu, the user can access:

◆ **Incomplete visit** processors for tracking the administrative functions of chart completion:

    ◆ **Consultations** - for patients referred to a consultant or specialist.

    ◆ **Occupational Medicine** - for employees injured on the job.

    ◆ **Orthopedic Visits** - for orthopedic medicine.

    ◆ **Patient responsibility** - for visits that will be paid by the patient, a guarantor, or patient's group health insurance.

    ◆ **Physicals** - for employee physical examinations and drug screen visits.

    ◆ **Rehab Services** - for physical therapy and occupational therapy visits.

◆ **Referrals,** including the referral dashboard and referral reminders.

◆ **Surgery/Procedure** authorizations needed, including the surgery/procedure dashboard and surgery/procedure reminders.

◆ **Appointments** needing authorization processor and authorization reminders.

◆ **Further Review Needed** processor for the healthcare facility.

◆ **Charts Needing Review** - these are encounters seen by physician's assistants and nurse practitioners that need to be reviewed by the supervising physician of the healthcare facilities before billing to the payer.

◆ **Employee Health** - this dashboard tracks the employee health needs by employer based on the care rules of the employer. Each employee of a healthcare facility needs to have a TB test on an annual basis. This is an example of a care rule.

◆ **Open Cases** - this processor tracks the open workers' compensation cases. The clinical staff uses this processor to administratively close cases where the patients did not return for their scheduled appointments.

◆ **On-line Open Cases Aging** - using this processor the clinical staff monitors the length of time that the workers' compensation cases have been open to ensure that the patients are receiving appropriate continuum of care.

◆ **RS Appts to Schedule** - using this processor the administrative staff manages the appointment authorization process for referrals to in-house rehab services.

◆ **Company Log Review** - using this processor the administrative staff reviews the demographic changes to the employer's information for accuracy and thoroughness. The billing module holds up billing for employers with demographic changes until the administrative staff completes the log review process.

In the example in this book, the physician ordered an overread for the left ankle x-ray. The x-ray overread is performed by a radiologist at another facility, and the results of the overread communicated back to the physician, either by mail, by fax, by secure email, or electronically through a data transfer between their respective EMR systems.

The physician also referred the patient to an orthopedic surgeon for additional examination, to treat the left ankle, and to communicate the findings and treatment back to the physician.

## Incomplete Visits

Typically, within a day or two, the radiologist will finish reading the x-ray and communicate the results back to the clinic. When the results arrive back at the clinic, the clinical staff enters the information in the x-ray overread order in MedTrak.

To locate the unfinished x-ray order, the clinical staff accesses the Pending Menu (shown two pages before this one) off the MedTrak Main Menu. Since this is a patient responsibility patient, the clinical staff then clicks the *Patient Responsibility* button in the **Incomplete Visits** section on the Pending Menu. The next screen to appear is the Incomplete Patient Responsibility screen (shown below).

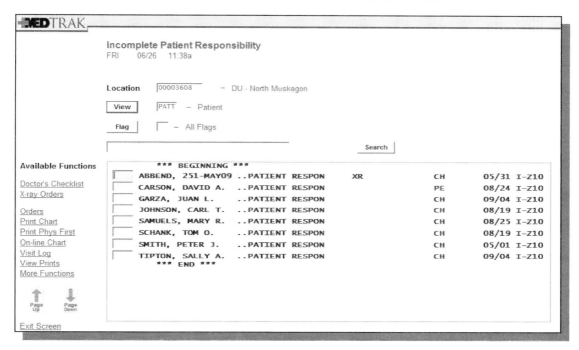

The initial view for this screen is alphabetical by the patient's last name for the location that the user signed in to. To find your patient, you can reset the **View** to be by date of service. The view by company is only for workers' compensation cases.

All of the incomplete visits screens list the patients, the employer (or patient responsibility), the flags representing what is still incomplete for the visit, the date of service, the type of visit (initial - I, or return - R) and the employee initials of the provider.

## Incomplete Flags

Each of the Incomplete Visits screens uses "flag" to indicate what is still pending for the visit. For example, **XR** is used to identify that an x-ray is incomplete for the visit. When these flags are used on multiple types of incomplete visit screens, they indicate the same reason for the visit being incomplete.

These flags represent the incomplete steps in the processing of the patient's visit. When the clerical staff completes a step represented by one of the flags, the flag clears from line. Once all of the flags clear, the patient drops off the processing screen because all of the steps are now done.

The following table lists the incomplete visit flags and what screens use them:

| Flag | Description | Where Used | | | | | |
|------|-------------|------------|---|---|---|---|---|
| | | Occ Med | PE | Con-sult | RS | Ortho | Patient Resp |
| AU | Visit still needs authorization | 📂 | 📂 | 📂 | 📂 | 📂 | 📂 |
| XR | X-ray (complete the x-ray orders) | 📂 | 📂 | 📂 | 📂 | 📂 | 📂 |
| LB | Laboratory (complete the lab orders) | 📂 | 📂 | 📂 | 📂 | 📂 | 📂 |
| OR | Orders (complete orders other than x-ray or lab) | 📂 | 📂 | 📂 | 📂 | 📂 | 📂 |
| CL | Complete the physician's history and exam questions | 📂 | 📂 | 📂 | 📂 | 📂 | 📂 |
| PF | Print the physician's first report | 🖨 | | | | | |
| CH | Print the patient's chart for filing | 🖨 | 🖨 | 🖨 | 🖨 | 🖨 | 🖨 |
| DS | Print the discharge summary | 🖨 | | | 🖨 | | 🖨 |
| PF | Print physician's first report | 🖨 | | | | | |
| P2 | Print physician's progress report | 🖨 | | | | | |
| PE | Print physical exam report | | 🖨 | | | | |
| MC | Print the medical clearance | | 🖨 | | | | |
| MH | Patient is on medical hold waiting further information | | 📂 | | | | 📂 |
| CN | Complete the referral order | | | 📂 | | | |
| PRCN | Print the consultant referral letter | | | 🖨 | | | |
| RN | Print the rehab services notes | | | | 🖨 | | |

📂 = Complete the order(s) or history and exam questions   🖨 = Print a report

As can be seen on the Incomplete Patient Responsibility screen (on the previous page), the patient in this example has two flags. The **XR** flag represents the incomplete overread of the left ankle x-ray. The **CH** flag represents that after completing the x-ray overread, the clinical staff needs to print the chart for the paper file.

Healthcare facilities whose goal is to be paperless do not use the **CH** flag to print the patient's chart. They eliminate this step in their chart processing because they do not have a paper file of information for the patient.

To enter the results of the overread by the radiologist, the clinical staff places the cursor in the command field for the patient and clicks the *X-ray Orders* button. The next screen to appear is the x-ray section of the <u>Orders</u> screen (shown below).

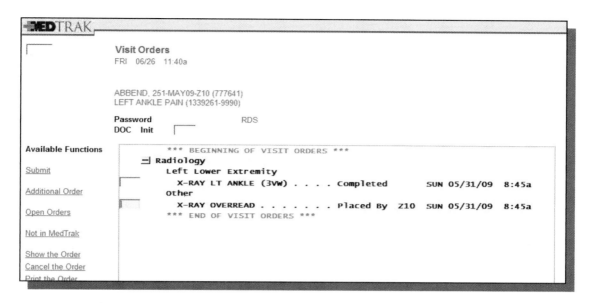

The **X-ray Lt Ankle** x-ray was completed while the patient was in the clinic. The **X-ray Overread** order is still incomplete and shows as being placed. The clerical staff places the cursor in the command field for the overread and clicks the *Show the Order* button. The next screen to appear is the <u>X-ray Overread</u> details screen (shown below).

```
MEDTRAK

              X-RAY OVERREAD (10830) - 05/31/09
              FRI    06/26   11:41a
              DU - North Muskegon

               PATIENT RESPONSIBILITY (2)
              ABBEND, 251-MAY09-Z10 (777641)
              LEFT ANKLE PAIN (1339261-9990)

              Password              RDS
              Function    [      ]

Available Functions            ***   X-RAY OVERREAD   ***
                               TECHNICIAN
Submit Answers      : [*     ] *    X-ray type:  X-Ray Lt Ankle (3vw)
                    : [464646]      X-ray number:  464646
Responsibility (*)  : [Acme Xray] *  X-ray sent to:  Acme Xray
                    * [*     ] *    X-ray prepared by:  Z10 - MEDTRAK - RDS
Procedure (x)                  CLERICAL
                    : [      ] *    Report return date:  n/a
Stored Resp (:)     : [      ] *    Narrative:  n/a
                    : [      ] *    Summary:  n/a
Expanded Answer                RADIOLOGIST
                    * [      ] *    Radiologist:  n/a
View Prints                    PHYSICIAN
                    * [      ] *    Reviewed By:  n/a
Info                                ***  END OF ORDER  ***

      ↑        ↓
    Page     Page
     Up      Down
Exit Screen
```

The clerical staff enters information on this screen and presses the *ENTER* key (as shown on the next page).

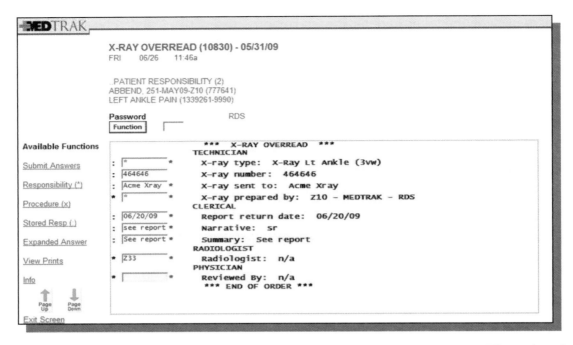

The clerical staff enters the date the radiologist report arrived back at the clinic. Then the clerical staff scans the radiologist report and attaches it to the patient's case. In the **Narrative** and **Summary** data entry fields, the clerical staff enters **sr** (the trigger for **See report**). Then they enter **Z33** for the initials of the radiologist. If the clinical staff did not know the radiologists initials, they would use the *F1* key in the data input field to display the help screen. After entering the data, the clerical staff clicks the *Submit Answers* button to accept the answers. The X-ray Overread details screen (shown below) refreshes with the answers showing to the right of the questions.

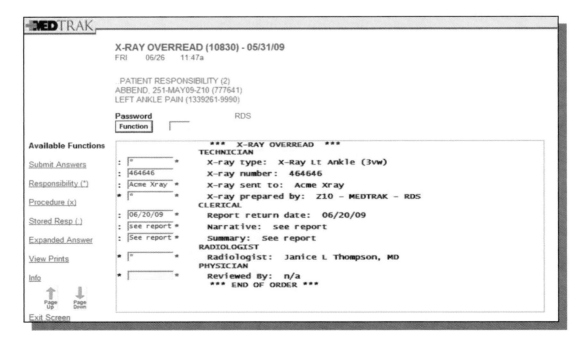

The remaining step in the clinical workflow is for the ordering physician to review the narrative and summary from the radiologist.

The clerical staff exits the X-ray Overread details screen and returns to the x-ray section of the Orders screen (shown below). The **X-ray Overread** order is still incomplete because the ordering physician needs to review the radiologist report.

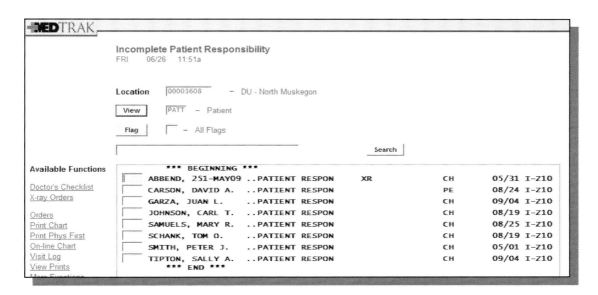

The clerical staff exits the Visit Orders screen to return to the Incomplete Patient Responsibility screen (shown below) to process the next results report that the clinic received.

Once the physician reviews the radiologist's report, the **XR** flag will automatically clear and the clerical staff will print the chart to clear the patient from the incomplete processing screen.

---

**Do This ▶** **22.01** - Sign in to MedTrak

　　　　　　**22.02** - Click the *Pending* tab at the top of the screen
　　　　　　　　　　　(you should be on the Pending Menu)

---

**Do This** ▶ **22.03** - Click the *Incomplete Visits/Patient Responsibility* button
(you should be on the Incomplete Patient Responsibility screen)

**22.04** - Place the cursor next to your patient

**22.05** - Click the *X-ray Orders* button

**22.06** - Place the cursor next to the **X-ray Overread** order

**22.07** - Click the *Show the Order* button

**22.08** - Type in the following answers to the **X-ray Overread** questions:

**Report return date** - type in today's date

**Narrative** - type the **sr** trigger (for **See report**)

**Summary** - type the **sr** trigger (for **See report**)

**Radiologist** - type the **Z33** radiologist's initials

(do not answer the **Reviewed by** at this time)

**22.09** - Click the *Submit Answers* button
(review your answers)

**22.10** - Click the *Exit Screen* button
(you should be on the Visit Orders screen for x-rays)

**22.11** - Click the *Exit Screen* button
(you should be on the Incomplete Patient Responsibility)

**22.12** - Click the *Exit Screen* button
(you should be on the Pending Menu)

The clinical workflow disciplines for the overread of the x-ray called for the clinical staff to prepare the x-ray to be sent out to the radiologist, then the clerical staff to record the results of the radiologist's read of the x-ray. The final step is for the ordering physician to read the radiologist's report.

## Further Review Needed

MedTrak alerts the ordering physician that the overread of the x-ray by the radiologist is back and ready for them to review by placing an entry on the physician's Further Review Needed processor.

To access the Further Review Needed processor, the physician can click the *Further Review* button on the Clinic Status screen or click the *Further Review Needed* button on the Pending Menu.

For this example, the physician clicks the *Further Review Needed* button on the Pending Menu to display the Further Review Needed processor (shown on the next page).

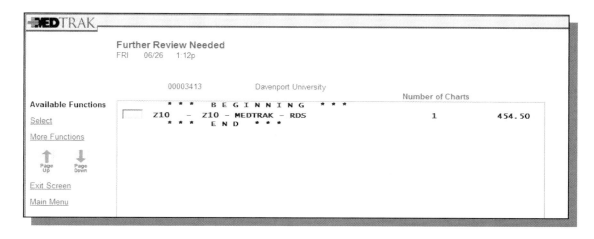

This processor displays the names of all of the staff of the medical facility that have action items that need further review. These items could involve one of the following:

♦ X-ray overread results

♦ Lab results

♦ Referring treatment results

♦ Questions about a referral

♦ Questions concerning the billing

♦ Any other question about a case from another staff member

In this example, the ordering physician has only one chart representing a billing of $454.50 to review. To review the chart, the physician places the cursor in the command field next to his or her name and clicks the *Select* button. The next screen to appear is the Further Review Needed detail listing screen (shown below).

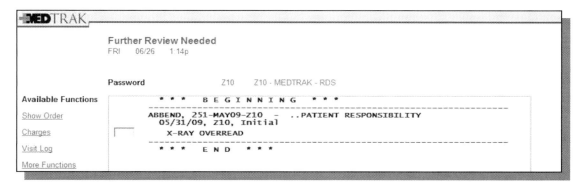

To review the **X-ray Overread** order, the physician places the cursor in the command field next to it and clicks the *Show Order* button.

The next screen to appear is the X-ray Overread details screen (shown on the next page).

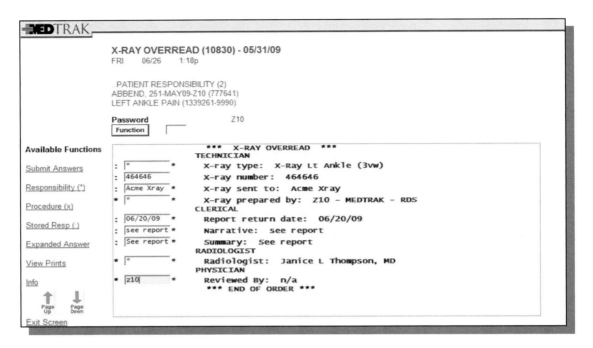

After reviewing the radiologist report by pulling up the scanned document, the physician enters his or her initials in the **Reviewed By** data entry field and clicks the *Submit Answers* button (as shown above).

The X-ray Overread order details screen refreshes with the physician's name next to the **Reviewed By** question. After reviewing the screen, the physician clicks the *Exit Screen* button to return to the Further Review Needed details processor (shown below).

Since this was the only further review needed by the physician, the Further Review Needed screen is clear.

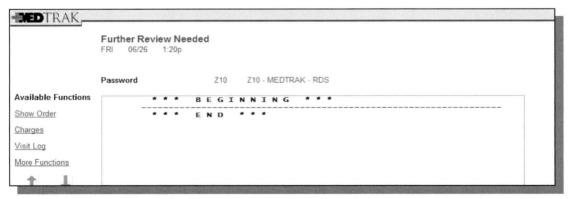

The physician clicks the *Exit Screen* button on this screen to return to the Further Review Needed summary screen. Since the physician only had one entry, this screen does not display his or her name.

The physician clicks the *Exit Screen* button again to return to the Pending Menu.

**Do This** ▶ **22.13** - Click the *Further Review Needed* button

(from the Pending Menu)

**22.14** - Place the cursor next to your physician

**22.15** - Click the *Select* button

**22.16** - Place the cursor next to the **X-ray Overread** order

**22.17** - Click the *Show Order* button

**22.18** - Type in the following answer to the **X-ray Overread** questions:

**Reviewed By** - type your initials

**22.19** - Click the *Submit Answers* button

(review your answer - this clears the **XR** flag)

**22.20** - Click the *Exit Screen* button

(you should be on Further Review Needed details)

**22.21** - Click the *Exit Screen* button

(you should be on Further Review Needed summary)

**22.22** - Click the *Exit Screen* button

(you should be on the Pending Menu)

## *Referrals to Specialists*

When a physician refers a patient to see a specialist or to have a scheduled test (like an MRI or Cat scan), an order is placed for a referral.

In this order, the physician documents:

- ◆ the body part or parts needing examination and/or treatment

- ◆ any special notes about the patient's referral that the specialist should know about

- ◆ how soon the visit to the specialist needs to happen

- ◆ whether the referral is for evaluation only, for evaluation and treatment, or to have the specialist take over the patient's care

Once the physician places the referral, the order appears on the Referrals Dashboard (shown on the next page) for processing by the clinical staff. To access the Referrals Dashboard, the clinical staff clicks the Pending Menu tab on the MedTrak Main Menu and then the *Dashboard* button in the **Referrals** section of the Pending Menu.

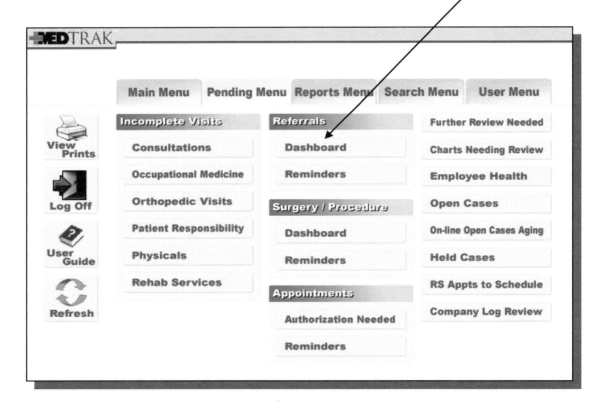

**Do This** ▶ **22.23** - Click the *Pending* tab at the top of the MedTrak Main Menu screen
(you should be on the Pending Menu)

**22.24** - Click the *Referrals Dashboard* button

The totals on the <u>Referrals Dashboard</u> (shown below) represent the total number of referrals that are:

- ◆ **Pending** - awaiting approval or denial by the payer
- ◆ **Approved** - approved by the payer and now needing to be scheduled
- ◆ **Denied** - denied by the payer; the clinical staff will record the denial reason
- ◆ **Scheduled** - scheduled to see the specialist and waiting for the specialist's report
- ◆ **Completed** - patient has seen the specialist and the report is ready for review
- ◆ **Reviewed** - the physician reviewed the specialist's report and the referral can be closed

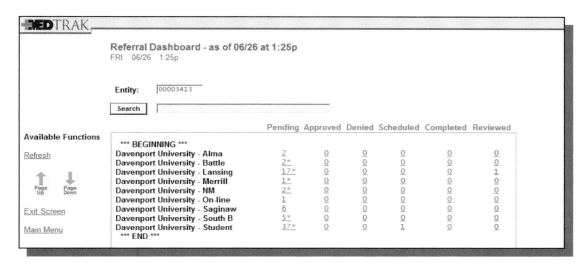

To display the individual referrals that make up the total, the clinical staff clicks on the number. The next screen to appear is the <u>Referrals</u> detail screen (shown on the next page), listing the referrals. This screen displays:

- ◆ **Location** - this can be changed by selecting a different location on the dashboard
- ◆ **Status** - this can be changed to display a different status
- ◆ **View** - the view of the referral can be by date ordered, scheduled date, company, patient, and type of consultant.
- ◆ **Search** - to quickly search for a referral based on the type of view
- ◆ **Date ordered** - based on the date that the physician ordered the referral
- ◆ **Patient name** - name of the patient
- ◆ **Type of referral** - type of specialist the patient is to see
- ◆ **Referral status** - the current status of the referral

From this screen the clinical staff can use the buttons to:

- ◆ **Select -** displays the questions for the referral
- ◆ **Visit Log** - displays the visit log for the patient's encounter
- ◆ **Case** - displays the case information
- ◆ **Visit** - displays the visit information
- ◆ **Notes** - displays the notes about the referral
- ◆ **Reminders** - displays the reminders about the referral

In this example, the physician placed the orthopedic referral while working at the North Muskegon (NM) clinic location. To display the two individual referrals for that location (shown below), the clinical staff clicks the **2*** in the **Pending** column for the **Davenport  -  NM** location on the Referral dashboard (shown on the previous page). The asterisk (*) next to the number indicates to the clinical staff that there is a referral that needs immediate (stat) attention.

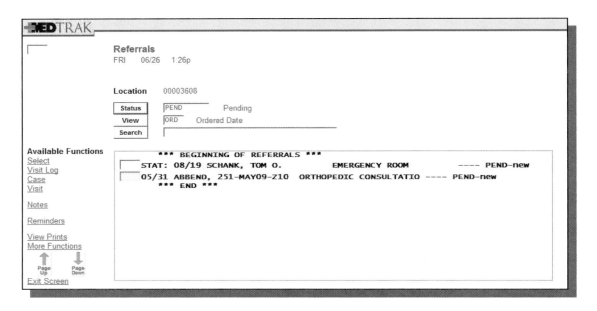

Then the clinical staff places the cursor in the command field next to the patient's orthopedic consultation order and clicks the *Select* button. The next screen to appear is the Orthopedic Consultation details screen (shown below). This is the first detail screen that displays the individual questions that need answering to process and complete the referral.

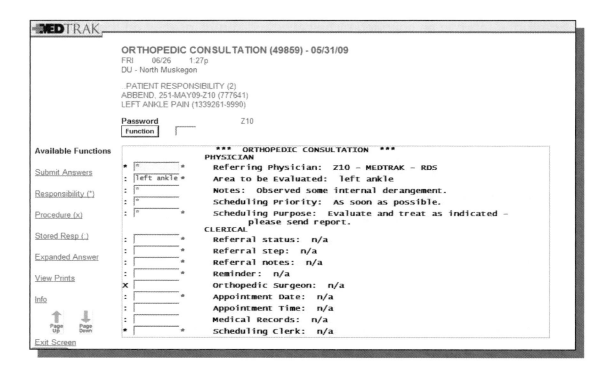

The referral order detail screen displays:

- Header - the header contains the:
    - Referral order name
    - Date ordered
    - Clinic location
    - Company name (if workers' compensation)
    - Patient name
    - Chief complaint
- Function field - this command field allows access to many other functions
- Order details:

    Physician questions:
    - **Referring physician** - name of the physician who ordered the referral.
    - **Notes** - any special notes about the referral from the physician.
    - **Scheduling priority** - when the physician wants the patient to be seen.
    - **Scheduling purpose** (must be one of these options)
        - evaluation only
        - or, evaluation and treatment
        - or, the physician is transferring the patient's care to the specialist

    Clinical staff questions:
    - **Referral status** - either the referral is awaiting authorization, is approved, or is denied.
        - Answering **approved** to this question moves the referral to the **Approved** column on the Referral Dashboard.
        - Answering **denied** to this question moves the referral to the **Denied** column on the Referral Dashboard.
        - Answering **awaiting authorization** leaves the referral in the **Pending** column as you wait for authorization action.
    - **Referral step** - allows staging of the referrals that are in the **Pending** column.
        - Additional information is required before approval or denial by the payer.
        - Clinical assistance is needed to clarify something. The clinical staff uses the FRN (Further Review Needed) order to send a message back to the clinician.
        - A call to the employer is needed to clarify something.
        - A call to the payer is needed.
        - The clinical staff needs to contact the ordering provider.
        - Utilization review is needed.
        - This is a new referral with no steps toward approval taken as yet.
    - **Referral notes** - this field is used to record the notes related to obtaining approval.
    - **Reminder** - this field is used to set up a reminder (tickler) for follow-up for the referral. If the clinical staff enters a "**y**" in this field, the reminder note screen will appear for setting up the reminder.

- ◆ **Orthopedic surgeon** - the user selects the orthopedic surgeon from the list of consultants.

- ◆ **Appointment date** - once the appointment is set, the clinical staff records the date.

- ◆ **Appointment time** - the appointment time is recorded here.

- ◆ **Medical records** - used to indicate whether the patient needs to bring medical records to the appointment.

- ◆ **Scheduling clerk** - the clinical staff member who scheduled the appointment enters his or her employee initials in this field.

  Answering this question moves the referral to the **Scheduled** column on the Referral Dashboard.

- ◆ **Consultant report return** - the date the consultant sent the report back to the clinic

- ◆ **Consultant summary** - the results of the consultant examination are recorded in this question. The "**sr**" trigger is used if the consultant report is scanned and attached.

  Answering this question moves the referral to the **Completed** column on the Referral Dashboard.

Physician question:

- ◆ **Physician review** - the physician enters his or her initials in this field once the consultant report has been reviewed using the Further Review Needed processor.

  Answering this question moves the referral to the **Reviewed** column on the Referral Dashboard.

In this example, the clinical staff member entered the following on the detail screen (shown below).

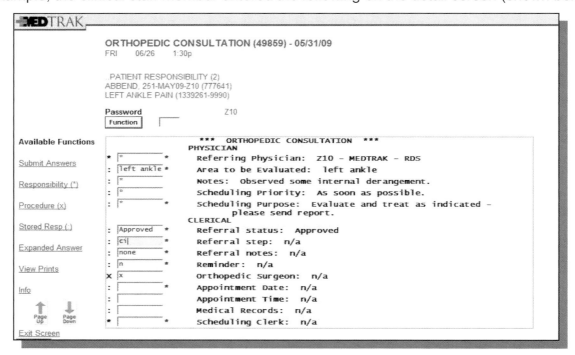

The "x" entered in the **Orthopedic Surgeon** data entry field will display the Consultant Select screen (shown on the next page).

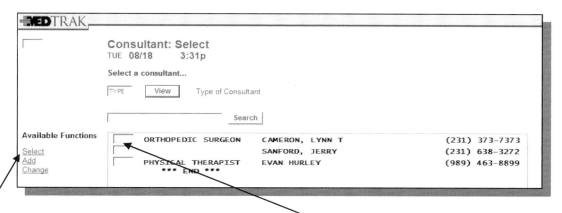

The clinical staff member places the cursor in the command field next to Cameron and clicks the *Select* button. The detail questions screen (shown below) refreshes with the consultant selected.

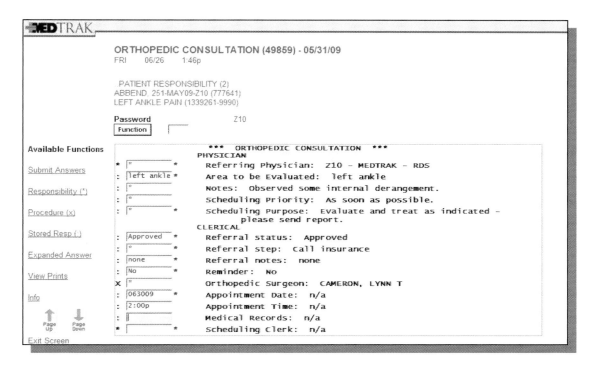

A member of the clinical staff enters an appointment date and time. Then he or she indicates in the **Medical Records** question that the patient is to bring his or her x-rays to the appointment. To finish their part of the questions, the clinical staff enters their employee initials in the **Scheduling Clerk** data entry field. This completes the questions for the clinical staff until the consultant sends their report back to the clinic.

After answering the **Scheduling Clerk** question, the referral moves to the **Scheduled** column on the Referral Dashboard.

**Do This** ▶ **22.25** - Click the total amount in the **Pending** column for your clinic location

**22.26** - Place the cursor next to your orthopedic consultation referral

**22.27** - Click the *Select* button

**22.28** - Answer these questions for the **Orthopedic Consultation** order:

Type **a** in the **Referral status** question (approved)

Type **ci** in the **Referral step** question (call insurance)

Type **none** in the **Referral notes** question

Type **n** in the **Reminder** question (no reminder needed)

Type **x** in the **Orthopedic surgeon** question

**22.29** - Click the *Submit Answers* button

**22.30** - Place the cursor next to the orthopedic consultant  -  **Lynn Cameron**

**22.31** - Type an **x** and press the *ENTER* key

(you should be on your orthopedic consultation referral)

**22.32** - Answer these questions for the **Orthopedic Consultation** order:

Type today's date in the **Appointment date** question

Type **12:00p** in the **Appointment time** question

Type **xr** in the **Medical records** question

Type your employee initials in the **Scheduling** clerk question

**22.33** - Click the *Submit Answers* button

(review your answers; this moves the referral to **Scheduled**)

**22.34** - Click the *Exit Screen* button

(you should be on the Referrals screen)

**22.35** - Click the *Exit Screen* button

(you should be on the Referral Dashboard)

**22.36** - Review the totals on the dashboard

(your referral should now be in the **Scheduled** column)

## *After the Referral Visit*

After the patient's referral visit for examination and possible treatment, the referral specialist will report back to the referring physician. When the report arrives back at the clinic, the clinical staff enters the information in the referral order in MedTrak.

To locate the unfinished orthopedic consultation order, the clinical staff accesses the Pending Menu off the MedTrak Main Menu. The clinical staff then clicks the *Referrals Dashboard* button on the Pending menu. The next screen to appear is the Referral Dashboard (shown below).

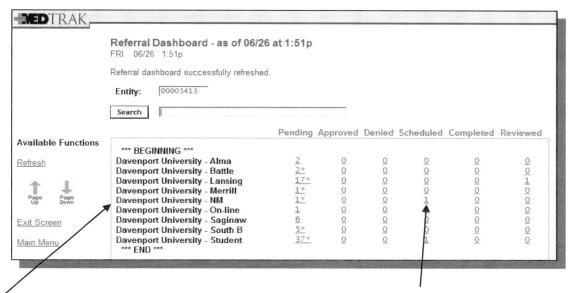

To display the orthopedic consultation order, the clinical staff clicks the **1** in the **Scheduled** column for the **NM** location. The next screen to appear is the Referrals screen (shown below) for the scheduled referrals for the NM location. In this example, there is only one.

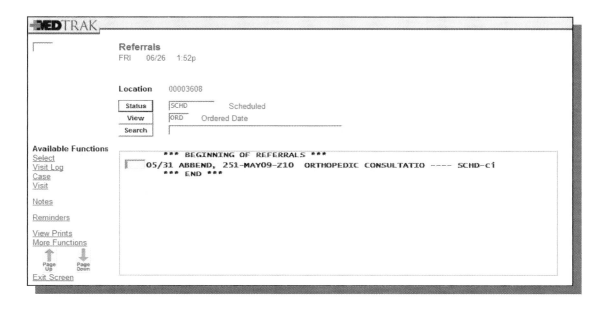

The clinical staff places the cursor next to the orthopedic consultation order and clicks the *Select* button to display the detail questions (shown below).

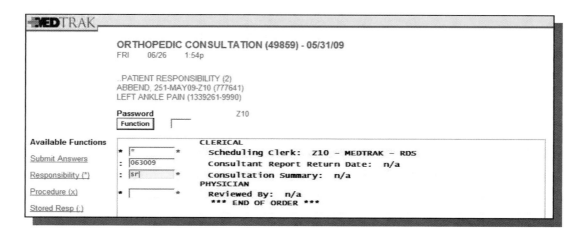

To display the next referral detail screen (shown below), the clinical staff clicks the *Page Down* button.

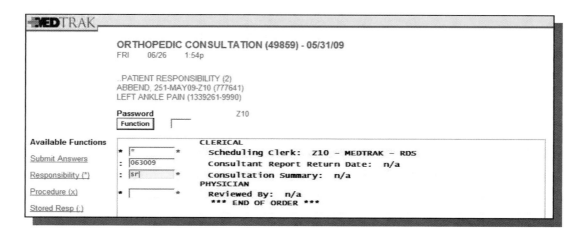

On this screen the clinical staff enters the date that the consultant report arrived at the clinic. Then they scan the report and attach the scanned report to the patient. In the **Consultant Summary** question's data entry field, the clinical staff types the **sr** trigger for the **See report** stored response, and then clicks the *Submit Answers* button.

The screen refreshes, with the answers to the two questions displaying. The clinical staff exits the screen to return to process the next referral. Answering the consultant report summary information automatically moves the referral to the **Completed** column on the Referral dashboard. The dashboard must be refreshed by clicking the *Refresh Totals* button for this to show.

**Do This** ▶ **22.37** - Click the total amount in the **Scheduled** column for your location

**22.38** - Place the cursor next to your orthopedic consultation referral

**22.39** - Click the *Select* button

**22.40** - Click the *Page Down* button

**22.41** - Answer these questions for the **Orthopedic Consultation** order
**Consultant Report Return Date** - type in today's date
**Consultant Summary** - type in **sr** (for **See report**)
(do not answer the **Reviewed by** at this time)

**22.42** - Click the *Submit Answers* button
(review your answers - this moves the referral to **Completed**)

**22.43** - Click the *Exit Screen* button
(you should be on the <u>Referrals</u> screen)

**22.44** - Click the *Exit Screen* button
(you should be on the <u>Referral Dashboard</u>)

**22.45** - Review the totals on the dashboard
(your referral should now be in the **Completed** column)

**22.46** - Click the *Exit Screen* button
(you should be on the <u>Pending Menu</u>)

## Further Review Needed

MedTrak alerts the ordering physician that the report from the orthopedic consultant is back and ready for review by placing an entry on the physician's <u>Further Review Needed</u> processor.

To access the <u>Further Review Needed</u> processor, the physician can click the *Further Review* button on the <u>Clinic Status</u> screen or click the *Further Review Needed* button on the <u>Pending Menu</u>.

For this example, the physician clicks the *Further Review Needed* button on the <u>Pending Menu</u> to display the <u>Further Review Needed</u> processor (shown below).

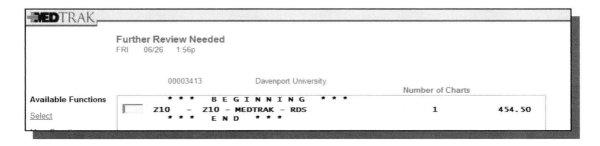

In this example, the ordering physician has only one chart representing a billing of $454.50 to review. To review the chart, the physician places the cursor in the command field next to the name and clicks the *Select* button. The next screen to appear is the Further Review Needed detail listing screen (shown below).

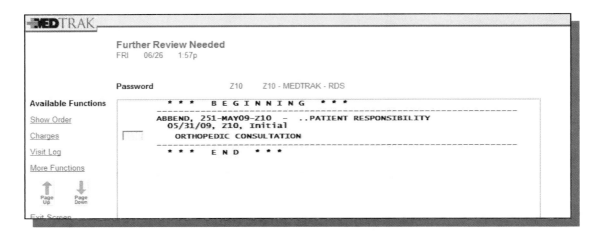

To review the **Orthopedic Consultation** order, the physician places the cursor in the command field next to it and clicks the *Show Order* button. The physician then clicks the *Page Down* button on the Orthopedic Consultation details screen to move to the second screen of questions.

The next screen to appear is the Orthopedic Consultation details screen (shown below).

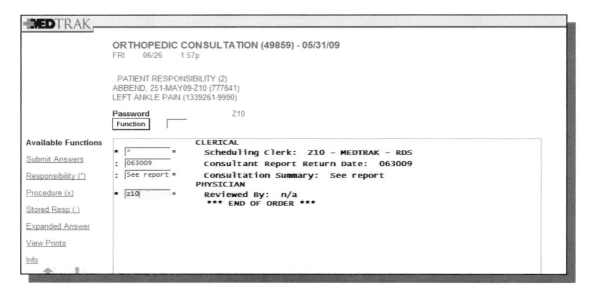

After reviewing the orthopedic surgeon's report by pulling up the scanned document, the physician enters his or her initials in the **Reviewed By** data entry field and clicks the *Submit Answers* button (as shown above).

The Orthopedic Consultation order details screen refreshes with the physician's name next to the **Reviewed By** question.

The physician then clicks the *Exit Screen* button to return to the Further Review Needed details processor (shown on the next page).

Since this was the only further review needed by the physician, the <u>Further Review Needed</u> screen is clear.

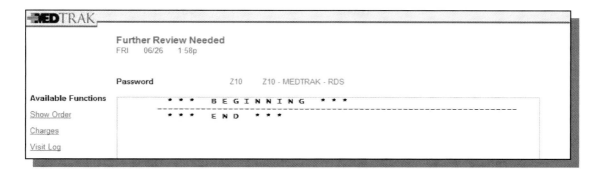

The physician clicks the *Exit Screen* button on this screen to return to the <u>Further Review Needed</u> summary screen. Because the physician only had one entry, this screen does not display his or her name.

The physician clicks the *Exit Screen* button again to return to the <u>Pending Menu</u>.

**Do This** ►

**22.47** - Click the *Further Review Needed* button
(from the Pending Menu)
(you should be on <u>Further Review Needed</u> summary screen)

**22.48** - Place the cursor next to your physician (it is your name)

**22.49** - Click the *Select* button

**22.50** - Place the cursor next to the **Orthopedic Consultation** order

**22.51** - Click the *Show Order* button
(you should be on the <u>Orthopedic Consultation</u> details screen)

**22.52** - Click the *Page Down* button

**22.53** - Type in the following answer for **Orthopedic Consultation**
(type your initials in the **Reviewed By** question)

**22.54** - Click the *Submit Answers* button
(this moves the referral to the **Reviewed** column)

**22.55** - Click the *Exit Screen* button
(you should be on the <u>Further Review Needed</u> details screen)

**22.56** - Click the *Exit Screen* button
(you should be on the <u>Further Review Needed</u> summary screen)

**22.57** - Click the *Exit Screen* button
(you should be on the <u>Pending Menu</u>)

## Closing the Referral

Once the physician has reviewed the consultant's report, the referral is now in the **Reviewed** column on the Referral Dashboard. The clinical staff can now close the referral because it is completed.

To close the referral, the clinical staff accesses the Referral Dashboard (shown below) off the Pending Menu. Then the clinical staff clicks on the totals number in the **Reviewed** column for the clinic location. In this example, there is only one referral in the **Reviewed** column.

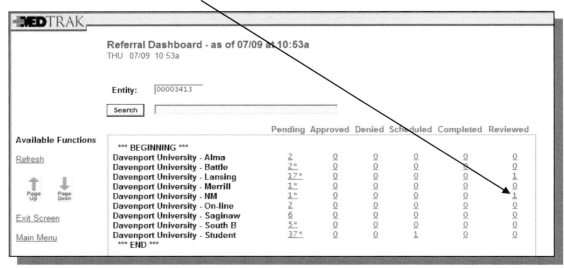

The next screen to appear is the Referrals screen (shown below) listing the referral from the **Reviewed** column.

To close the referral and clear it from the Referral Dashboard, the clinical staff types **clos** in the command field and presses the *ENTER* key.

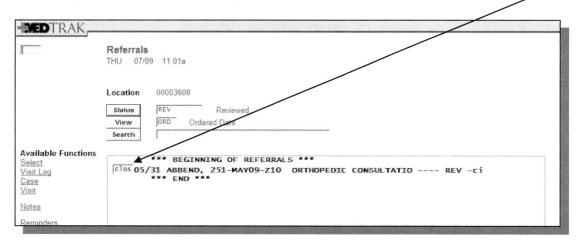

The Referrals screen refreshes with the orthopedic referral cleared off the screen. If the clinical staff has more referrals to close, they do so at this time. When done, the clinical staff exits the screen to return to the Referral Dashboard to continue processing other referrals. Refreshing the Referral dashboard clears the orthopedic referral from the dashboard.

**Do This** ▶ **22.58** - Click the *Dashboard* button in the **Referral** section

(from the Pending Menu)

(you should be on Referral dashboard)

**22.59** - Click the number in the **Reviewed** column for your clinic location

**22.60** - Place the cursor next to the **Orthopedic Consultation** order

**22.61** - Type the **clos** command in the command field for your referral

**22.62** - Press the *ENTER* key

(the screen refreshes with your referral removed)

**22.63** - Click the *Exit Screen* button

(you should be on Referral dashboard)

**22.64** - Review the totals on the dashboard

(your referral should be removed from the **Reviewed** column)

**22.65** - Click the *Exit Screen* button

(you should be on the Pending Menu)

## Printing the Chart

For this example, the last step in the pending results processing for this encounter is to print the patient's chart for placing it in the paper folder. Remember, electronic medical record systems (EMR) are set up to be paperless. Some medical facilities continue to print a paper chart for backup purposes and file it in the patient's folder.

The clinical staff clears the patient's encounter from the Incomplete Patient Responsibility processor by printing the chart to clear the **CH** flag.

From the Pending Menu, the clinical staff clicks the *Patient Responsibility* button in the **Incomplete Visits** section to display the processor (shown on the next page).

By answering the **X-ray Overread** question, the **XR** flag clears from the Incomplete Patient Responsibility screen. When the clinical staff accesses this screen, the only remaining flag is the **CH** flag, which represents printing the chart. The clinical staff types **prch** in the command field next to the patient and presses the *ENTER* key to print the chart and automatically clear the flag.

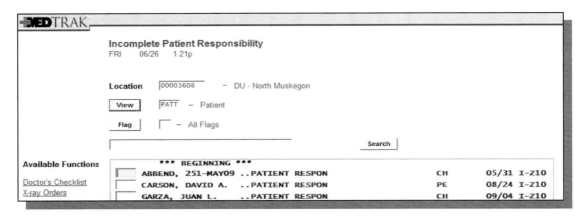

Because this was the last incomplete processing flag for this patient's visit, the patient drops off this screen. Once the patient no longer appears on the Incomplete Patient Responsibility screen, the clinical staff knows that there are no remaining items to complete for this patient's encounter. The pending results of both the overread of the x-ray and the orthopedic consultation are now complete, and the clinical portion of the chart is done.

**Do This ▶**

**22.66** - Click the *Incomplete Visits/Patient Responsibility* button
(from the Pending Menu)

**22.67** - Type the **prch** command in the command field next to your patient
(to print the patient's chart)

**22.68** - Press the *ENTER* key
(the patient's chart will be in your View Prints PDF queue)

**22.69** - Click the *View Prints* button
(this will open another window called Available User Reports)

**25.70** - Place the cursor in the command field next to the patient's chart

**25.71** - Click the *View Report* button
(this will open Adobe, displaying the PDF of the patient's chart)

**25.72** - Click the *diskette* icon at the top right of the PDF

**25.73** - Save this PDF to a folder for your class assignments

**25.74** - Close the *Adobe* window displaying your invoice

**25.75** - Close the Available User Reports window

**22.76** - Click the *Exit Screen* button
(you should be on Pending Menu)

# CHAPTER
# 23

# Unbilled Charges

**Estimated time needed to complete this chapter - 30** minutes

## What you need to know before doing this chapter

- ◆ How to log into MedTrak
- ◆ How to register a patient
- ◆ How to access Clinic Status off the Main Menu
- ◆ How to move a patient to a room and answer nursing notes
- ◆ How to use the Visit Documentation processor (Out the Door)
- ◆ How to discharge the patient from the back examination area
- ◆ How to collect the payment from the patient at the front desk

## Learning outcomes gained from this chapter

- ◆ How to review unbilled charges using the Unbilled Charges dashboard

## Key concepts in this chapter

*billable items*
*super bill*
*billing coders*
*rate tables*
*line item charge*
*billing editors*
*further review needed*
*incomplete visits*
*completed visits*
*needs authorization*
*demographics need review*
*provider notes are incomplete*
*charges available for review*
*further review done*
*transcriptionist*

## Unbilled Charges

### Major Categories of Clinical Workflow

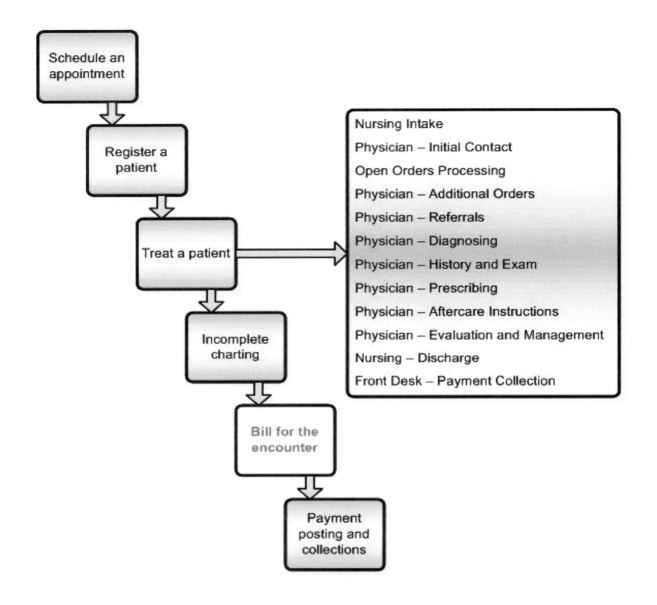

## Unbilled Charges

The first step in the medical billing process is to convert the clinical activities to *billable items* to present on the invoice to the payer. In medical facilities that use paper to document the clinical activities, the items listed on paper (typically called a *super bill*) need to be entered into the billing system. *Billing coders* use the information on the super bill plus any other clinical documentation (paper chart) to be sure that all billable items are accurately and completely coded. The coders enter the CPT (Current Procedural Terminology) codes into the billing system along with the appropriate HCPCS (Healthcare Common Procedure Coding System) codes and NDC (National Drug Codes) codes.

A billing system contains *rate tables* that add the rate to the billable item (*line item charge*) based on the type of visit, the location, and the payer. Different rate tables exist for Medicare, insurance companies, workers' compensation, employee health, and self-pay visits.

With the advent of clinical workflow systems like MedTrak, the first step in the medical billing process is automated. The line item charges including the rate based on the type of visit, location, and payer are automatically created during the clinical processing. This automatic line item charge creation eliminates the need for a coder to manually enter the charges for the visit. The coders now become *billing editors*. They review the billing information to see if the line item charges are reasonable and complete. The billing editor has the on-line chart for researching the billable items. If the billing editors have questions about the billable items, they can send a request for further information (*further review needed*) to the physician or clinical staff directly in the system. This enables the billing editor to work remotely and completely without paper. The billing editor can be sitting anywhere there is Internet access.

In MedTrak, all of the line item charges created during the clinical visit appear on the <u>Unbilled Charges</u> dashboard (shown on the next page). This dashboard is used by the billing editors to track their workflow and process the line item charges for the encounters (patient visits). The billing managers also use this dashboard to monitor the billing editor's workload.

To access the <u>Unbilled Charges</u> dashboard, the billing editor clicks the *Billing* button on the MedTrak <u>Main Menu</u> (shown below).

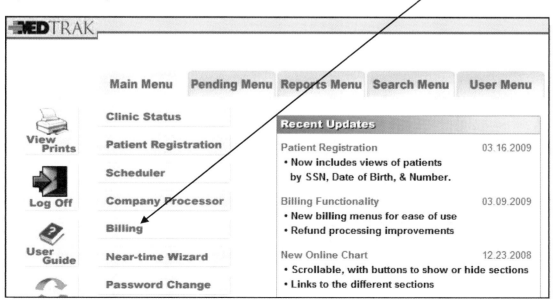

The next screen to appear is the <u>Billing Menu</u> (shown below). On the <u>Billing Menu</u>, the billing editor clicks the *Unbilled Dashboard* button.

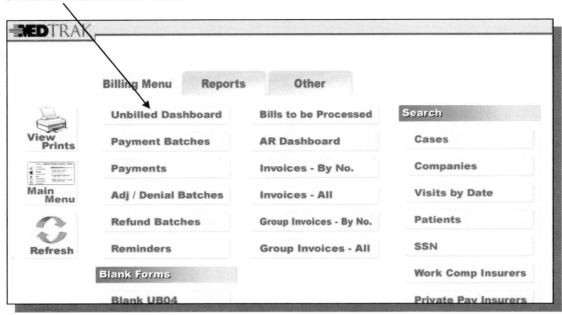

The next screen to appear is the <u>Unbilled Charges Dashboard</u> (shown below) for the location based on the billing editor's location sign-on information.

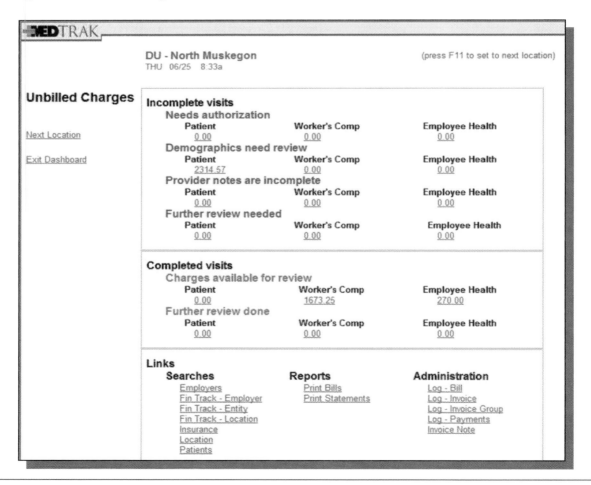

## *Unbilled Charges Dashboard*

The Unbilled Charges Dashboard (shown on the previous page) provides a consolidated view of all of the unbilled charges for a particular medical location. To save the billing editors time, MedTrak audits the clinical and billing data for visits and categorizes the visits as follows:

# Incomplete Visits

The top portion of the dashboard contains information about charts that need further information before they can be billed. Labeled in **red**, the visits (in dollars and cents) found are considered incomplete because the visits still need authorization, the patient or employer demographics need reviewing, the provider's history and exam notes are incomplete, or some other question about the visit is yet unanswered (Further review needed).

These *incomplete visits* are not ready to be posted to an invoice and will be blocked from posting by MedTrak until the issues holding up these visits from billing are removed. Once the issues are cleared up, these visits drop down into the **green** section for *completed visits*, in either the Charges available for review or Further review done, depending on the circumstances.

> *Needs authorization* for treatment – for example: a worker compensation injury where the worker is bleeding and needs immediate medical attention, but the employer contact is not available to authorize the visit either in person or by telephone. Or, the insurance company needs to authorize the visit before the patient can be seen, but it is an emergency.

> *Demographics need review* by billing personnel before posting the charges. This category results from name and/or address changes to the patient or the employer that need to be reviewed before the charges will be freed up for posting to an invoice.

> *Provider notes are incomplete* and need to be completed and/or reviewed before releasing the charges for posting to an invoice. The physician's notes concerning the patient's history and the physical exam conducted do not have to be completed while the patient is being seen in the medical facility. Once the clinical staff reviews that the physician's notes are complete, they will release the charges for posting off the Pending – Incomplete Visits screen.

> *Further review needed* charges result from the billing staff sending a further review needed request to the physician or other clinical staff asking a question about the charges related to the visit. Once the physician or clinical staff responds, the charges move down to the **Completed visits** category of **Further review done**.

## Completed Visits

> *Charges available for review* include all visits that are ready for posting to an invoice that have not had a FRN (**Further Review Needed**) on them.

> *Further review done* includes all visits that have had a **FRN (Further Review Needed)** on them completed by the physician or clinical staff.

## Links

> The bottom portion of the screen contains links to other information in MedTrak.

## Needs Authorization

The **Needs authorization** category provides access to visits that are not authorized yet. For workers' compensation initial visits and employee health initial visits, the authorization information is in the visit record and needs to be updated there. For patient responsibility visits, authorization records are attached to the patient record.

For this example, the visit did not need authorization, so the visit charges do not appear in this section of the dashboard.

## Demographics Need Review

The **Demographics need review** category on the Unbilled Charges Dashboard provides access to visits that need the demographic information (patient or employer name and address, etc.) reviewed before posting another invoice. For each patient and/or employer whose demographic information has changed since the last time the demographic log was reviewed and OK'd by an authorized person, MedTrak sets a **DR** flag (demographics need review).

Each visit that contains the **DR** flag (demographics need review) requires a review of the patient or company demographic change log. Once the demographic log is reviewed and OK'd by the billing editor, the **DR** flag for all visits for the patient or employer is cleared.

For this example, the patient's payer is Blue Cross/Blue Shield. Therefore, his visit charges are totaled in the **Patient** column of the **Demographics need review** section on the Unbilled Charges dashboard (shown below).

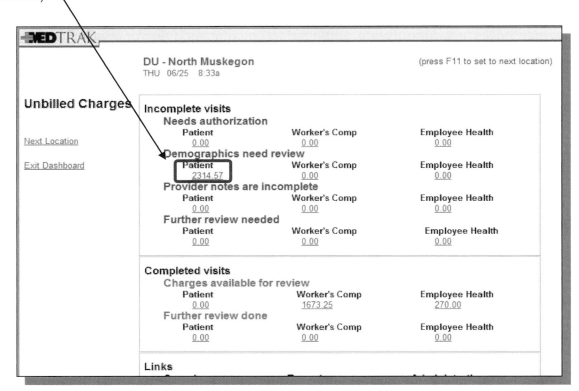

The billing editor clicks the amount field (it is represented as a Web link button) to access the visits represented by it. In this example, the user clicks the **2314.57** dollar amount.

Because this is a patient responsibility visit, the next screen to appear is the totals by Unbilled Charges financial class screen (shown below).

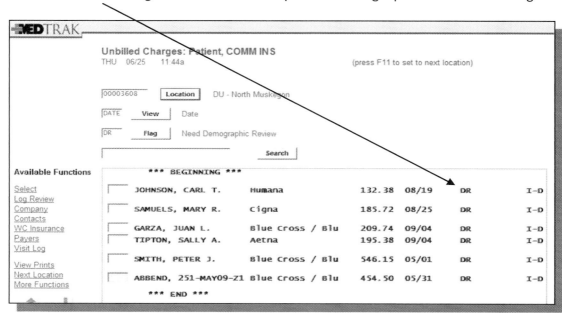

When processing unbilled charges, billing editors prefer to work one financial class at a time. That is why the **$2314.57** amount is broken down on this screen to the different financial classes that it represents.

Our patient has **Blue Cross/Blue Shield** as his insurance company. **Blue Cross/Blue Shield** is a commercial insurance carrier, so the billing editor places the cursor in the input field next to **Comm Ins** and clicks the *Select Class* button.

The next screen to appear is the Unbilled Charges: Patient, COMM INS screen (shown below). This screen lists all of the visits with unbilled charges that need their demographics reviewed for that medical facility for patient responsibility patients with a financial class of commercial insurance. These visits are marked with a **DR** flag to indicate that the patient demographics need reviewing.

To review the demographic changes log, the billing editor places the cursor in the command field next to the patient's visit and clicks the *Log Review* button to see the demographic log (shown below).

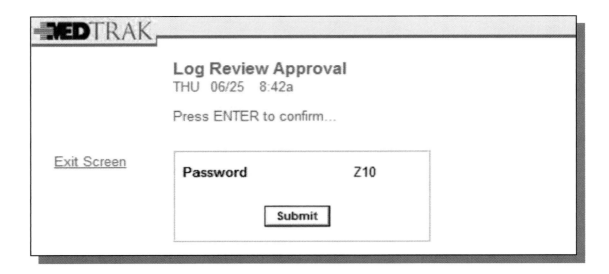

The purpose of tracking and reviewing demographic changes to the patient's or employer's records is to be sure that no one has made a change that would adversely affect the billing in any way. If an invoice is sent to the wrong address or to the wrong payer, it will be a long drawn-out process to learn of the mistake, correct it, and then invoice the right payer or payer address. This type of mistake is costly and could result in never receiving payment for the services.

After reviewing the demographic changes for accuracy, the billing editor clicks the *Log is OK* button to clear the **DR** flag (demographic review flag).

The Log Review Approval screen (shown below) appears for confirmation that the demographic changes are correct. If the password is not automatically filled in on this screen, the billing editor enters the password, then clicks the *Submit* button to approve the demographic changes.

The <u>Unbilled Charges: Patient, COMM INS</u> screen (shown below) reappears with the patient whose demographic log was just reviewed not showing since the **DR** flag is now cleared.

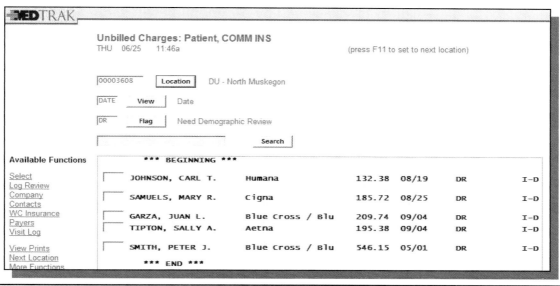

**Do This** ▶ **23.01** - Sign into **MedTrak**

**23.02** - Click the *Billing* button on the MedTrak <u>Main Menu</u>
> (you should be on the <u>Billing Menu</u>)

**23.03** - Click the *Unbilled Dashboard* button
> (you should be on the <u>Unbilled Charges</u> dashboard)

**23.04** - Click the *Patient* amount under **Demographics need review**

**23.05** - Place the cursor in the command field next to **Comm Ins**

**23.06** - Click the *Select Class* button
> (you should be on the <u>Unbilled Charges</u> by patient screen)

**23.07** - Locate your patient; you can change the view if you need to

**23.08** - Place the cursor in the command field next to your patient

**23.09** - Click the *Log Review* button
> (you should be on the <u>Log Review</u> screen for your patient)

**23.10** - Review your demographic information

**23.11** - Click the *Log is OK* button
> (you should be on the <u>Log Review Approval</u> screen)

**23.12** - Click the *Submit* button
> (you should be on <u>Unbilled Charges: Patient, COMM INS</u>)
> (you should not see your patient listed)

The billing editor continues to review demographic logs for the rest of the visits on the screen to clear their **DR** flags.

In this example, the billing editor exits this screen by clicking the *Exit Screen* button. The <u>Unbilled Charges: Patient, Need Demographic Review</u> screen by financial class (shown below) reappears.

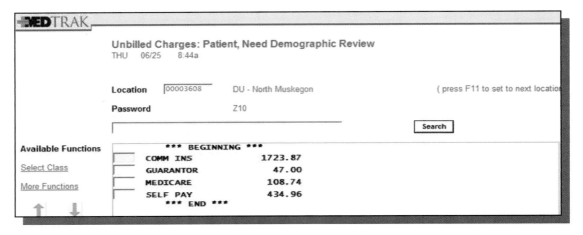

The billing editor also exits this screen without reviewing the other visits represented by the totals by clicking the *Exit Screen* button. The <u>Unbilled Charges Dashboard</u> (shown below) reappears.

In the **Incomplete Visits** box for **Demographics need review**, the **Patient** amount of charges reduces by the amount of charges for the visit. In the **Completed Visits** box for **Charges available for review**, the **Patient** amount of charges increases by the amount for this visit.

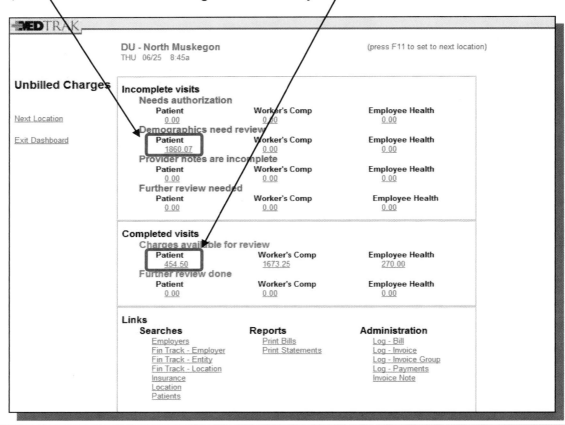

**Do This** ▶ **23.13** - Click the *Exit Screen* button

(you should be on the financial class summary screen)

**23.14** - Click the *Exit Screen* button

(you should be on Unbilled Charges Dashboard)

(the **Demographics need review** value is reduced)

(the **Charges available for review/Patient** value is increased)

## Provider Notes are Incomplete

The **Provider notes are incomplete** section includes visits that need the **CL** flag cleared (provider's checklist containing history and exam questions). This flag is removed in the Pending - Incomplete Visits. This flag (**CL**) removal is the responsibility of the clinical staff and not the billing department. For workflow purposes, this same visit appears on a pending screen for the clinical staff to work and contains the **CL** flag.

Each visit that contains the provider notes are incomplete flag **CL** and requires someone on the clinical staff to work with the physician to complete the history and exam questions on the doctor's checklist. The physician could dictate the notes and have a *transcriptionist* enter the information in the checklist. After verifying that the notes are complete, the clinical staff use the **cmcl** command (it stands for completed checklist) on the pending screen next to the visit to clear the flag. See the Pending – Incomplete documentation for more information on **Pending** processing.

For the purposes of this textbook, the patient encounter does not need the **CL** flag cleared.

## Further Review Needed

The **Further review needed** section contains visits that the billing department had additional questions about before they could post the charges to an invoice. The billing department creates the further review needed status by placing a *Further Review Needed* order on the visit.

For the purposes of this textbook, the patient encounter does not use the further review needed functionality.

## Charges Available for Review

Colored in green, the visits found in the second box on the dashboard are considered "completed" and ready to post to an invoice. Visits are broken down into two categories: Charges available for review and Further review done.

The Charges available for review visits flow from the Incomplete visits area for **Needs authorization, Demographics need review**, and **Provider notes are incomplete** .

The Further review done visits flow from the Further review needed category.

In this example, the only flag that needed clearing was the **Demographics need review** (**DR**) flag. Once that flag cleared, the visit moved down to the **Completed visits** category for billing.

During the processing of the charges ready for posting to an invoice, the billing editor either posts the charges or sends a further review needed message to the physician asking for clarification of some of the billing information.

Because MedTrak is real-time, the Unbilled Charges Dashboard constantly updates to reflect the current status of the unbilled charges for the medical facility.

# CHAPTER

# 24

# Posting Charges to a Bill

**Estimated time needed to complete this chapter  -  20** minutes

## What you need to know before doing this chapter

- How to log into MedTrak
- How to register a patient
- How to access Clinic Status off the Main Menu
- How to move a patient to a room and answer nursing notes
- How to use the Visit Documentation processor  (Out the Door)
- How to discharge the patient from the back examination area
- How to collect the payment from the patient at the front desk
- How to review unbilled charges

## Learning outcomes gained from this chapter

- How to post unbilled charges to an invoice

## Posting Charges to a Bill

**Major Categories of Clinical Workflow**

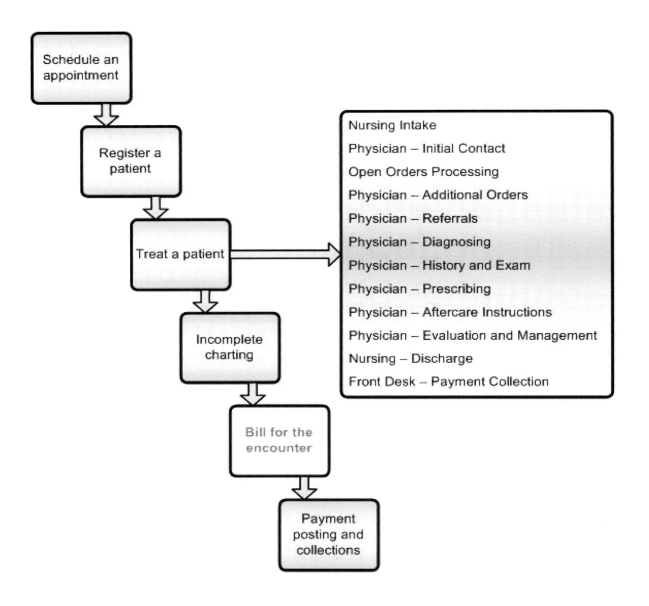

## Posting Charges to a Bill

The <u>MedTrak Unbilled Charges Dashboard</u> displays the total amount of charges for the patient visits that are ready for posting to an invoice.

The billing editor, working with the collaboration of the clinical staff, has:

+ cleared the encounters needing authorization
+ reviewed the demographic changes to the patient and the companies
+ reminded the physicians of the encounters still needing the history and exam completed
+ sent **Further Review Needed** messages to the clinical staff asking for clarification

The encounters ready for billing are in the following categories:

### Completed Visits

> **Charges available for review** includes all visits that are ready for posting that have **not** had an **FRN** (further review needed) on them.

> **Further review done** includes all visits that have had an **FRN** (further review needed) on them completed by the clinical staff.

To access the <u>Unbilled Charges Dashboard</u> (shown below), the billing editor accesses the <u>Billing Menu</u> off the MedTrak <u>Main Menu</u> then clicks the *Unbilled Dashboard* button.

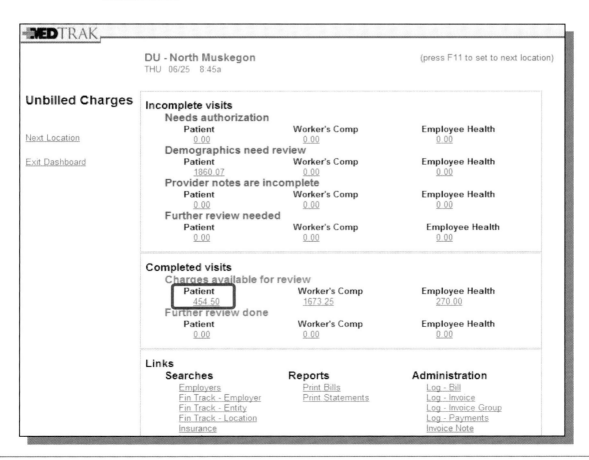

If you are already on the <u>Unbilled Charges</u> dashboard (shown on the previous page), then skip the next Do This section. If you are not on the <u>Unbilled Charges</u> dashboard, then do the next steps.

---

**Do This** ▶    **24.01** -   Sign into **MedTrak**

          **24.02** -   Click the *Billing* button on the MedTrak <u>Main Menu</u>
                 (you should be on the <u>Billing</u> menu)

          **24.03** -   Click the *Unbilled Dashboard* button
                 (you should be on the <u>Unbilled Charges Dashboard</u>)

---

## Charges Available for Review

In this example, the billing editor clicks the Charges available for review/Patient amount (**$454.50**) in the **Completed visits** category. The next screen to appear is the <u>Unbilled Charges: Patient, Ready to Post</u> screen (shown below).

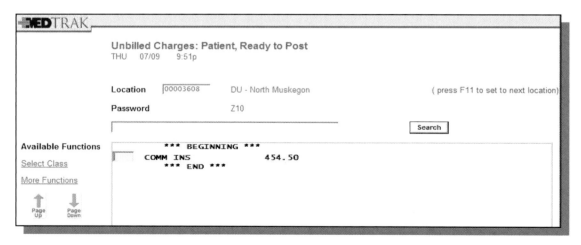

When processing unbilled charges, billing editors like to work one financial class at a time. For this example, the only encounters ready for billing are in the **COMM INS** (commercial insurance) financial class.

Our patient has Blue Cross/Blue Shield as his insurance company. Blue Cross/Blue Shield is a commercial insurance carrier, so the billing editor places the cursor in the command field next to **COMM INS** and clicks the *Select Class* button.

The next screen to appear is the <u>Unbilled Charges: Patient, COMM INS</u> screen (shown below). This screen lists all of the encounters for that clinic location for patient responsibility patients with a financial class of commercial insurance.

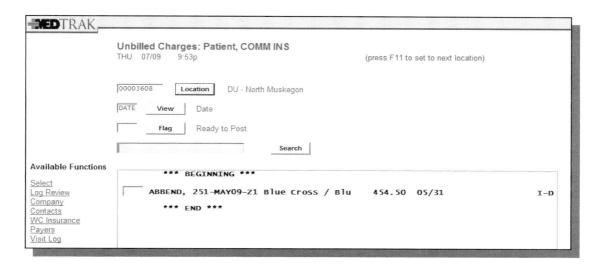

In this example, the only patient visit on this screen that is ready for charge posting is our visit (as shown above). This screen displays:

♦ **Location**  -  this can be changed by entering a different location number and pressing the *ENTER* key.

♦ **View**  -  the view of the encounters can be by date of service, patient, and company.

♦ **Flag**  -  selecting the completed visits total automatically sets the flag to Ready to Post.

♦ **Search**  -  to quickly search for an encounter based on the type of view.

The billing editor places the cursor in the command field next to the patient's visit and clicks the *Select* button to see the billing information about this visit (shown below).

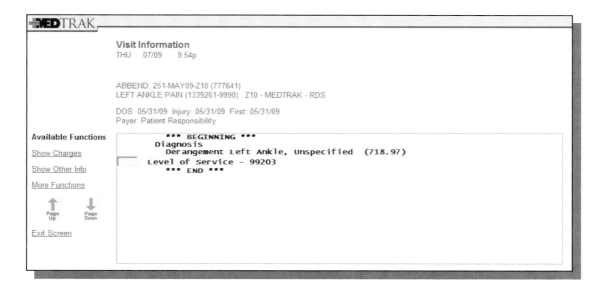

In the body of the screen, the following information displays:

- ◆ Any special notes about the billing (if available – for workers' compensation and employee health)
- ◆ Diagnoses including ICD-9 code (all will list if there is more than 1)
- ◆ Level of service CPT code

After reviewing this information, the user clicks the **Show Charges** button. The line item charge information screen (shown below) for the patient's visit appears.

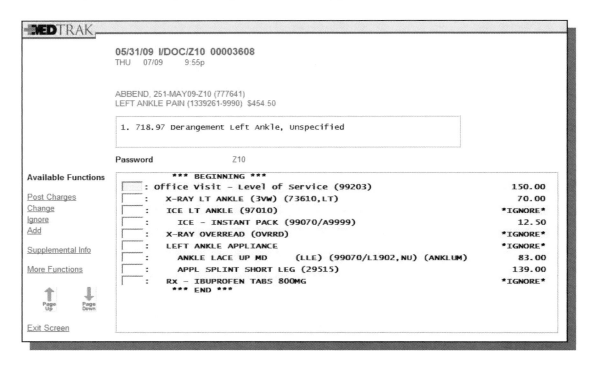

Information about the patient's visit shows at the top of the screen:

- ◆ Date of service  -  **05/31/09**
- ◆ Type of visit  -  **I/DOC** (initial visit to see a doctor)
- ◆ Provider's initials  -  **Z10**
- ◆ Medical facility location identifier  -  **00003608**
- ◆ Name of the patient  -  **Abbend, 251-May09-Z10**
- ◆ Reason for the visit  -  **Left ankle pain**
- ◆ Total charges for the visit  -  **$454.50**
- ◆ Diagnoses appear in the box  -  **718.97  -  Derangement Left Ankle, Unspecified**

In the body of the screen, the following information displays about the line items for posting to the bill:

- ◆ Line item description
- ◆ CPT code
- ◆ CPT modifier (if needed)
- ◆ HCPCS code (if needed)
- ◆ NDC code (if needed)
- ◆ Amount of the charge for the line item

## Reviewing the Line Items

Several of the line items appear with an *IGNORE* in the charge amount field. MedTrak automatically ignores header information and prescriptions, because these are not billable. The ignored line items provide additional billing information for the billing editor.

Sometimes line items appear with a zero charge amount associated with them. This is also intentional. MedTrak provides line item information with zero charge amounts to notify the billing editor of certain procedures performed for the patient to indicate how involved the visit was. The billing editor manually ignores these zero amount line items before posting the bill.

In this example, the following line items appear automatically ignored by MedTrak:

- ◆ Header line item for the ice to the left ankle
- ◆ X-ray overread (the charge for this is included in the left ankle x-ray line item)
- ◆ Header line item for the left ankle appliance
- ◆ Prescription line item for the Ibuprofen

The encounter's line items are a direct result of the clinical activity documented by the physician and the clinical staff. To fix a line item that contains an erroneous code, the billing editor places the cursor in the command field next to the line item and clicks the *Change* button. If this occurs, the billing editor will fix this one and send a message to the billing rules manager to correct the rule. That way, the next time this line item is selected, the code will be correct.

## Assigning Diagnoses to the Line Items

This example only had one diagnosis. MedTrak, therefore, automatically assigns it to each line item. If the visit had several diagnoses, each line item would need the appropriate diagnoses attached to it for presentation to the payer on the **CMS1500**.

To associate a line item with a diagnosis, use the following diagnosis numbers in the command field next to the line item and press the *ENTER* key.

| | | | |
|---|---|---|---|
| **1** | only associated with the 1st | **2** | only associated with the 2nd |
| **12** | associated with the 1st and 2nd | **23** | associated with the 2nd and 3rd |
| **123** | associated with the 1st, 2nd, and 3rd | **234** | associated with the 2nd, 3rd, and 4th |
| **124** | associated with the 1st, 2nd, and 4th | **24** | associated with the 2nd and 4th |
| **1234** | associated with all four | **3** | only associated with the 3rd |
| **13** | associated with the 1st and 3rd | **34** | associated with the 3rd and 4th |
| **134** | associated with the 1st, 3rd, and 4th | **4** | only associated with the 4th |
| **14** | associated with the 1st and 4th | | |

## Posting the Charges

Additionally, other supplemental information is needed for some invoices. MedTrak provides access to these supplemental fields through the use of the *Supplemental Info* button.

In this example, the billing editor will not be inputting any of the supplemental information fields.

After reviewing all of the charges for accuracy and relevancy, the billing editor posts the charges to an invoice. To post the charges, the user can place the cursor in any one of the line item input fields and click the *Post Charges* button.

MedTrak performs a number of edits to check the line item charge posting for accuracy and completeness of data. If any of the edits fail, MedTrak will refresh the charges screen with the error message presented in red right under the date and time at the top of the screen. If there are no errors, MedTrak will post the invoice. Some of these line item edits include:

- ◆ Line item amount is not zero.
- ◆ CPT codes exist for each line item (or HCPCS or NDC codes).
- ◆ If multiple diagnoses, each line item is associated with a diagnosis.

The Unbilled Charges:  Patient, COMM INS screen (shown below) will reappear, and your patient visit will not be on the screen, because the charges are now posted to an invoice.

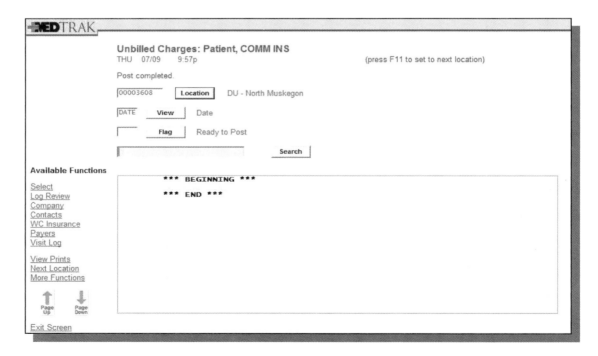

The billing editor will continue to process the visits on this screen. When finished, the billing editor clicks the *Exit Screen* button to return to the Unbilled Charges: Patient - Ready to Post screen. From that screen the billing editor can choose another financial class to process, or exit to the Unbilled Charges dashboard.

In this example, the billing editor clicks the *Exit Screen* button to return to the <u>Unbilled Charges</u> dashboard (shown below). The **Patient** amount in the Charges available for review section of the **Completed Visits** is reduced by the **$454.50** amount.

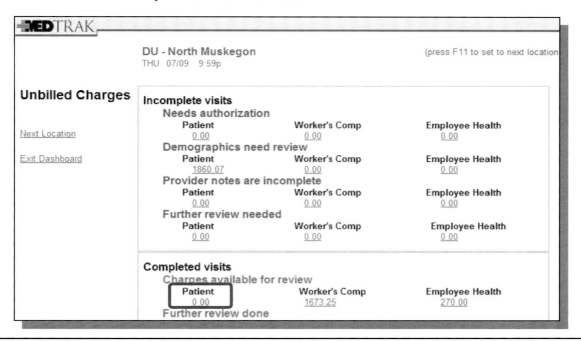

**Do This** ▶ **24.04** - Click the *Patient* amount for **Charges available for review**

**24.05** - Place the cursor in the command field next to **Comm Ins**

**24.06** - Click the *Select Class* button
(you should be on <u>Unbilled Charges: Patient, COMM INS</u>)

**24.07** - Locate your patient; you can change the view if you need to

**24.08** - Place the cursor in the command field next to your patient

**24.09** - Click the *Select* button
(you should be on the <u>Visit Information</u> screen for your patient)

**24.10** - Review the information on this screen

**24.11** - Click the *Show Charges* button
(review the line items on this screen)

**24.12** - Click the *Post Charges* button
(you should be on <u>Unbilled Charges: Patient, COMM INS</u>)

**24.13** - Click the *Exit Screen* button
(you should be on <u>Unbilled Charges: Patient, Ready to Post</u>)

**24.14** - Click the *Exit Screen* button
(you should be on the <u>Unbilled Charges Dashboard</u>)

# CHAPTER
# 25

# Printing Bills

**Estimated time needed to complete this chapter  -  15** minutes

**What you need to know before doing this chapter**

- ◆ How to log into MedTrak
- ◆ How to register a patient
- ◆ How to access Clinic Status off the Main Menu
- ◆ How to move a patient to a room and answer nursing notes
- ◆ How to use the Visit Documentation processor (Out the Door)
- ◆ How to discharge the patient from the back examination area
- ◆ How to collect the payment from the patient at the front desk
- ◆ How to review unbilled charges
- ◆ How to post charges to create an invoice

**Learning outcomes gained from this chapter**

- ◆ How to print a bill (invoice)

## *Printing Bills*

### Major Categories of Clinical Workflow

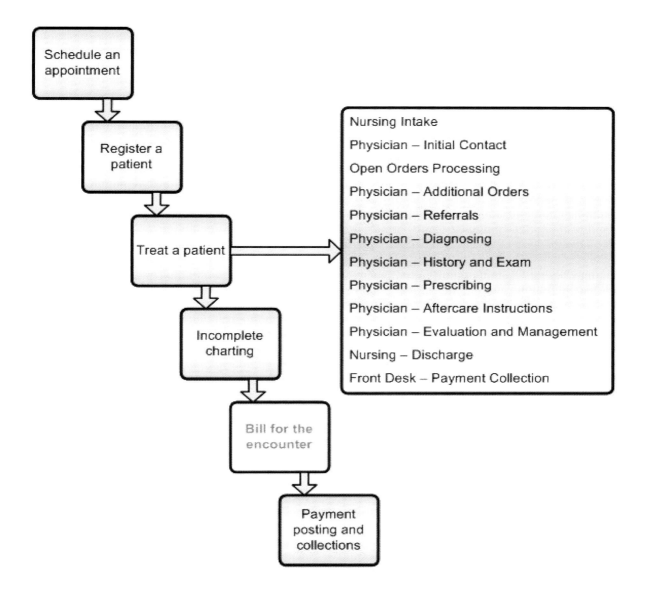

## *Printing Bills*

After the billing editor creates the bill for the encounter, MedTrak accumulates the bill along with all of the bills that have not been printed (or electronically transmitted) on the <u>Bills ready to be Processed</u> dashboard. MedTrak allows the user to print bills in batches, individually, or send them electronically to a clearing house for transmission to the payer.

To print a bill or transmit it to a payer, the billing staff uses the <u>Bills ready to be Processed</u> dashboard (shown below). The billing staff accesses the <u>Billing Menu</u> off the MedTrak <u>Main Menu</u> then clicks the *Bills to be Processed* button. This dashboard displays the totals for all of the bills for all clinic locations for the entity, not just one clinic location.

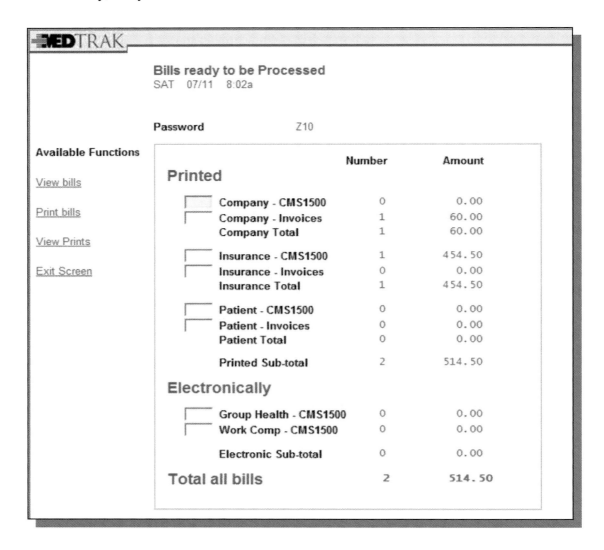

If you are already on the <u>Bills ready to be Processed</u> dashboard (shown above), then skip the next **Do This** section. If you are not on the <u>Bills ready to be Processed</u> dashboard, then do the next steps.

**Do This ▶**   **25.01** - Sign into **MedTrak**

**25.02** - Click the ***Billing*** button on the MedTrak <u>Main Menu</u>
(you should be on the <u>Billing Menu</u>)

**25.03** - Click the ***Bills to be Processed*** button
(you should be on the <u>Bills ready to be Processed</u> dashboard)

This screen is divided into the different types of bills that a medical entity could send out to payers.

Bills will either be printed for mailing or transmitted for electronic submission. Additionally, bills can be mailed to companies (employers), insurance companies, and patients either on a CMS1500 or the MedTrak invoice format.

Bills can be electronically sent to clearing houses that handle group health or workers' compensation. Workers' compensation requires sending additional supporting information attached to the CMS1500, the patient's chart, and any required forms based on state regulations. For example, the State of California requires that the patient's chart and a DFR (Doctor's First Report) accompany the CMS1500 for an initial injury patient visit.

In this example, the payer for the Abbend invoice is Blue Cross/Blue Shield and the electronic submission flag is not set on for the payer (in the payer profile). So, Abbend's bill will be in the **Insurance – CMS1500** category of the **Printed** section on the <u>Bills ready to be Processed</u> dashboard.

Typically, the billing staff will print all of the bills in one category at a time or transmit all of the bills in one category at the same time. However, for this chapter, you will print just your bill.

To locate the bill to print, the billing staff places the cursor in the input field next to the **Insurance – CMS1500** category and clicks the ***View bills*** button. The next screen that appears is the <u>Invoices, Unprinted, CMS1500's, Not Bill Elec</u> screen (shown below).

This screen lists just the one invoice for this example. Your screen could list many more invoices. Using the **Search** field and the different display options at the top of the screen, locate your invoice.

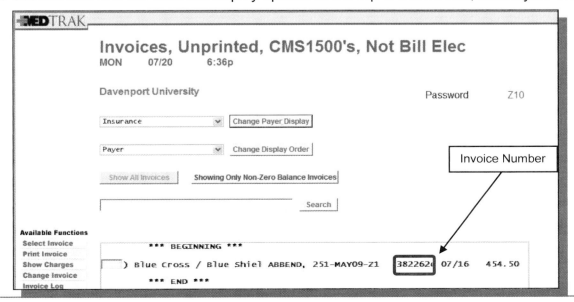

This processor is used for all invoice processors. That is why it has the following options available:

- ◆ **Payer Display -** invoices can be displayed by:
  - ◆ All payers
  - ◆ Patient name
  - ◆ Insurance company name
  - ◆ Employer name
  - ◆ Other payer group name

- ◆ **Display Order** - the view of the invoices can be sorted by:
  - ◆ Date of service
  - ◆ Payer name
  - ◆ Patient name
  - ◆ Employer name
  - ◆ Invoice number
  - ◆ Case number
  - ◆ Social security number

- ◆ **Show All Invoices** - regardless of whether the balance owed by the payer is zero or not

- ◆ **Show Only Invoices with Non-Zero Balances** - only positive or negative balances

- ◆ **Search** - to quickly search for an invoice based on the type of view

To print just this one invoice, the billing staff places the cursor in the command field next to the invoice and clicks the *Print Invoice* button. The invoice for this example and for your processing prints to the PDF queue and is printed from there by accessing it using the *View Prints* button.

---

**Do This** ▶ **25.04** - Place the cursor in the command field for **Insurance—CMS1500**

**25.05** - Click the *View Bills* button

**25.06** - Locate your invoice
(use the drop-down menus above the search field, if necessary)

**25.07** - Record your invoice number here: _____
(just use the number; the "c" next to it indicates CMS1500)

**25.08** - Place the cursor next to your invoice

**25.09** - Click the *Print Invoice* button

---

The <u>Invoices, Unprinted, CMS1500's, Not Bill Elec</u> screen (shown below) refreshes with the message at the top in red "**Report sent to printer.**" The invoice is now in the PDF queue for you to print as a work product for this class.

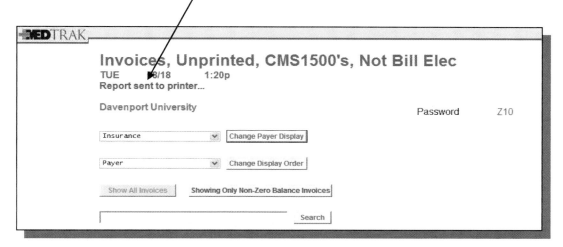

The billing staff clicks the *Exit Screen* button to return to the <u>Bills ready to be Processed</u> screen (shown below). Notice that the number of invoices to print is now reduced by 1 and the dollar amount is also reduced.

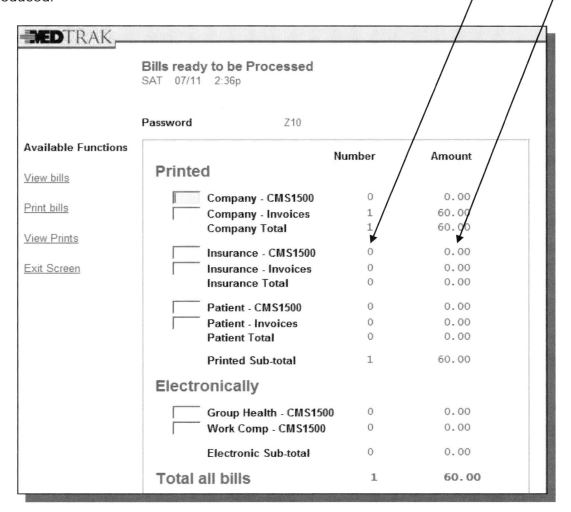

**Do This** ▶ **25.10** - Click the *Exit Screen* button

(you should be on <u>Bills ready to be Processed</u>)

(the **Insurance - CMS1500** value is reduced)

**25.11** - Click the *View Prints* button

(this will open another window displaying your PDF print queue)

(this screen is called <u>Available User Reports</u>)

**25.12** - Place the cursor in the command field next to the **CMS1500**

**25.13** - Click the *View Report* button

(this will open Adobe displaying the PDF of your **CMS1500**)

**25.14** - Click the *diskette* icon at the top right of the PDF

**25.15** - Save this PDF to a folder for your class assignments

**25.16** - Attach this saved PDF to your assignment

**25.17** - Close the *Adobe* window displaying your invoice

**25.18** - Close the <u>Available User Reports</u> window

**25.19** - Click the *Exit Screen* button

(you should be on the <u>Billing Menu</u>)

# CHAPTER 26

# Payment Processing

**Estimated time needed to complete this chapter  -  45** minutes

## What you need to know before doing this chapter

- How to log into MedTrak
- How to register a patient
- How to access Clinic Status off the Main Menu
- How to move a patient to a room and answer nursing notes
- How to use the Visit Documentation processor (Out the Door)
- How to discharge the patient from the back examination area
- How to collect the payment from the patient at the front desk
- How to review unbilled charges
- How to post charges to create an invoice
- How to print a bill (invoice)

## Learning outcomes gained from this chapter

- How to process a payment and post it to an invoice

## Key concepts in this chapter

*batched totaled*

*weekly deposit*

*daily deposit*

*lock box*

*auditing and control*

*unapplied payment amounts*

*tax identification number*

*payment processing*

*explanation of benefits*

*balance bill*

## Payment Processing

### Major Categories of Clinical Workflow

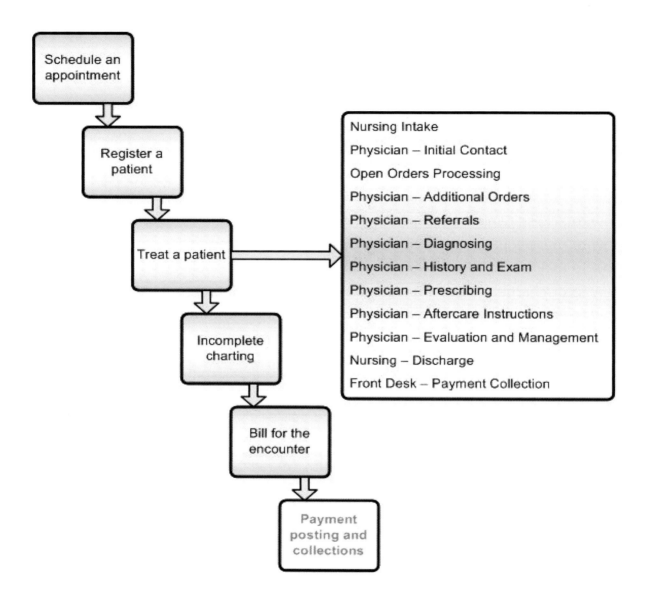

## *Payment Processing*

Medical facilities receive payments for services in several ways:

♦ Some patients pay for services at the front desk. These payments could be for all of the charges for the visit, the co-payment amount required by the insurance company, or the co-insurance amount required by the insurance company.

♦ Some payments arrive in the mail from patients, insurance companies, employers, and other payers.

♦ Some payments are made electronically by the insurance company.

The payments received at the front desk are typically *batch totaled* for a *weekly deposit* to the bank. Depending on the procedures for the medical facility, the front desk payments could be batched on a daily basis.

The payments that arrive in the mail are typically batch totaled for a *daily deposit* to the bank.

Some medical facilities use a service from the bank called a "*lock box*." Lock box services involve the bank opening mail containing checks from patients and other payers and depositing the checks to the medical facilities account. The bank will make a copy of the check and send the check copy to the medical facility along with any remittance documentation that the payer included with the check. Using this service facilitates faster access to payments for the medical facility.

The MedTrak Payment Batches screen records and tracks the payment batches for the medical facility. A new batch record is added for each deposit made to the bank. For *auditing and control* purposes, the total money in the bank deposit must match the total of the payments in the batch.

The payment entry staff accesses the Billing Menu from the MedTrak Main Menu. On the Billing Menu, the user clicks the *Payment Batches* button to display the Payment Batches screen for that medical entity.

If you are already on the Payment Batches screen (shown on the next page), then skip the next Do This section. If you are not on the Payment Batches screen, then do the next steps.

---

**Do This** ► **26.01** - Sign into **MedTrak**

**26.02** - Click the *Billing* button on the MedTrak Main Menu
(you should be on the Billing Menu)

**26.03** - Click the *Payment Batches* button
(you should be on the Payment Batches screen)

---

## Payment Batches

The <u>Payment Batches</u> screen (shown below) defaults to displaying only payment batches with *unapplied payment amounts*. Those are batches with a remaining balance that will be applied to invoices or refunded to the payer. To see all of the payment batches (including closed batches whose balances are zero), the payment entry staff clicks the *Show all balances* button.

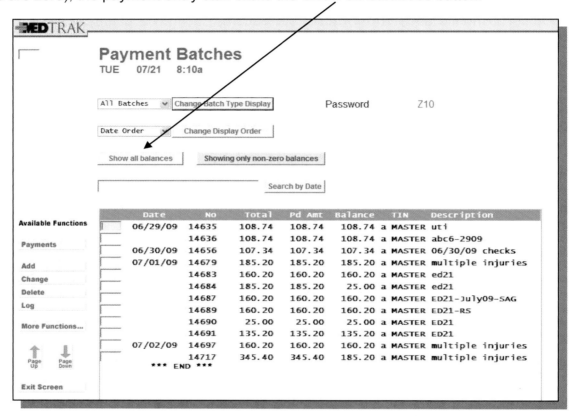

This <u>Payment Batches</u> processor (shown above) has the following options available:

- **Batch Type** - payment batches can be displayed by:
  - **Unsubmitted** - batches that are not ready for review by a supervisor
  - **Submitted** - batches that are ready for review by a supervisor
  - **Approved** - batches that have been reviewed and approved by a supervisor for payment posting to invoices
  - **All** - all types of payment batches (unsubmitted, submitted, and approved)
- **Display Order** - the view of the invoices can be sorted by:
  - Payment batch date
  - Payment batch number
- **Show all balances** - regardless of whether the balance on the batch is zero or not
- **Show only non-zero balances** - only positive or negative balance payment batches
- **Search** - to quickly search for a payment batch based on the sort order

Some medical facilities separate the *payment processing* functions for control purposes. They have one group of employees open checks, total them for the bank deposit, and record them in batches in MedTrak. The supervisor then reviews the bank deposit and compares it to the batch totals in MedTrak. If they are in balance, the supervisor approves the batch for application of the payments to the open invoices and the bank deposit for delivery to the bank. Then, another group of employees applies the payments to the open invoices. Only approved payment batches can be applied to open invoices.

For purposes of this book, the payment batches will automatically be approved for payment posting and not require the supervisor to approve them.

For this example, the payment batch total is **$236.50** and contains two payments:

1. The **$25.00** co-payment from the patient collected by the front desk person when the patient was done with the visit.

2. A check from Blue Cross/Blue Shield of Michigan for **$211.50**.

To add a new batch of payments, the payment entry staff clicks the *Add* button. The Payment Batch add screen (shown below) appears.

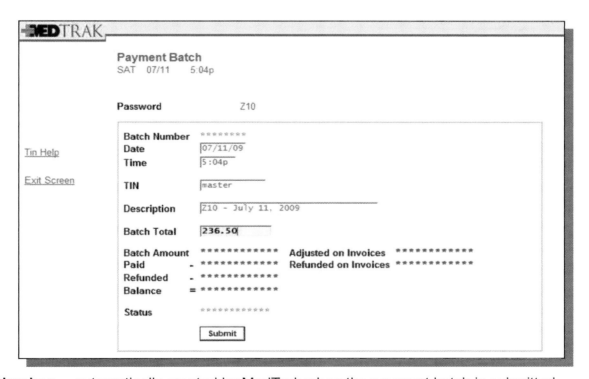

**Batch Number** - automatically created by MedTrak when the payment batch is submitted.

**Date and Time** - MedTrak also automatically puts in the current date and time. The payment entry staff will change these to match the bank deposit.

**TIN** - this field is for the *tax identification number* for tax reporting purposes. Every medical facility has at least one. A medical facility could have multiple TIN's depending on the legal structure of the business. Income must be reported to the government based on business ownership; medical facilities therefore batch their payments by date and TIN. For this example, the TIN is "**master**."

**Description** - this contains a description of the batch made up by the payment entry staff.

**Do This** ▶   **26.04** - Click the *Add* button

         (you should be on the <u>Payment Batches</u> screen)

      **26.05** - Leave the payment batch **Date** and **Time** as MedTrak loaded them

      **26.06** - Enter the **TIN**

         (**master** is the tax identification number)

      **26.07** - Enter the payment batch **Desc** (description)

         (type your employee initials and today's date)

      **26.08** - Enter the **Batch Total** amount

         (**$236.50** is the batch total)

      **26.09** - Click the *Submit* button

         (you should be on the individual <u>Payment</u> screen)

## Adding a Payment

The next screen to appear is the <u>Payment</u> screen (shown below) for adding individual payments.

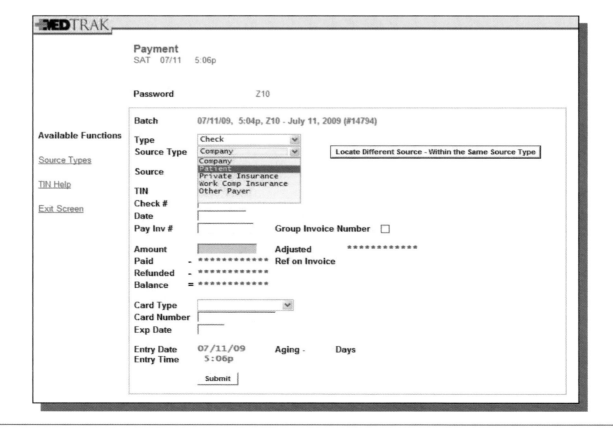

MedTrak automatically sets the **Type** of payment to **Check** (because most payments come in the form of a check). If the payment is made another way (cash, credit card, or money order), the payment staff uses the type of payment drop-down menu to select the other type of payment.

For the **Source Type** field, MedTrak automatically sets this field to **Company**. The payment entry person uses the drop-down menu as shown on the screen on the previous page to select the type of payment source. For this example, the first payment source type will be **Patient**, and the second payment from Blue Cross/Blue Shield of Michigan will have a source type of **Private Insurance**.

The **Pay Inv #** is an important field. To save time, MedTrak allows the payment entry staff to enter the invoice number that the payment is paying. Many times the payer will either record the invoice number on the check or enclose an *explanation of benefits* with the check.

The explanation of benefits (EOB) is exactly what its name implies. The EOB explains exactly what the payer is paying and why. Insurance companies do not typically pay the full amount of line items on an invoice, unless the medical facility bills exactly what the payer is expecting to pay.

On the individual payment screen, the payment entry staff records all of the information about the payment:

- **Type** of payment - check, cash, credit card, etc.
- **Source Type** – source of the payment will be one of the following:
    - Company - the patient's employer
    - Patient
    - Private Insurance - Blue Cross or Medicare, or other private insurance company
    - Work Comp Insurance - the employer's insurance company
    - Other Payer - a drug screen third party administrator or drug screen consortium
- **TIN** - this will automatically be filled in from the payment batch information
- **Check #**
- **Date** of the check
- **Pay Inv #** - this is the invoice number that the payment is paying (if the payer records it on the EOB)
- **Amount** of the payment
- **Credit card** information (if the payer used a credit card) is at the bottom of the screen

After recording the payment information, the user clicks the *Submit* button.

For the first payment, the payment entry staff records the payment from the patient for the **$25.00** co-payment amount. The patient wrote check number **476** on **May 31, 2009** to pay for invoice number **380927**. This is the invoice number recorded in Chapter 25, Printing Bills.

- **Type** - Check
- **Source Type** - Patient
- **TIN** - master
- **Check #** - 476
- **Date** - 053109
- **Pay Inv #** - 380927
- **Amount** - 25

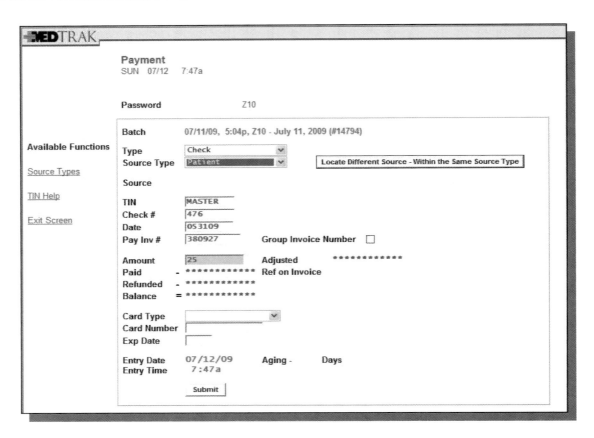

The next screen to appear is the Patient: Select screen (shown below). The payment entry staff places the cursor in the command field next to the patient **Abbend** and clicks the *Select* button.

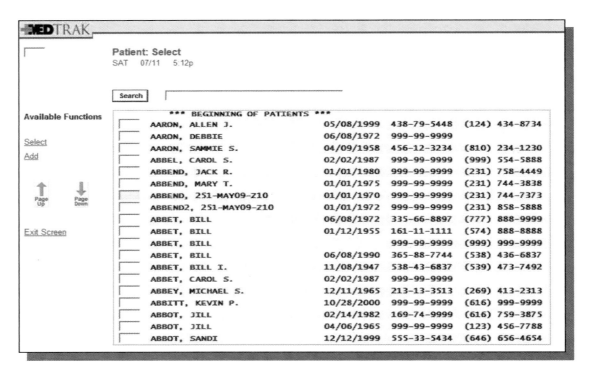

**Do This ▶**

**26.10** - Select **Patient** from the **Source Type** drop down menu

**26.11** - Leave the **TIN** as loaded from the payment batch

**26.12** - Enter the **Check #**

(type the check number recorded by the front desk)

**26.13** - Enter the **Date** of the check

(use the date of service)

**26.14** - Enter the **Pay Inv #**

(type the invoice number for your invoice - **not 380927**)

**26.15** - Skip the **Group Invoice Number** check box

**26.16** - Enter the **Amount** of the check

(type 25 - do not enter the $ sign or cents)

**26.17** - Click the *Submit* button

(you should be on the Patient: Select screen)

**26.18** - Place the cursor in the command field next to your patient

**26.19** - Click the *Select* button

(you should be on the Payment Posting screen for your invoice)

## Posting the Payments to the Line Items

After selecting the payer, the next screen to appear is the Payment Posting screen (shown on the next page) for the invoice.

This screen is broken down as follows:

♦ The invoice information is in the top frame in green

♦ The payment information is in the top frame in blue

♦ The line item information is in the bottom frame and presents up to four line items on one screen

♦ There are columns of numbers for each **line item** for:

♦ Billed amount

♦ Total paid by all payments

♦ Total adjusted by all payments

♦ Amount paid by this payment

♦ Up to five adjustment, denial, and write-off codes and amounts

♦ Balance owed

♦ Totals at the bottom for the entire invoice

The buttons are used as follows:

- *Submit Payment* - transmits the payment posting information to MedTrak.
- *Paid in Full* - automatically enters the paid amount equal to the billed amount for each line item. Use this button only when the total payment amount equals the total of the invoice.
- *Adjustment Codes* - displays the list of adjustment, denial, and write-off codes available to the medical facility.
- *Line Item Log* - displays the history of all of the payment and adjustment activity for the line items for this invoice.

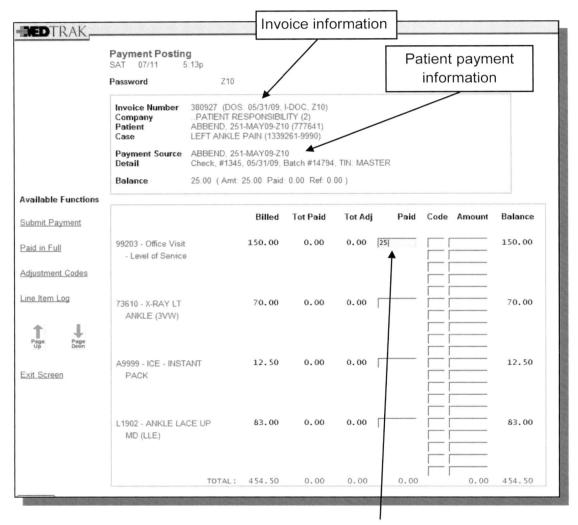

For this example, the payment entry staff enters the patient's **$25.00** payment (without the dollar sign or cents included) for the co-payment for the office visit and clicks the *Submit Payment* button.

The <u>Payment Posting</u> screen (shown below) refreshes, showing the payment information recorded.

The payment information at the top shows the balance left on the payment is **zero**.

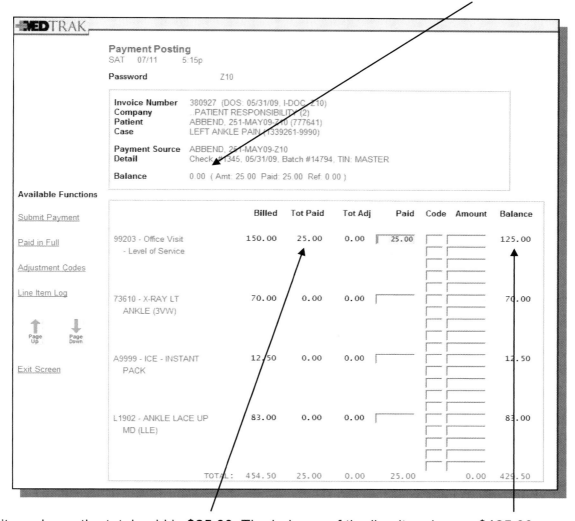

The line item shows the total paid is **$25.00**. The balance of the line item is now **$125.00**.

After reviewing the application of the payment to this invoice, the payment staff clicks the *Exit Screen* button to add the next payment to the payment batch. The <u>Payment</u> entry screen (shown below) reappears with the message in red at the top of the screen: **Successful add - ready to add another. . .**

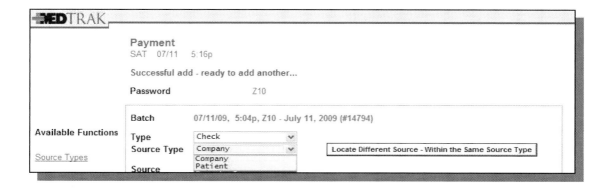

**Do This** ▶ **26.20** - Place the cursor in the **Paid** field for the **Office Visit** line item

(type **25** - do not enter the $ sign or cents)

**26.21** - Click the **Submit Payment** button

(the Payment Posting screen refreshes)

**26.22** - Check that your payment information recorded properly

**26.23** - Click the **Exit Screen** button

(you should be on the Payment entry screen)

For the second payment, the payment entry staff records the payment from the private insurance company (Blue Cross/Blue Shield of Michigan) for **$211.50**. Blue Cross enclosed an EOB with check number **75464** to pay for invoice number **380927**. After entering the payment information, the payment entry staff clicks the **Submit** button to record the payment.

- ◆ **Type** - check
- ◆ **Source Type** - Private Insurance
- ◆ **TIN** - MASTER
- ◆ **Check #** - 75464
- ◆ **Date** - 061509
- ◆ **Pay Inv #** - 380927
- ◆ **Amount** - 211.50

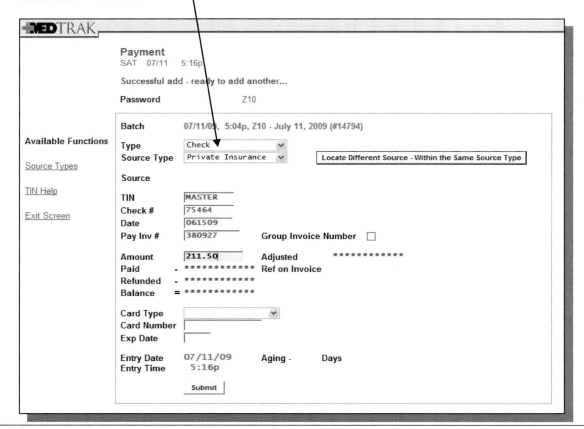

The next screen to appear is the <u>Entity/Payers: Select</u> screen (shown below). The payment entry staff places the cursor in the command field next to **Blue Cross** and clicks the *Select Payer* button.

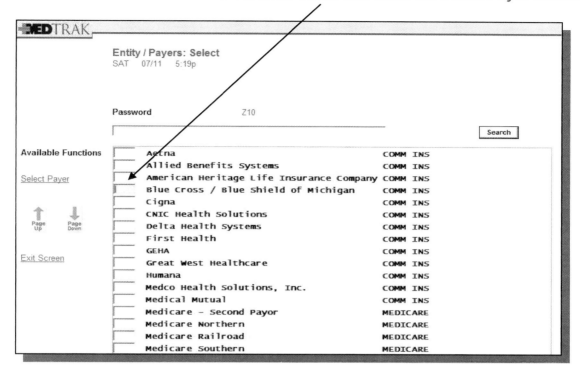

**Do This** ▶ **26.24** - Select **Private Insurance** from the **Source Type** drop-down menu

**26.25** - Leave the **TIN** as loaded from the payment batch

**26.26** - Enter the **Check Number**
> (make up a check number)

**26.27** - Enter the **Date** of the check
> (use yesterday's date)

**26.28** - Enter the **Pay Inv #**
> (type the invoice number for your invoice - **not 380927**)

**26.29** - Enter the **Amount** of the check
> (type 211.50 - do not enter the $ sign)

**26.30** - Click the *Submit* button
> (you should be on the <u>Entity/Payers: Select</u> screen)

**26.31** - Place the cursor in the command field next to **Blue Cross**

**26.32** - Click the *Select Payer* button
> (you should be on the <u>Payment Posting</u> screen for your invoice)

## Posting the Payments to the Line Items

After selecting the payer, the next screen to appear is the Payment Posting screen (shown below).

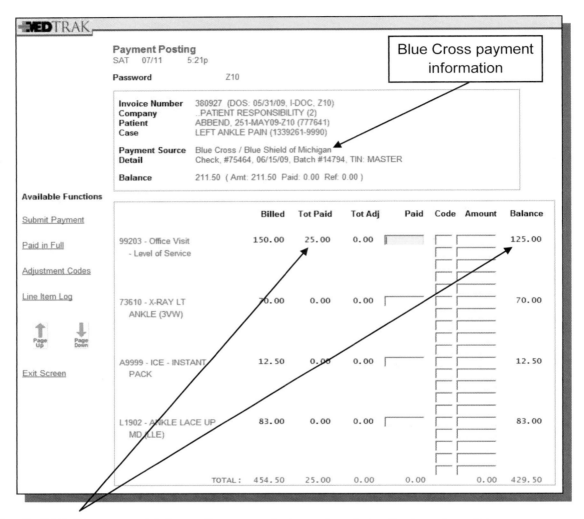

This patient's $25.00 payment information recorded previously is displayed on this screen.

For this example, the payment entry staff enters Blue Cross's payment information based on the EOB enclosed with the check. On the EOB from Blue Cross, they applied the following to the line items:

- ◆ **Office Visit**
  paid $25.00.
  credited $25.00 for the patient's co-payment.
  credited the patient's deductible for $100.00.
  payment entry staff will balance bill the secondary payer.

- ◆ **X-ray lt ankle**
  paid $50.00.
  adjusted $20.00 for belonging to the PPO (code a01).

- ◆ **Ice instant pack**
  paid $5.00.
  adjusted $7.50 for belonging to the PPO (code a01).

- ◆ **Ankle lace up**
  paid $51.50.
  adjusted $31.50 for belonging to the PPO (code a01).

- ◆ **Appl splint short leg**
  paid $80.00.
  adjusted $59.00 for belonging to the PPO (code a01).

When the payment entry staff places the cursor in a **Code** field for a line item and clicks the *Adjustment Code* button, the Adjustment Codes screen (shown below) appears. The first five codes are standard codes that MedTrak provides for everyone to use. After the **DD** code, the codes are specific to the medical facility.

- ◆ **BB** - for balance billing the line item to the next payer
- ◆ **RB** - for rebilling the line item to the current payer
- ◆ **CP** - to indicate that the amount next to the code field is the patient's co-payment amount
- ◆ **CI** - to indicate that the amount next to the code field is the patient's co-insurance amount
- ◆ **DD** - to indicate that the amount next to the code field is applied to the patient's deductible

MEDTRAK

**Adjustment Codes**
SUN 07/12 2:23p

**Available Functions**

Submit Selection

*** BEGINNING ***
- ☐ BB - Balance Bill
- ☐ RB - Re-Bill
- ☐ CP - Co-Payment
- ☐ CI - Co-Insurance
- ☐ DD - Deductible
- ☐ A01 - Adjustment PPO reduction
- ☐ A02 - Multiple procedure reduction
- ☐ A04 - Billed over fee schedule
- ☐ A05 - Penalty and interest adjustment

↑ Page Up    ↓ Page Down

Exit Screen

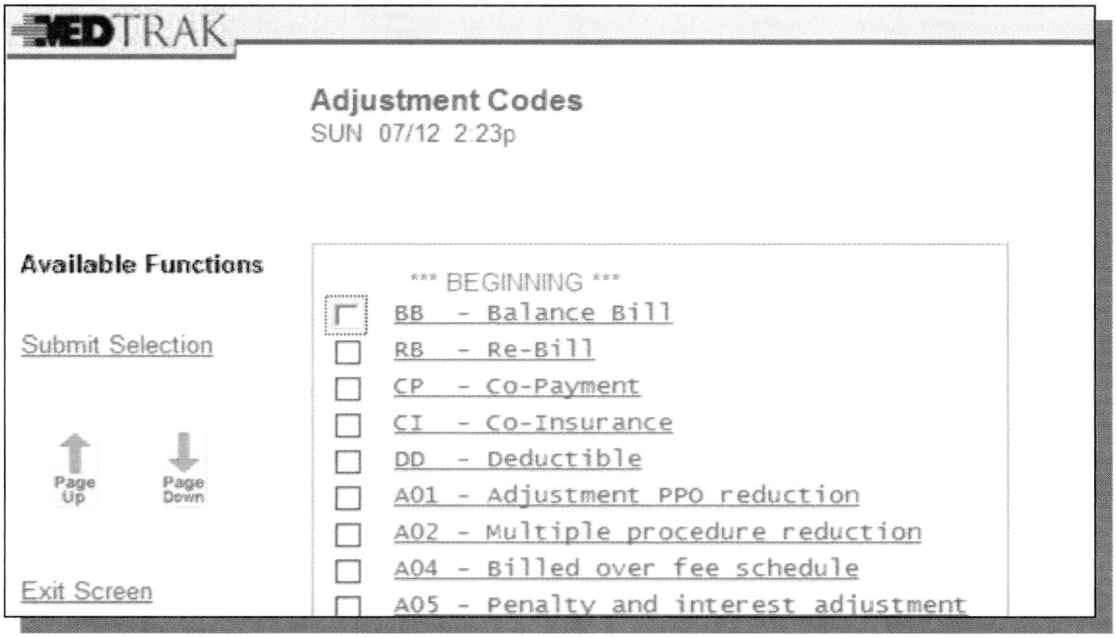

If a patient has multiple payers (in this example, Blue Cross is the primary payer and Nationwide is the secondary payer), the payment entry staff can *balance bill* the office visit line item to the next payer using the **bb** command in the **Code** field for the line item. Notice that codes are not case sensitive, and therefore, can be entered in lower case.

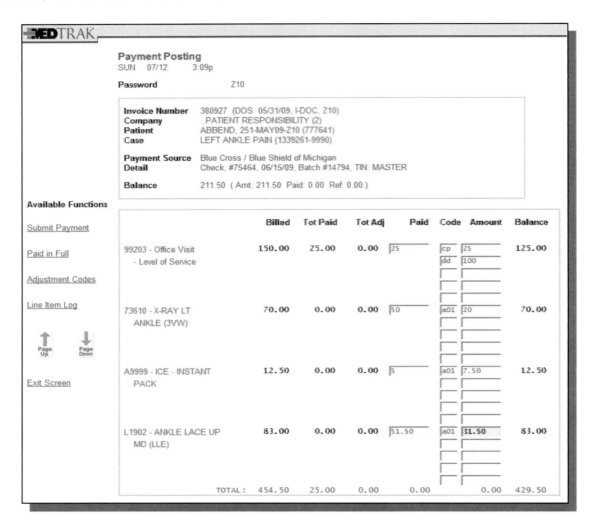

The payment entry staff enters the above information and clicks the *Page Down* button to advance to the second Payment Posting screen (shown on the next page) to view the rest of the line items for this invoice. There are five line items on this invoice. Each payment posting screen only has room for four at a time.

The *Page Down* and Page Up buttons act just like the *Submit Payment* button, and they move up a screen or down a screen after recording the data that is on the screen. This saves time.

After entering the payment and adjustment information for the application of the short leg splint line item, the payment entry staff clicks the *Submit Payment* button to record the data.

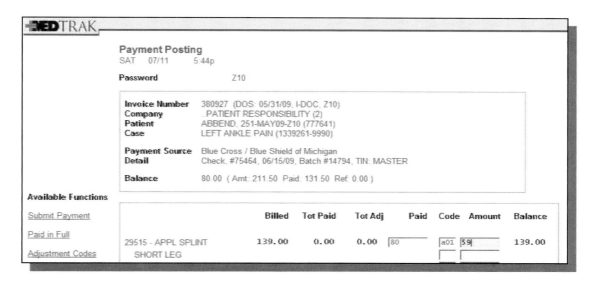

The Payment Posting screen refreshes with the payment information updated. The **$211.50** payment from Blue Cross is applied to each line item including the associated adjustments. The payment balance is **zero**. The **$100.00** invoice balance will now be billed to Nationwide insurance.

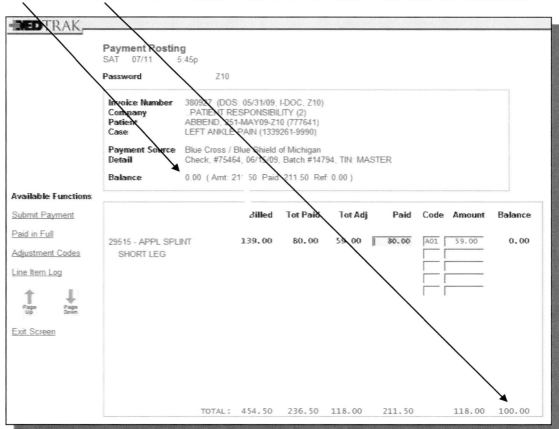

The payment entry staff clicks the *Exit Screen* button to return to the Payment screen (not shown).

After reviewing the **Blue Cross** payment information, the payment entry staff clicks the *Exit Screen* button to return to the <u>Payment</u> add screen. For this example, the payment entry staff added both payments for this batch of payments.

**Do This ▶**  **26.33** - Place the cursor in the **Paid** field for the **Office Visit** line item
(type **25** - do not enter the $ sign or cents)

**26.34** - Place the cursor in the first **Code** field for the **Office Visit**
(type **cp** - for co-payment)

**26.35** - Place the cursor in the first **Amount** field for the **Office Visit**
(type **25** - for the co-payment amount)

**26.36** - Place the cursor in the second **Code** field for the **Office Visit**
(type **dd** - for deductible)

**26.37** - Place the cursor in the second **Amount** field for the **Office Visit**
(type **100** - for the amount applied to the patient's deductible)

**26.38** - Place the cursor in the **Paid** field for the **X-ray** line item
(type **50** - do not enter the $ sign or cents)

**26.39** - Place the cursor in the first **Code** field for the **X-ray**
(type **a01** - for the PPO adjustment)

**26.40** - Place the cursor in the first **Amount** field for the **X-ray**
(type **20** - do not enter the $ sign or cents)

**26.41** - Place the cursor in the **Paid** field for the **Ice** line item
(type **5** - do not enter the $ sign or cents)

**26.42** - Place the cursor in the first **Code** field for the **Ice**
(type **a01** - for the PPO adjustment)

**26.43** - Place the cursor in the first **Amount** field for the **Ice**
(type **7.50** - do not enter the $ sign)

**26.44** - Place the cursor in the **Paid** field for the **Lace Up** line item
(type **51.50** - do not enter the $ sign)

**26.45** - Place the cursor in the first **Code** field for the **Lace Up**
(type **a01** - for the PPO adjustment)

**26.46** - Place the cursor in the first **Amount** field for the **Lace Up**
(type **31.50** - do not enter the $ sign)

**(go to the Do This box on the next page)**

**Do This** ▶ **26.47** - Click the *Page Down* button

**26.48** - Place the cursor in the **Paid** field for the **Appl Splint** line item
(type **80** - do not enter the $ sign or cents)

**26.49** - Place the cursor in the first **Code** field for the **Appl Splint**
(type **a01** - for the PPO adjustment)

**26.50** - Place the cursor in the first **Amount** field for the **Appl Splint**
(type **59** - do not enter the $ sign or cents)

**26.51** - Click the *Submit Payment* button

**26.52** - Check that your payment information recorded properly
(use the *Page Up* and *Page Down* buttons to switch screens)
(the invoice balance should be $100.00)

**26.53** - Click the *Exit Screen* button
(the Payment add screen appears again)

The payment posting staff then clicks the *Exit Screen* button.

The next screen to appear is the Batch Payments screen (shown below). This screen lists all of the payments in a batch.

For this example, the Batch Payments screen lists both the patient payment for $25.00 and the Blue Cross payment for $211.50.

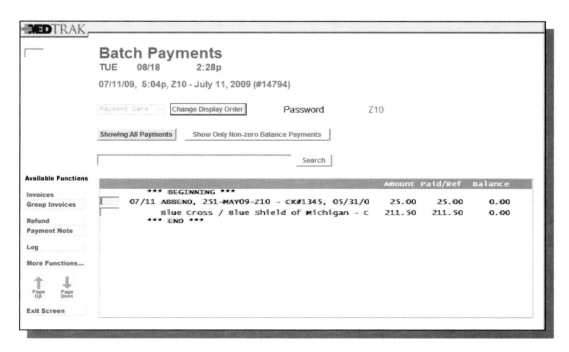

Both of these payments have payment balances on them of zero, meaning that all of the payments are applied to invoices. The payment entry staff clicks the *Exit Screen* button to return to the <u>Payment Batches</u> screen (shown below) to add another payment batch.

The default view on the <u>Payment Batches</u> screen is to display only payment batches that do not have a zero balance. This means that any payment batches that have all of their associated payments fully applied to invoices will not initially display. To view the payment batch in this example, the payment entry staff clicks the *Show all balances* button on the <u>Payment Batches</u> screen (shown below), and then uses the **Search** field to reset to the date of the payment batch.

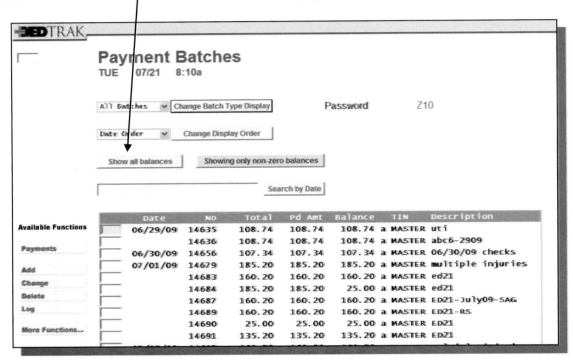

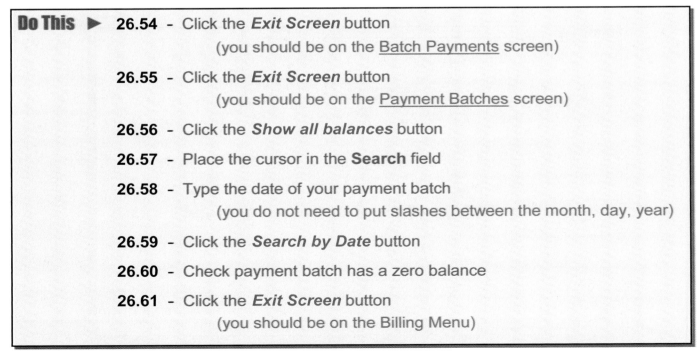

**Do This** ▶    **26.54** – Click the *Exit Screen* button

            (you should be on the <u>Batch Payments</u> screen)

        **26.55** – Click the *Exit Screen* button

            (you should be on the <u>Payment Batches</u> screen)

        **26.56** – Click the *Show all balances* button

        **26.57** – Place the cursor in the **Search** field

        **26.58** – Type the date of your payment batch

            (you do not need to put slashes between the month, day, year)

        **26.59** – Click the *Search by Date* button

        **26.60** – Check payment batch has a zero balance

        **26.61** – Click the *Exit Screen* button

            (you should be on the Billing Menu)

# CHAPTER
# 27

# Accounts Receivable

**Estimated time needed to complete this chapter  -  20** minutes

## What you need to know before doing this chapter

- How to log into MedTrak
- How to register a patient
- How to access Clinic Status off the Main Menu
- How to move a patient to a room and answer nursing notes
- How to use the Visit Documentation processor (Out the Door)
- How to discharge the patient from the back examination area
- How to collect the payment from the patient at the front desk
- How to review unbilled charges
- How to post charges to create an invoice
- How to print a bill (invoice)
- How to process a payment and post it to an invoice

## Learning outcomes gained from this chapter

- How to use the AR Dashboard

## Key terms used in this chapter

*no payments*
*underpaid*
*overpaid*
*denied*
*no follow-up*
*with follow-up*
*payments not yet applied*
*unidentified*

## Accounts Receivable

### Major Categories of Clinical Workflow

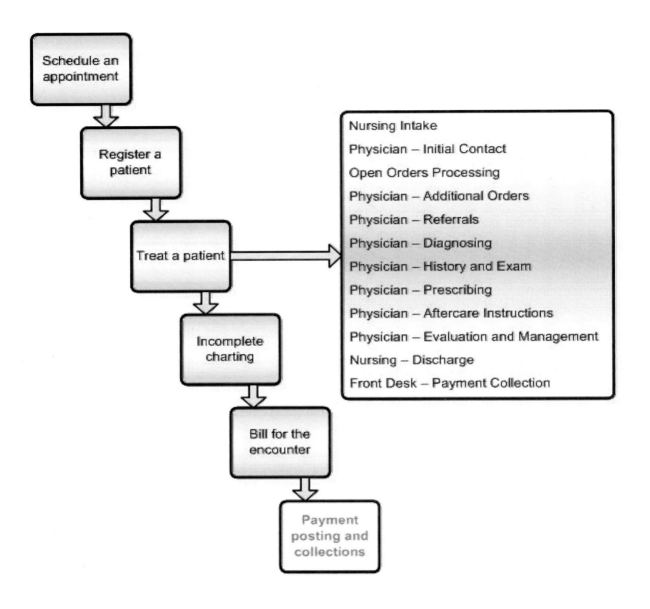

## Accounts Receivable Aging

To access the <u>Accounts Receivable Aging</u> (shown below), the user signs into MedTrak, clicks the *Billing* button, and then clicks the *AR Dashboard* button. This dashboard tracks invoices and payments with non-zero balances:

- ◆ Invoices with *no payments*
- ◆ Partially paid invoices (*underpaid*)
- ◆ *Overpaid* invoices where the payer paid more than they owed or two payers paid for the same invoice
- ◆ *Denied* invoices where the payer denies that they owe for the charge(s)
- ◆ Invoices with *no follow-up* (no collection activities started yet)
- ◆ Invoices *with follow-up* (collection activities started)
- ◆ *Payments not yet applied* to invoices (where the payer is known to the medical facility)
- ◆ Payments received from *unidentified* sources (where the payer is not known)

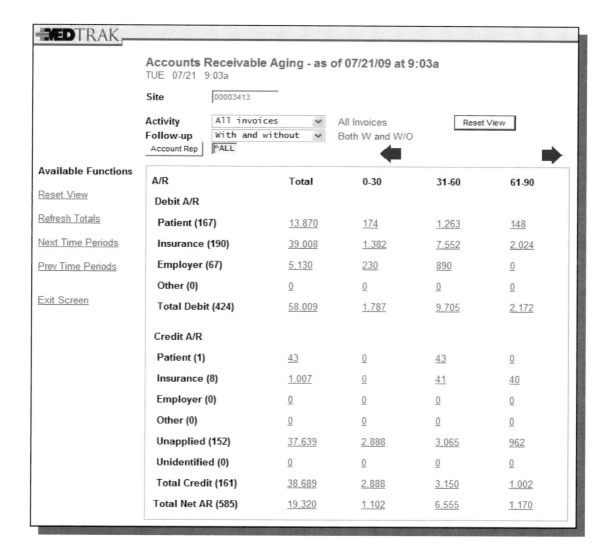

**Accounts Receivable Aging - as of 07/21/09 at 9:03a**
TUE 07/21 9:03a

**Site** `00003413`

**Activity** `All invoices` ▾  All Invoices   [Reset View]
**Follow-up** `With and without` ▾  Both W and W/O
[Account Rep] `*ALL`

**Available Functions**

Reset View

Refresh Totals

Next Time Periods

Prev Time Periods

Exit Screen

| A/R | Total | 0-30 | 31-60 | 61-90 |
|---|---|---|---|---|
| **Debit A/R** | | | | |
| Patient (167) | 13,870 | 174 | 1,263 | 148 |
| Insurance (190) | 39,008 | 1,382 | 7,552 | 2,024 |
| Employer (67) | 5,130 | 230 | 890 | 0 |
| Other (0) | 0 | 0 | 0 | 0 |
| Total Debit (424) | 58,009 | 1,787 | 9,705 | 2,172 |
| | | | | |
| **Credit A/R** | | | | |
| Patient (1) | 43 | 0 | 43 | 0 |
| Insurance (8) | 1,007 | 0 | 41 | 40 |
| Employer (0) | 0 | 0 | 0 | 0 |
| Other (0) | 0 | 0 | 0 | 0 |
| Unapplied (152) | 37,639 | 2,888 | 3,065 | 962 |
| Unidentified (0) | 0 | 0 | 0 | 0 |
| Total Credit (161) | 38,689 | 2,888 | 3,150 | 1,002 |
| Total Net AR (585) | 19,320 | 1,102 | 6,555 | 1,170 |

The <u>Accounts Receivable Aging</u> dashboard has two main sections (rows of information):

> **Debit A/R** - separated by the type of payer and includes all unpaid invoices whether under paid or with no payments. The total number of invoices included in each row displays in parentheses next to the category title.

> **Credit A/R** - separated by the type of payer and includes all overpaid invoices, unapplied payments, and unidentified payments. The total number of invoices or payments included in each displays in parentheses next to the category title.

> **Total Debit, Total Credit, and Total Net AR** - MedTrak displays totals for the debit and credit sections, with the total net accounts receivable in the last row. Again, the total number of invoices and payments displays in parentheses next to the category title.

The <u>Accounts Receivable Aging</u> dashboard breaks down into *aging periods* (columns of information):

| | |
|---|---|
| **Total** | total in that category |
| **0-30** | total in that category that are 30 days old or less |
| **31-60** | total in that category that are between 31 and 60 days old |
| **61-90** | total in that category that are between 61 and 90 days old |
| **91-120** | total in that category that are between 91 and 120 days old |
| **121-150** | total in that category that are between 121 and 150 days old |
| **151-180** | total in that category that are between 151 and 180 days old |
| **181-270** | total in that category that are between 181 and 270 days old |
| **271-360** | total in that category that are between 271 and 360 days old |
| **361+** | total in that category that are over 360 days old (in essence one year) |

Filters are set up to display just the invoices for one medical facility or the entire entity. You can also filter the dashboard based on the activity (no payment, underpaid, overpaid, and denied), and by invoices with follow-up and without. For invoices with follow-up, you can filter by the account representative responsible for collecting payment for the invoice.

The <u>Accounts Receivable</u> dashboard totals reflect the amounts based on the last time that the dashboard was refreshed by the user. Typically, users refresh the <u>Accounts Receivable</u> dashboard each morning to reflect all of the previous day's activity. To refresh the <u>Accounts Receivable</u> dashboard, the user clicks the *Refresh Totals* button.

To display the invoices (or payments) in that category for that aging period, the user clicks the appropriate amount field.

To display the different aging periods, click the **blue arrow** buttons at the top of the screen, or use the *Next Time Periods* and *Prev Time Periods* buttons.

The Accounts Receivable dashboard (shown below) is now set to the next set of aging periods from the previously shown screen.

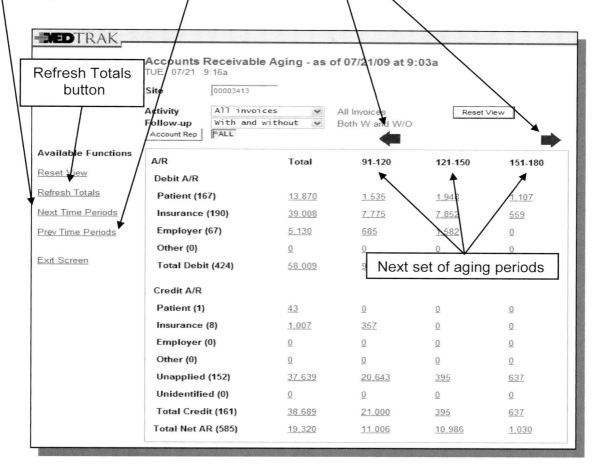

Refresh Totals button

Next set of aging periods

Do This ▶ **27.01** - Sign into MedTrak

**27.02** - Click the *Billing* button on the Main Menu

**27.03** - Click the *AR Dashboard* button
(you should be on Accounts Receivable Aging dashboard)

**27.04** - Review the totals
(your invoice is included)

**27.05** - Click the right **blue arrow** button once at the top of the screen
(you should be on the 91-120 aging period screen)

**27.06** - Click the *Prev Time Periods* button
(you should be on the 0-30 aging period screen)

## *Invoice Activity Filter*

The **Activity** filter at the top of the screen is a drop-down selection menu. The user clicks the drop-down menu, selects the invoice activity filter, and then clicks the *Reset View* button at the top of the screen or the *Reset View* button on the left side of the screen.

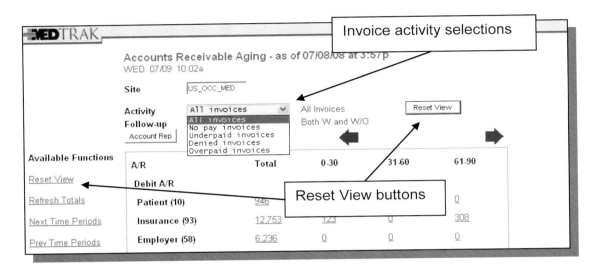

**Do This** ▶ **27.07** - Click the *Activity* drop-down menu

**27.08** - Select the *Underpaid invoices* option

**27.09** - Click the *Reset View* button
(you should be viewing the aging for underpaid invoices only)

**27.10** - Click the *Activity* drop-down menu

**27.11** - Select the *All invoices* option

**27.12** - Click the *Reset View* button
(you should be viewing the aging for all invoices again)

## Invoice Follow-Up Filter

The **Follow-up** filter at the top of the screen is also a drop-down selection menu. The user clicks the drop-down menu, selects the follow-up filter, and then clicks the *Reset View* button at the top of the screen or the *Reset View* button on the left side of the screen.

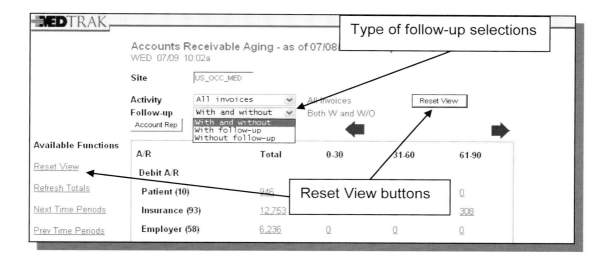

---

**Do This** ▶ **27.13** - Click the *Follow-up* drop-down menu

**27.14** - Select the *With follow-up* invoices option

**27.15** - Click the *Reset View* button
(you should be viewing the aging for follow-up invoices only)

**27.16** - Click the *Follow-up* drop-down menu

**27.17** - Select the *With and without* option

**27.18** - Click the **Reset View** button
(you should be viewing the aging for all invoices again)

## *Selecting an Accounts Receivable Category and Aging Period*

To view the invoices in a category, the user clicks the number that represents the category and aging period.

On the <u>Accounts Receivable</u> dashboard (shown below), the billing staff clicks the **Debit A/R - Insurance** category for the **0-30** day aging period to locate the **Abbend** invoice from the last chapter.

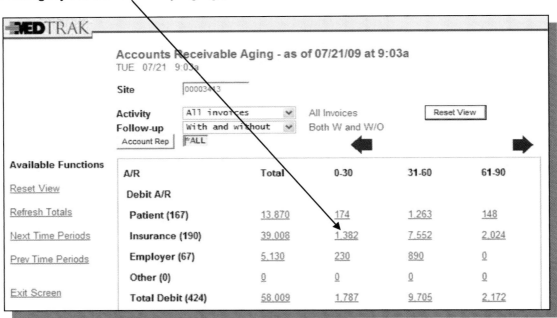

The first screen to appear is the <u>A/R by Balance: Insurance</u> screen that displays the payers in total balance owed order. Because the **Abbend** invoice's primary payer is Blue Cross/Blue Shield of Michigan, the collector clicks the **Blue Cross/Blue Shield of Michigan** name.

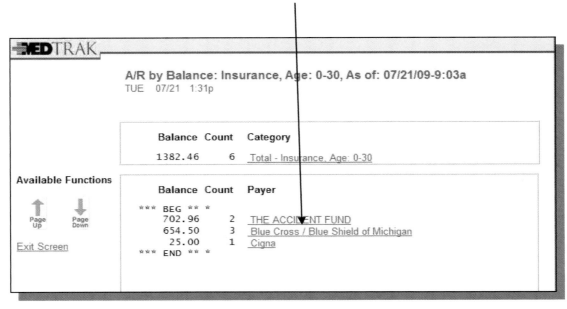

The Invoices screen displaying the **0-30** day invoices for **Blue Cross** displays (shown below).

The **Abbend** invoice appears on the first screen. If the patient's invoice did not appear on the screen, the collector would change the *Payer Display* to be by patient and then use the **Search** field to locate the patient.

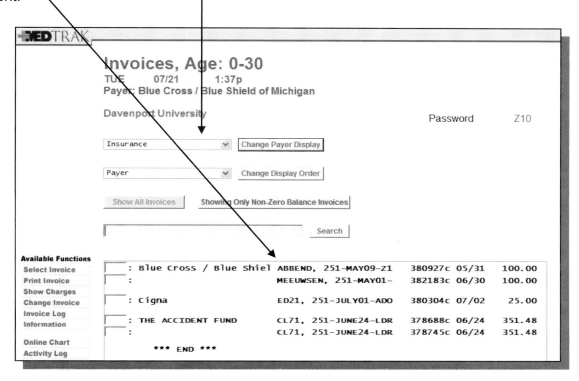

The Invoices screen accessed from the Accounts Receivable Aging screen only displays invoices with a non-zero balance.

At the top of the Invoices screen (shown below), there is a drop-down menu for resetting the **Payer Display**. The billing staff selects a different payer display and clicks the *Change Payer Display* button.

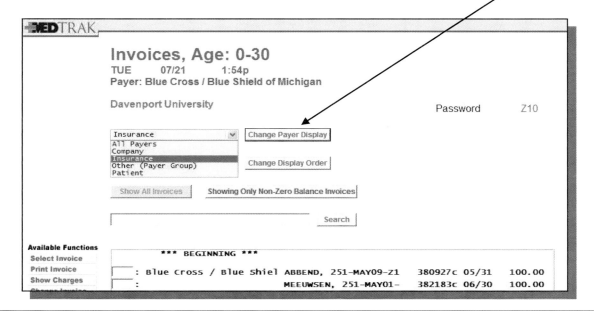

Also at the top of the <u>Invoices</u> screen (shown below) is drop-down menu for resetting the **Display Order**. The billing staff selects a different display order and clicks the *Change Display Order* button.

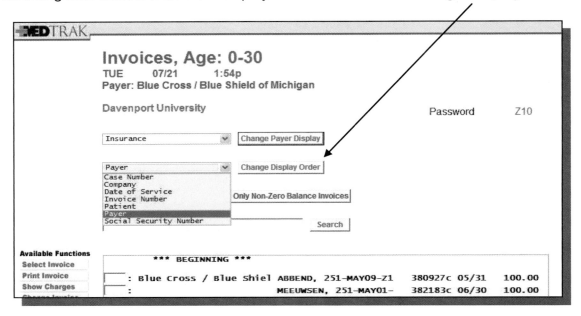

The Invoices screen (shown below) also has a search field to locate an invoice. The billing staff types in the search parameter and clicks the *Search* button to reset the display.

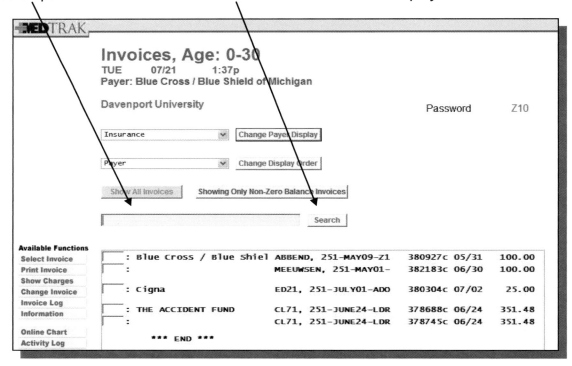

## *Balance Billing to the Secondary Payer*

In this example, the patient has a secondary payer (Nationwide Insurance). Because Blue Cross/Blue Shield applied $100.00 of the office visit to the patient's deductible, this balance is still owing on the invoice.

The billing department is going to balance bill the $100.00 to Nationwide. The payment poster could have balance billed the invoice by using the **bb** command on the line item when posting the Blue Cross payment, but in this example the billing staff will balance bill the invoice using the Invoices screen.

To balance bill the next payer, the billing staff enters the balance billing command **bb** in the command field next to the patient's invoice on the Invoices screen (shown below) and presses the *ENTER* key.

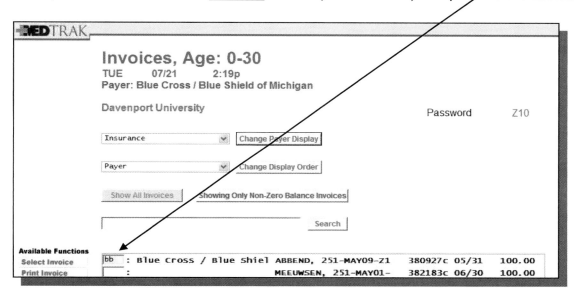

The Invoices screen refreshes with the message at the top - **Balance Billed to COMM INS— Nationwide Insurance** and the invoice is not appearing anymore for Blue Cross.

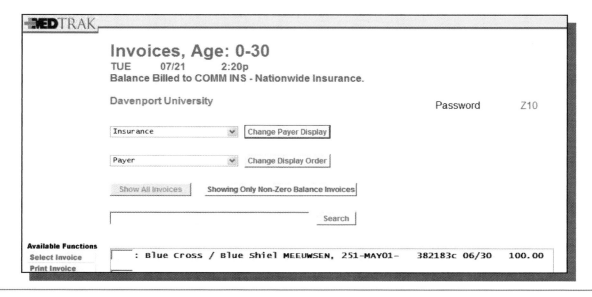

The billing staff clicks the *Exit Screen* button on the <u>Invoices</u> screen and then clicks the *Exit Screen* button on the <u>A/R by Balance</u> screen to return to the <u>Accounts Receivable Aging</u> dashboard.

After refreshing the totals on the AR Dashboard (shown below), the next time that the billing staff accesses the **Debit AR - Insurance** for the **0-30** day range, the **Abbend** invoice balance of $100.00 is now owed by **Nationwide**.

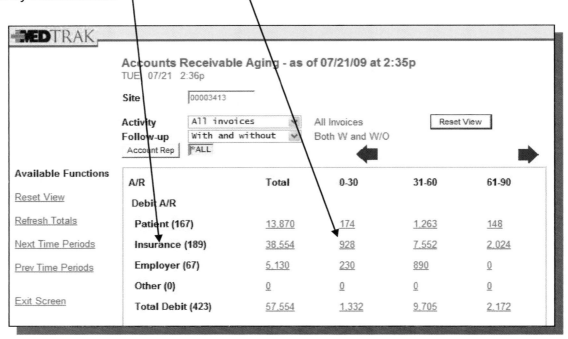

The next time the billing department sends out bills, **Nationwide** will receive the invoice.

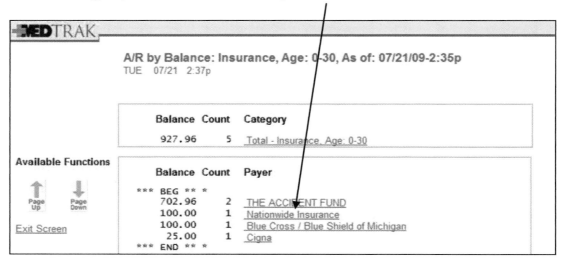

Selecting Nationwide Insurance displays the Invoices screen (shown below) showing the **Abbend** invoice with a balance of $100.00.

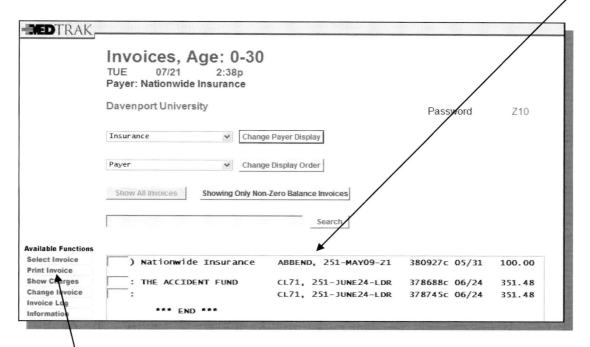

For this example the billing staff places the cursor in the command field next to the **Abbend** invoice and clicks the *Print Invoice* button.

**Do This** ▶ **27.19** - Click the *0-30* category for **Debit AR - Insurance** invoices

(you should be on the Accounts Receivable Aging screen)

**27.20** - Click the **Blue Cross/Blue Shield of Michigan** name

**27.21** - Locate your invoice on the Invoices screen

(change the display if needed and use the **Search** function)

**27.22** - Place the cursor next to your invoice

**27.23** - Type **bb** (for balance billing) and press the *ENTER* key

(your invoice is balance billed to Nationwide Insurance)

**27.24** - Click the *Exit Screen* button

(you should be on the A/R by Balances screen)

**27.25** - Click the *Exit Screen* button

(you should be on the Accounts Receivable Aging screen)

**27.26** - Review the totals on the dashboard

**(go to the Do This box on the next page)**

**Do This** ▶   **27.27** - Click the *0-30* category for **Debit AR - Insurance** invoices

                  (you should be on the <u>A/R by Balance</u> screen)

**27.28** - Click the **Nationwide Insurance** name

                  (you should be on the <u>Invoices</u> screen)

**27.29** - Locate your invoice on the <u>Invoices</u> screen

                  (change the display if needed and use the **Search** function)

**27.30** - Place the cursor next to your invoice

**27.31** - Click the *Print Invoice* button

                  (your invoice will be in the *View Prints* PDF queue)

**27.32** - Click the *View Prints* button

                  (this will open another window displaying your PDF print queue)

                  (this screen is called <u>Available User Reports</u>)

**27.33** - Place the cursor in the command field next to the **CMS1500**

**27.34** - Click the *View Report* button

                  (this will open Adobe, displaying the PDF of your **CMS1500**)

**27.35** - Click the *diskette* icon at the top right of the PDF

**27.36** - Save this PDF to a folder for your class assignments

**27.37** - Attach this saved PDF to your assignment

**27.38** - Close the *Adobe* window displaying your invoice

**27.39** - Close the <u>Available User Reports</u> window

**27.40** - Click the *Exit Screen* button

                  (you should be on the <u>A/R by Balance</u> screen)

**27.41** - Click the *Exit Screen* button

                  (you should be on the <u>Accounts Receivable Aging</u> screen)

**27.42** - Click the *Exit Screen* button

                  (you should be on the <u>Billing Menu</u>)

# CHAPTER

# 28

# Collection Activity

**Estimated time needed to complete this chapter - 20** minutes

**What you need to know before doing this chapter**

- How to log into MedTrak
- How to register a patient
- How to access <u>Clinic Status</u> off the <u>Main Menu</u>
- How to move a patient to a room and answer nursing notes
- How to use the <u>Visit Documentation</u> processor (Out the Door)
- How to discharge the patient from the back examination area
- How to collect the payment from the patient at the front desk
- How to review unbilled charges
- How to post charges to create an invoice
- How to print a bill (invoice)
- How to process a payment and post it to an invoice
- How to use the <u>AR Dashboard</u>

**Learning outcomes gained from this chapter**

- How to record collection activity

## Collection Activity

### Major Categories of Clinical Workflow

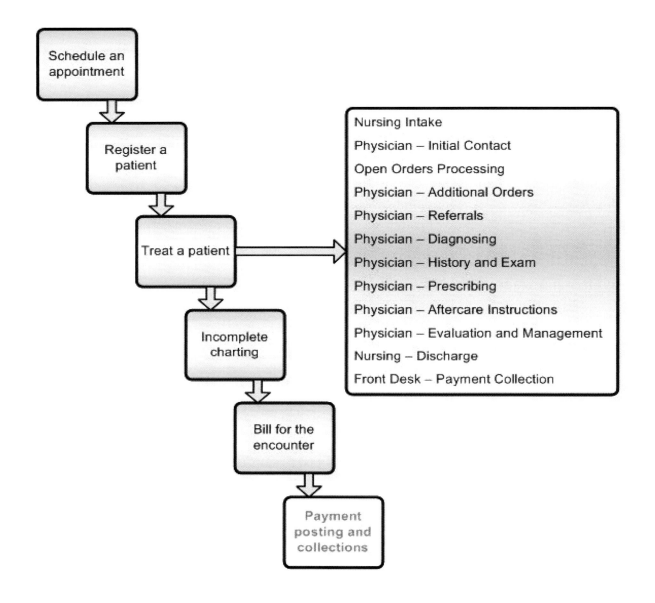

## Case/Billing Activity Log

MedTrak provides collection activities to be logged through the use of an **Activity Log**. Collectors access the case/billing activity log off the <u>Invoices</u> processor. In this example, the collector uses the <u>Accounts Receivable Aging</u> dashboard (shown below) to find the invoice to record collection activity.

Collector activities include:

♦ Recording follow-up *notes* based on conversations or emails or letters from payers related to paying outstanding invoices.

♦ Setting up *reminders* for further follow-up activity.

♦ Attaching *scanned or emailed documents* related to the collection activity.

In this example, the collector:

♦ records a follow-up note related to an attempted phone conversation with the payer (Nationwide)

♦ sets up a reminder to call the payer again

♦ attaches a document sent by Nationwide denying responsibility for paying the invoice

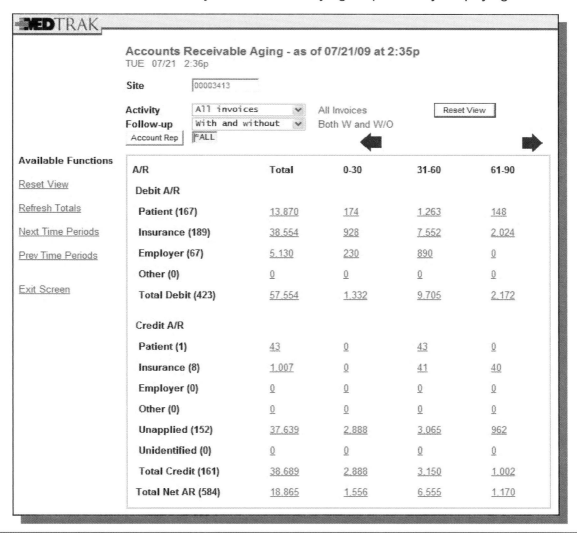

Accounts Receivable Aging - as of 07/21/09 at 2:35p
TUE 07/21 2:36p

**Site** 00003413

**Activity** All invoices — All Invoices — Reset View
**Follow-up** With and without — Both W and W/O
Account Rep *ALL

**Available Functions**

Reset View

Refresh Totals

Next Time Periods

Prev Time Periods

Exit Screen

| A/R | Total | 0-30 | 31-60 | 61-90 |
|---|---|---|---|---|
| **Debit A/R** | | | | |
| Patient (167) | 13,870 | 174 | 1,263 | 148 |
| Insurance (189) | 38,554 | 928 | 7,552 | 2,024 |
| Employer (67) | 5,130 | 230 | 890 | 0 |
| Other (0) | 0 | 0 | 0 | 0 |
| **Total Debit (423)** | 57,554 | 1,332 | 9,705 | 2,172 |
| | | | | |
| **Credit A/R** | | | | |
| Patient (1) | 43 | 0 | 43 | 0 |
| Insurance (8) | 1,007 | 0 | 41 | 40 |
| Employer (0) | 0 | 0 | 0 | 0 |
| Other (0) | 0 | 0 | 0 | 0 |
| Unapplied (152) | 37,639 | 2,888 | 3,065 | 962 |
| Unidentified (0) | 0 | 0 | 0 | 0 |
| **Total Credit (161)** | 38,689 | 2,888 | 3,150 | 1,002 |
| **Total Net AR (584)** | 18,865 | 1,556 | 6,555 | 1,170 |

In this example, the collector locates the invoice by selecting the **Debit A/R - Insurance 0-30** aging category on the Accounts Receivable Aging dashboard (shown on the previous page).

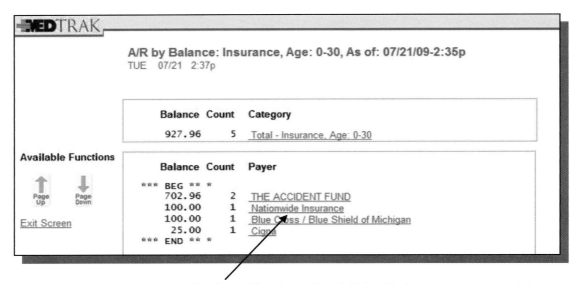

Then the collector selects the payer (Nationwide) from the A/R by Balance processor (shown above).

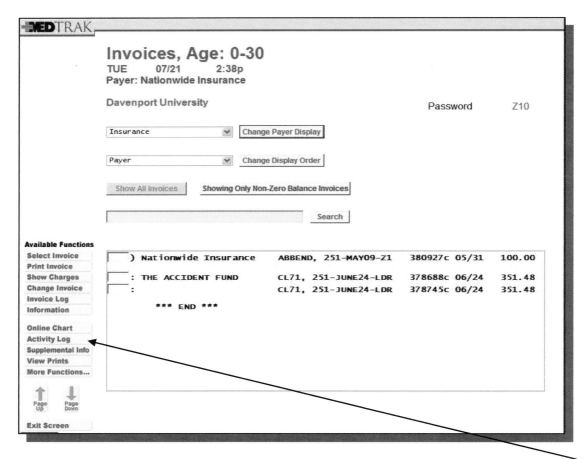

The collector places the cursor in the command field next to the invoice and clicks the *Activity Log* button.

The next screen to appear is the Case/Billing Activity Log (shown below). Because this is the first time the collector is accessing this processor, there are no log entries on the screen.

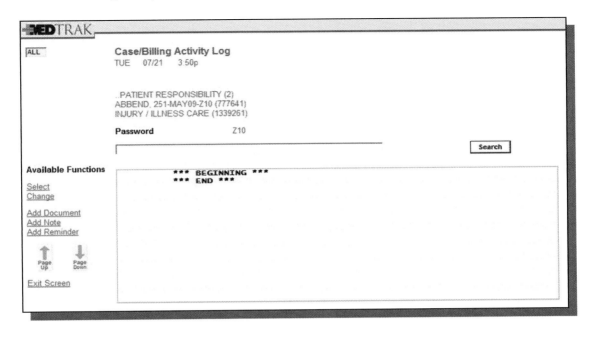

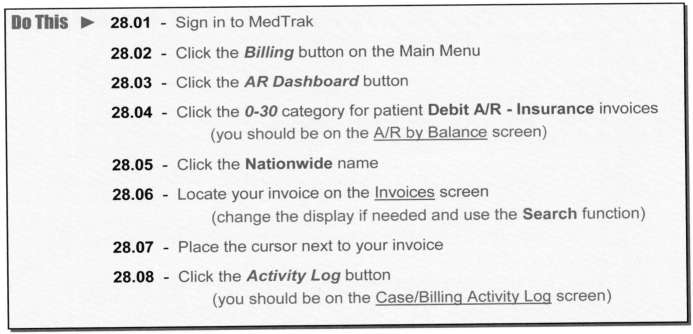

**Do This ▶** **28.01** - Sign in to MedTrak

**28.02** - Click the *Billing* button on the Main Menu

**28.03** - Click the *AR Dashboard* button

**28.04** - Click the *0-30* category for patient **Debit A/R - Insurance** invoices
(you should be on the A/R by Balance screen)

**28.05** - Click the **Nationwide** name

**28.06** - Locate your invoice on the Invoices screen
(change the display if needed and use the **Search** function)

**28.07** - Place the cursor next to your invoice

**28.08** - Click the *Activity Log* button
(you should be on the Case/Billing Activity Log screen)

## Billing Notes

When a collector records a follow-up billing note in the activity log for the patient's case, the invoice is automatically considered in follow-up and can be filtered using the **Follow-up** filter on the Accounts Receivable Aging dashboard.

To place the invoice into the **Follow-up** category, the collector clicks the *Add Note* button on the Case/Billing Activity Log screen to display the Case/Billing Note add screen (shown below).

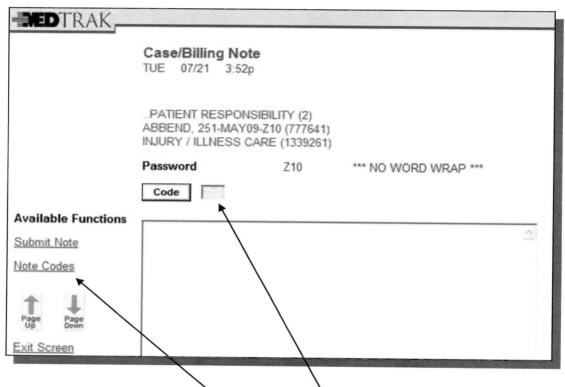

Each note requires a three-character code in the **Note Code** field. To view the available codes (shown below), the collector clicks the *Note Codes* button.

There are <u>three</u> types of billing note codes:

♦ Follow-up notes - these will put in the invoice in the **With Follow-up** category

♦ General notes - these are just comment notes about the case of billings

♦ Refund notes - these notes relate to refunds of payments on the case

In this example, the collector records a follow-up note regarding a phone call made to Alice Johnson at Nationwide Insurance about the denial letter received from the payer. The collector did not reach Alice and marked the note with a follow-up code of **F01 - Left Voice Message**. After selecting the note code and entering the note, the collector clicks the *Submit Note* button.

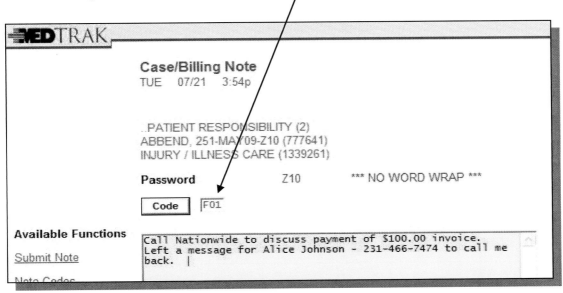

The <u>Case/Billing Activity Log</u> reappears, showing the follow-up note. The invoice is now in the **With Follow-up** accounts receivable category.

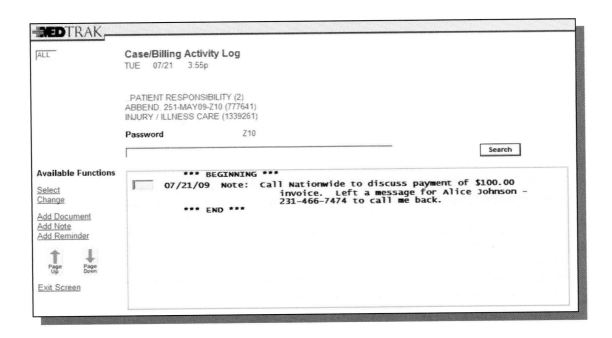

**Do This** ▶ **28.09** - Click the *Add Note* button

(you should be on the <u>Case/Billing Note</u> add screen)

**28.10** - Click the *Note Codes* button

(you should be on the <u>Note Codes</u> screen)

**28.11** - Click on the **F01 - Left Voice Message** note to select it

**28.12** - Enter a note about the collection activity

**28.13** - Click the *Submit Note* button

(you should be on the <u>Case/Billing Activity Log</u> screen)

(there should be a record of your note)

## Attaching Documents

MedTrak allows the attaching of foreign documents (documents received from outside the clinic) to a case. These could be the scanned insurance and ID card at the front desk. They could also be scanned denial letters or other billing correspondence from payers.

To attach a document to the <u>Case/Billing Activity Log</u>, the collector clicks the *Add Document* button. The next screen to appear is the <u>Add Document</u> screen (shown below).

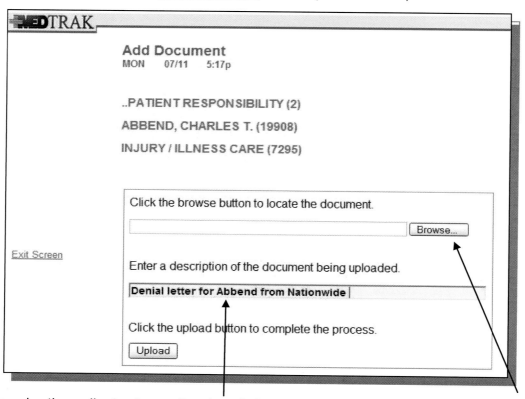

In this example, the collector types the description of the document and clicks the *Browse* button to locate the document in the local network.

After locating the document in the local network, the collector clicks the *Open* button to record the document's local address.

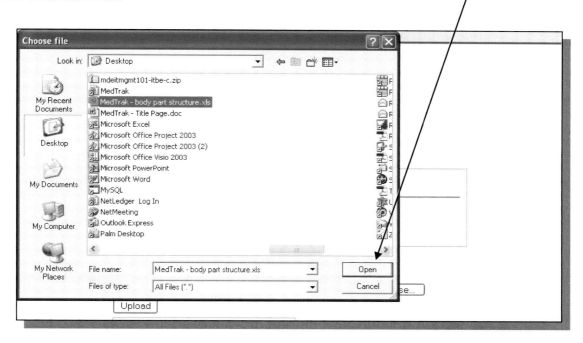

The Add Document screen refreshes with the address of the document in the **Upload document** field (shown below). The collector clicks the *Upload* button to store the document in MedTrak's server.

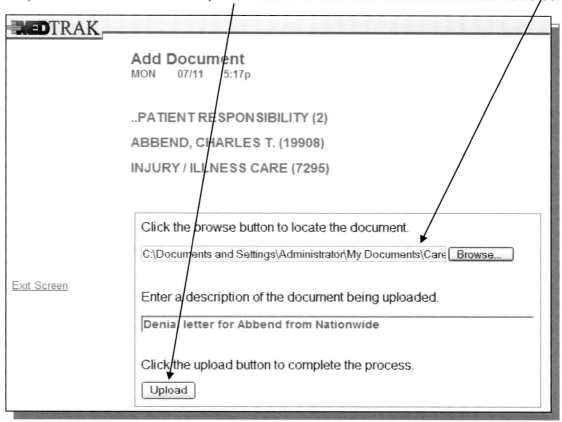

The <u>Case/Billing Activity Log</u> screen refreshes with the record of the document now appearing.

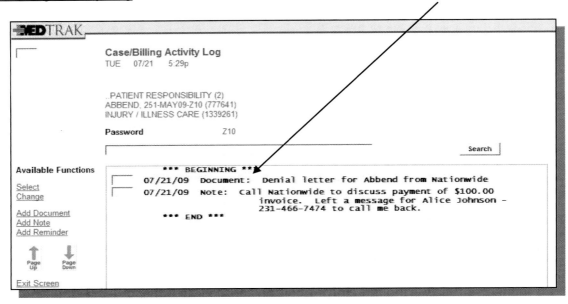

To view the document, the collector places the cursor in the command field next to the document and clicks the **Select** button. The attached document will appear in another window.

**Do This** ▶ **28.14** - Click the **Add Document** button

(you should be on the <u>Add Document</u> screen)

**28.15** - Type in a description of the document

**28.16** - Click the **Browse** button

(you should be on the <u>Choose File</u> screen on your local computer)

**28.17** - Locate a document to upload to MedTrak

**28.18** - Click the **Open** button

(you should be on the <u>Add Document</u> screen)

(your document's address should be in the **Upload** field)

**28.19** - Click the **Upload** button

(you should be on the <u>Case/Billing Activity Log</u> screen)

(there should be a record of your document)

**28.20** - Place the cursor in the command field next to your document

**28.21** - Click the **Select** button

(a window should appear displaying your document)

**28.22** - Close your document window

## Reminders (Ticklers)

In this example, the collector decides to set up a reminder to call Alice at Nationwide. To set up the reminder, the collector clicks the *Add Reminder* button. The Case/Billing Reminder screen appears (shown below).

The collector changes the date to the next day, sets the time to **03:00p**, and types the reminder (as shown below).

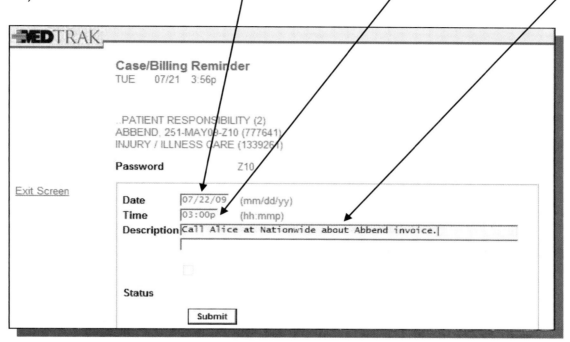

The collector clicks the *Submit* button. The Case/Billing Reminder screen refreshes in the event the collector wants to create a second reminder (and third, and ...) on the case.

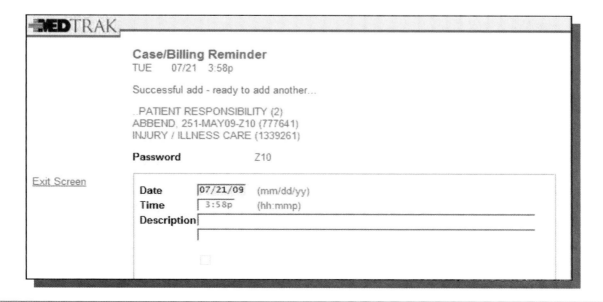

The collector clicks the *Exit Screen* button to return to the Case/Billing Activity Log screen (shown below). The reminder is now part of the log.

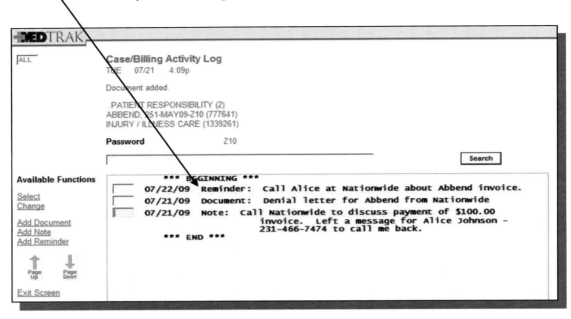

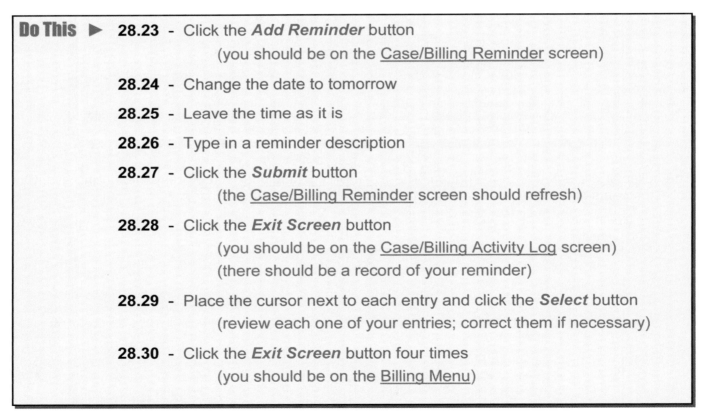

**Do This ▶**  **28.23** - Click the *Add Reminder* button
(you should be on the Case/Billing Reminder screen)

**28.24** - Change the date to tomorrow

**28.25** - Leave the time as it is

**28.26** - Type in a reminder description

**28.27** - Click the *Submit* button
(the Case/Billing Reminder screen should refresh)

**28.28** - Click the *Exit Screen* button
(you should be on the Case/Billing Activity Log screen)
(there should be a record of your reminder)

**28.29** - Place the cursor next to each entry and click the *Select* button
(review each one of your entries; correct them if necessary)

**28.30** - Click the *Exit Screen* button four times
(you should be on the Billing Menu)

## Reviewing Reminders

To review reminders, the collector accesses the reminders that pertain to them by clicking the *Reminders* button on the Billing Menu (shown below).

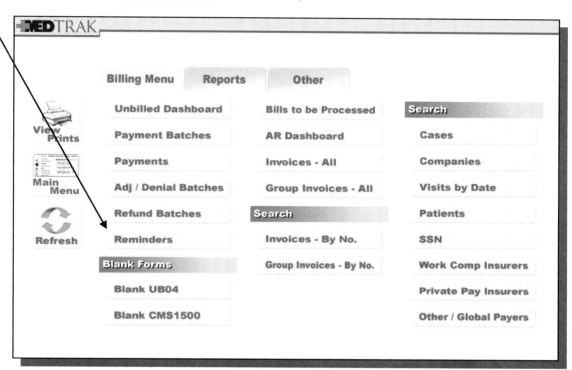

This example shows the reminder to call Alice at Nationwide.

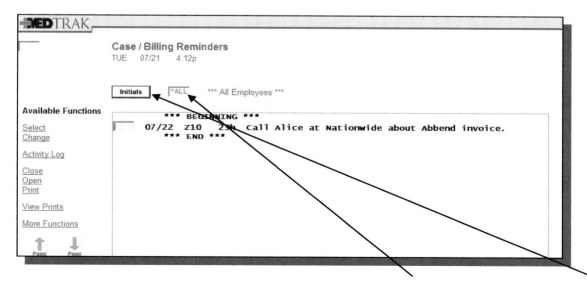

To filter the reminders, the collector types his or her initials in the **Initials** field and clicks the *Initials* button.

The collector can select a reminder and change it. He or she can close the reminder when it is done. The collector can also access the Case/Billing Activity Log to record more information about the collection activity.

When reminders are closed, they do not appear on this screen anymore, but they do remain on the Case/Billing Activity Log as a record of the collector's actions.

---

**Do This** ▶   **28.31** - Click the *Reminders* button on the Billing Menu
        (you should be on the Case/Billing Reminders screen)

**28.32** - Type your initials in the **Initials** field

**28.33** - Click the *Initials* button
        (you should see just your reminders)

**28.34** - Place the cursor next to your reminder

**28.35** - Click the *Activity Log* button
        (review the activity log)

**28.36** - Create a screen print of the Activity Log

**28.37** - Press the *Print Screen* (*Prt Scr*) key
        (located at the upper right of your keyboard)

**28.38** - Open a new **Word** document

**28.39** - Paste the screen print into the **Word** document

**28.40** - Save this **Word** document in a folder for your class assignments

**28.41** - Attach the Word document to your assignment

**28.42** - Click the *Exit Screen* button
        (you should be on the Case/Billing Reminders screen)
        (the cursor should be next to your reminder)

**28.43** - Click the *Close* button
        (your reminder should not appear anymore)

**28.44** - Click the *Exit Screen* button
        (you should be on the Billing Menu)

---